THE STROKE BOOK

Designed for use by busy professionals who need quick answers, **The Stroke Book** is a concise and practical reference for anyone involved in managing critically ill cerebrovascular patients. Contributors from leading stroke centers cover a wide range of common conditions and provide focused protocols for assessing and treating patients in the emergency room, intensive care unit, or on the hospital floor. Chapters are written in bulleted format and are packed with algorithms, tables, and summary boxes to provide immediate access to key information. This essential companion will help readers navigate stroke-related clinical situations successfully and make informed decisions about treatment.

THE STROKE BOOK

Michel T. Torbey, MD, MPH, FAHA

Associate Professor of Neurology and Neurosurgery
Director, Stroke Critical Care Program
Director, Neurointensive Care Unit
Medical College of Wisconsin
Milwaukee, WI

Magdy H. Selim, MD, PhD, FAHA

Assistant Professor of Neurology
Harvard Medical School
Co-Director, Stroke Center
Co-Director, Vascular Neurology Fellowship Training
Program
Beth Israel Deaconess Medical Center
Boston, MA

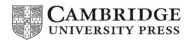

CAMBRIDGE UNIVERSITY PRESS
Cambridge, New York, Melbourne, Madrid, Cape Town, Singapore, São Paulo

Cambridge University Press
32 Avenue of the Americas, New York, NY 10013-2473, USA

www.cambridge.org
Information on this title: www.cambridge.org/9780521671606

© Cambridge University Press 2007

First published 2007

Printed in the United States of America

A catalog record for this book is available from the British Library.

Library of Congress Cataloging in Publication Data

The Stroke book / edited by Michel T. Torbey, Magdy H. Selim.
     p. cm.
Includes bibliographical references and index.
ISBN 978-0-521-67160-6 (pbk. : alk. paper)
1. Cerebrovascular disease – Handbooks, manuals, etc. I. Torbey, Michel T.
II. Selim, Magdy H.
[DNLM: 1. Cerebrovascular Accident – Handbooks.   WL 39 S921 2007]
RC388.5.S85226   2007
616.8′1-dc22   2007005300

ISBN 978-0-521-67160-6 paperback

Contents

List of contributors

Mark Alberts, MD
Professor of Neurology
Northwestern University Medical School
Director, Stroke Program
Northwestern Memorial Hospital
Chicago, IL

Andrei V. Alexandrov, MD
Professor of Neurology
University of Alabama
Director, UAB Comprehensive Stroke Research Center
Birmingham, AL

Ammar Alkawi, MD
University of Medicine & Dentistry of New Jersey
Department of Neurology
Newark, NJ

Eric Bershad, MD
Chief Resident, Department of Neurology
Case Western Reserve University
Cleveland, OH

James S. Castle, MD
Resident, Department of Neurology
Johns Hopkins University School of Medicine
Johns Hopkins Hospital
Baltimore, MD

Marc Fisher, MD
Professor of Neurology
University of Massachusetts Medical School
Vice Chairman, Department of Neurology
UMass Memorial Medical Center
Worcester, MA

Romergryko G. Geocadin, MD
Assistant Professor of Neurology, Neurosurgery, and Anesthesiology /
Critical Care Medicine
Johns Hopkins University School of Medicine
Chief, Neuroscience Critical Care Unit
Johns Hopkins Hospital and Bayview Medical Center
Baltimore, MD

Philip B. Gorelick, MD, MPH, FACP
Professor of Neurology
Chief, Neurology Service
University of Illinois at Chicago
Chicago, IL

Ann K. Helms, MD
Assistant Professor of Neurology
Medical College of Wisconsin
Milwaukee, WI

Nazli Janjua, MD
Assistant Professor of Neurology, SUNY Downstate Medical Center
Director, Department of Neurology
Long Island College Hospital
Brooklyn, NY

Angelos Katramados, MD
Henry Ford Health Sciences Center
Department of Neurology
Detroit, MI

Jawad Kirmani, MD
Assistant Professor of Neurology and Neurosciences
University of Medicine & Dentistry of New Jersey
Director, Stroke Center
Newark, NJ

Annabelle Lao
College of Nursing and Healthcare Innovation
Arizona State University
Barrow Neurological Institute
St Joseph's Hospital
Phoenix, AZ

Denise Lemke, APNP
Department of Neurology
Medical College of Wisconsin
Milwaukee, WI

Michael H. Lev, MD
Associate Professor of Radiology
Harvard Medical School

Director, CT and Neurovascular Laboratory
Massachusetts General Hospital
Boston, MA

Rafael H. Llinas, MD
Assistant Professor of Neurology
Johns Hopkins University School of Medicine
Associate Director of Johns Hopkins Neurology Residency
Director of Cerebrovascular Neurology
Johns Hopkins Bayview Medical Center
Baltimore, MD

Stephan A. Mayer, MD
Associate Professor of Clinical Neurology and Neurological Surgery
Columbia University
Director, Critical Care Neurology
Columbia-Presbyterian Medical Center
New York, NY

Santiago Ortega-Gutierrez, MD
Department of Neurology
Medical College of Winconsin
Milwaukee, WI

Laura Pedelty, MD
Assistant Professor of Neurology
University of Illinois at Chicago
Chicago, IL

Adnan Qureshi, MD
Professor of Neurology, Neurosurgery, and Radiology
University of Minnesota Medical School
Executive Director, Stroke Center
Associate Head, Department of Neurology
University of Minnesota Medical Center
Minneapolis, MN

Sean I. Savitz, MD
Assistant Professor of Neurology
Harvard Medical School
Beth Israel Deaconess Medical Center
Boston, MA

Magdy H. Selim, MD, PhD, FAHA
Assistant Professor of Neurology
Harvard Medical School
Co-Director, Stroke Center
Co-Director, Vascular Neurology Fellowship Training Program
Beth Israel Deaconess Medical Center
Boston, MA

Vijay Sharma, MBBS, MRCP
Associate Consultant
National University Hospital
Division of Neurology
Singapore

Sanjay K. Shetty, MD
Instructor in Radiology
Harvard Medical School
Beth Israel Deaconess Medical Center
Boston, MA

Jose I. Suarez, MD
Associate Professor of Neurology
Baylor College of Medicine
Houston, TX

Viktor Szeder, MD, PhD
Department of Neurology
Medical College of Wincosin
Milwaukee, WI

Andrew W. Tarulli, MD
Clinical Fellow in Neurology
Harvard Medical School
Beth Israel Deaconess Medical Center
Boston, MA

Michel T. Torbey, MD, MPH, FAHA
Associate Professor of Neurology and Neurosurgery
Director, Stroke Critical Care Program
Director, Neurointensive Care Unit
Medical College of Wisconsin
Milwaukee, WI

Panayiotis Varelas, MD, PhD
Henry Ford Health Sciences Center
Department of Neurology
Detroit, MI

Marta Lopez Vicente, MD
Department of Family Medicine
Medical College of Wisconsin
Milwaukee, WI

Katja Elfriede Wartenberg, MD
New York Presbyterian Hospital / Columbia University Medical Center
Department of Neurology
New York, NY

Thomas J. Wolfe, MD
Chief Resident
Department of Neurology
Medical College of Wisconsin
Milwaukee, WI

Osama O. Zaidat, MD, MS
Associate Professor of Neurology and Neurosurgery
Director, Neuro-interventional Program
Medical College of Wisconsin and Froedtert Hospital
Milwaukee, WI

Foreword

The field of cerebrovascular disorders has grown rapidly over the past few years with many advances in the areas of diagnosis, patient evaluation/management and therapy. It is increasingly important for general physicians and nonneurologists to be aware of these advances and implement them in practice. In *The Stroke Book*, Drs. Selim and Torbey have provided an excellent introductory book that overviews all of the burgeoning aspects of cerebrovascular medicine in a comprehensive but an easily understood manner. The list of contributors is distinguished and their contributions uniformly excellent. Readers of this book will find it user-friendly and a reliable source for introductory information about a wide range of cerebrovascular topics. It will especially be helpful for medical students, physicians in training and busy generalists, as the book provides a ready source of information that will be useful in daily practice when seeing patients with cerebrovascular disorders. The editors have demonstrated vision and care in the production of this book and should be congratulated for a job well done.

Marc Fisher, MD
Professor of Neurology
University of Massachusetts Medical School
Vice Chairman, Department of Neurology
UMass Memorial Medical Center
Worcester, MA

Introduction

Patients with cerebrovascular diseases can be complex to manage, especially for general neurologists and nonneurologists who often have a hard time keeping up with the rapid pace of recent advances in diagnosis and management. Most available textbooks in this field are voluminous and highly specialized. *The Stroke Book* has been produced to provide all healthcare professionals caring for stroke patients with a straightforward, concise, and practical reference to help them with management decisions. The book is intended to be limited in depth, while comprehensive in its scope. We have selected experienced contributors from major stroke centers to provide a logical approach to the diagnosis and management of a wide range of common cerebrovascular conditions. We make no attempt to reiterate the details of neurological examination and localization, but discuss particularly important or difficult differential diagnosis points when appropriate. We use tables, algorithms, and lists throughout the book in order to reduce the volume of the text without compromising the content. It is our hope that *The Stroke Book* will help readers better determine the immediate needs of stroke patients and make informed decisions about treatment. We are indebted to our contributors, families, and, particularly, our patients who stimulate our interest in stroke.

Michel T. Torbey and Magdy H. Selim

Assessment of Stroke Patients

1 Emergency medical services (EMS): First line of defense against stroke

Denise Lemke and Michel T. Torbey

Acute stroke management begins the moment the emergency response system is activated. Immediate triage and dispatch of appropriate emergency medical services (EMS) are essential for improving long-term survival. Each minute in which a large vessel ischemic stroke is untreated an average patient loses 1.9 million neurons. On average, it takes prehospital EMS 17–35 min to reach the emergency department (ED) with stroke patients. Hence, an estimated 32–66 million neurons can be lost during transport alone. The concept of the "Chain of Recovery" was developed to improve the care of stroke patients by incorporating prehospital and hospital management. The Chain of Recovery has five distinct components

1. identification of stroke patients;
2. dispatch system by emergency service activation;
3. EMS providers;
4. alert ED and stroke specialists; and
5. diagnosis and treatment.

Each component is essential for the appropriate management of a "brain attack." The first four components are based in the prehospital setting.

Qualification and classification of EMS personnel

Classification of EMS personnel is related to the extent of training and the direction of the National Registry of Emergency Medical Technicians (NREMT), the Department of Transportation (DOT), the National Highway and Traffic Safety Administration (NHTSA), and emergency physicians. There are some variations between states but the categories of emergency medical technicians (EMTs) include first responders, basic, intermediate, and paramedic. All programs utilizing EMTs have a physician director who is responsible for the medical direction and education of the EMTs. NREMT is the organization responsible for the national examinations, which incorporates a written and practical exam for all levels.

First responders

The first responder course is the EMT – basic course, with the exception of the transportation and equipment section, which is intended for public service (fire and law enforcement) and EMS rescue agencies that may or may not transport patients. The focus of the program is based on assessment, not diagnosis.

EMT – basic

EMT basic training for entry level EMTs incorporates

1. basic life support skills including CPR;
2. principles of general first aid;
3. nonvisualized advanced airway training; and
4. administration of epinephrine, albuterol, aspirin, and glucagons.

EMT – intermediate

EMT intermediate training is for personnel with skills above the basic level. This training incorporates

1. patient assessment;
2. triage principles;
3. management of shock;
4. airway management (comitube and entotracheal intubation after additional training and approval of the medical director);
5. intravenous infusion;
6. performing blood draws; and
7. administration of subcutaneous and selected intravenous medications (epinephrine, 50 percent dextrose, narcan, and albuterol)

Forty-eight hours of continuing education, verified by the medical director, is needed for biennial recertification renewal.

EMT – paramedic

Personnel with skills above the EMT intermediate level are trained for EMT paramedic. Training includes

1. advanced life support;
2. rescue resuscitation and emergency care;
3. administration of IV solutions and parenteral medications;
4. perform CPR and defibrillation of a pulse less nonbreather;
5. gastric and entotracheal intubation (rapid sequence intubation); and
6. EKG interpretation.

Forty-eight-hour DOT curriculum–based continuing education, active ACLS, and CPR status needed for biennial recertification.

Key assessment and management skills for EMS

EMS provides rapid assessment aimed at triaging the individual at home or at the scene of an accident to determine the urgency of the medical condition. In individuals suffering from "brain attack," the time to the ED is critical.

1. Individuals who are seen in the ED within a 3-hr window are candidates for intravenous (IV) tPA.
2. Reduced time interval from the onset of symptom to arrival at the ED of an individual suffering from stroke will increase the number of probable candidates for IV tPA and potentially reduce disability, institutionalization, and lifetime dollars spent on poststroke-related health care.

EMS routinely rapidly assesses, diagnoses, and prioritizes transport of the individual with a medical condition. Transportation of individuals suffering from trauma and heart attack to the ED is prioritized based on medical necessity for urgent treatment. A similar approach needs to be taken with the individual suffering from a "brain attack" to reduce the time interval from initial call received by the dispatch (detection) to arrival of EMS to the scene (dispatch), to transport to ED (delivery).

1. Any individual with an acute onset of unilateral weakness or speech difficulty warrants triaging as an acute stroke from the initial call to the dispatcher to the arrival of EMS at the scene.
2. Preliminary data collected by the dispatcher will potentially improve time to response and after neurological assessment at the scene confirms the diagnosis, reduce the time to the ED.

Stroke assessment and the concept of the seven Ds of stroke management (Table 1.1) are now integrated into the American Heart Association (AHA) basic life support classes, though continued education is needed nationally for EMS to improve assessment skills and reinforce the necessity for urgency in transport. This will ultimately decrease the time to arrival to the ED. Public education is an additional variable as only 38–50 percent of individuals access the emergency response system at the time of "stroke-like" symptoms.

The goals of the education include

1. EMS dispatchers
   a. preliminary neurological assessment via phone interview at the time of the initial call in
      i. key questions
         • acute unilateral weakness
         • acute confusion
         • acute change in speech pattern or quality of speech
         • symptoms under 24 hr
   b. high-priority status to individuals suffering from "brain attack"

Table 1.1: The seven Ds of stroke management

Responsibility	Task
General public, Basic Life Support (BLS) providers, EMS	Detection
	Dispatch
	Delivery
ED	Door
	Data
	Decision
	Drug

2. EMS/paramedics
   a. education of stroke symptoms, assessment, and current treatment trends
   b. use of simplified neurological assessment tools aimed at rapid identification of an individual suffering an acute stroke
   c. documentation
      i.   time of onset
      ii. time of initial call
   d. general assessment
      i.   airway
      ii. glucose evaluation
      iii. blood pressure
   e. advance notification of the ED prior to the arrival of the individual.

Assessment tools

Multiple scales have been developed to aid in the rapid diagnosis of stroke. Current tools are a modification of the hospital-based National Heart Institute Stroke Scale (NHISS). Key areas of assessment include face symmetry and motor function (80–90 percent of individuals suffering from a stroke demonstrate unilateral motor weakness) and abnormal speech. In addition, history of event (time of symptoms onset), blood pressure, review of medications, recent events, and blood sugar assist in the differential diagnosis (alcohol or drug intoxication, hypoglycemic states, postictal states, migraine, dementias, and metabolic encephalopathies).

Prehospital assessment tools

The Los Angeles Prehospital Stroke Screen (LAPSS)

The LAPSS is composed of four key history items, blood sugar measurement, and three areas of motor assessment. It was developed in the 1990s

Table 1.2: Los Angeles Prehospital Stroke Scale (LAPPS)

Screening criteria

1. Age > 45
2. History of seizures absent
3. Symptom duration < 24 hr
4. At baseline, patient is not wheelchair bound or bedridden
5. Blood sugar between 60 and 400
6. Obvious asymmetry (right versus left)
7. Facial smile/grimace
9. Grip
10. Arm strength

If 1–5 are yes with asymmetry on exam then LAPS criteria are met

(Table 1.2). The four key history items are aimed at ruling out potential stroke mimics and consist of

1. age > 45
2. absent history of seizure
3. duration of symptoms < 24 hr
4. determines that at baseline the individual was not wheelchair bound or bedridden.

Blood glucose is obtained and a reading of 60–400 eliminates hypoglycemia as a differential diagnosis. On physical exam, LAPSS evaluates for the presence and symmetry of

1. facial droop
2. grip strength
3. arm drift.

LAPPS demonstrated a sensitivity of 91 percent and a specificity of 97 percent for the identification of acute stroke patients. The test can be performed in less than 3 min.

The Cincinnati Prehospital Stroke Scale (CPSS)

The CPSS is a three-item scale based on the National Institutes of Health Stroke Scale (NIHSS). The presence of three components of the NIHSS in the CPSS are

1. facial palsy
2. arm weakness
3. dysarthria

CPSS identified 100 percent of stroke patients (Table 1.3). The scale rates the specific activity as normal versus abnormal and can be performed in less

Table 1.3: cincinnati prehospital stroke scale (CPSS)

Facial droop: Have patient smile, show teeth
  Normal: Both sides of face move equally
  Abnormal: One side of face does not move or does not move as well as
  the other

Arm drift: Arms held out straight in front of body with eyes closed for 10 s
  Normal: Both arms more equally or not at all
  Abnormal: One arm unable to maintain position or drifts compared to
  the other

Speech: Have patient repeat a phrase
  Normal: Patient uses correct words, no slurring
  Abnormal: Slurred words, inappropriate words, or unable
  to speak

Table 1.4: Face Arm Speech Test (FAST)

Speech impairment	Yes	No	Uncertain
Facial palsy	Yes	No	Uncertain
	Left	Right	
Arm weakness	Yes	No	Uncertain
Affected side	Right	Left	

Note: Speech: Assess quality of speech for difficulty articulating (slurring of words) or expressing oneself (word finding difficulties, object identification). Facial movements: Observe for symmetry of movement (ask patient to smile) and document side of asymmetry. Arm movements: Observe for symmetry of movement – ask patient to simultaneously raise arms 90° while sitting/supine; monitor for 5 s. Document the side of drift/weakness.

than 2 min. The test has a sensitivity of >95 percent when performed by EMS. CPSS identifies anterior circulation stroke more accurately than posterior circulation stroke.

The Newcastle Face Arm Speech Test (FAST)

The FAST was developed in the United Kingdom in 1998 and contains three key elements (facial weakness, arm weakness, and speech disturbances) from the CPSS, but avoids the need to repeat a sentence as a measure of speech, using instead an assessment of language ability by EMS during normal conversation with the patient. FAST was designed for assessment of a seated subject and hence does not assess leg weakness (Table 1.4). Inter-rater reliability between EMS and stroke physician was the best for assessment of arm weakness (95 percent).

Medical management on the scene

Blood pressure, fluid, and blood sugar management are the most common issues facing EMS on the scene. Persistently elevated blood pressure may preclude the use of thrombolytics. Systolic blood pressure less than 185 mmHg and diastolic blood pressure less than 110 mmHg are desirable prior to rt-PA infusion.

Intravenous fluid should be administered cautiously. D5W or D5/0.45 saline solution should be avoided. Hypoglycemia in the stroke patient should be diagnosed and managed expeditiously. Administration of glucose to a suspected stroke patient without documented hypoglycemia should be avoided. There is some increasing evidence that hyperglycemia may be associated with worsened neurological outcome.

Summary

Stroke management requires a multidisciplinary approach that starts with dispatch of EMS and goes all the way to rehabilitation. EMS providers are the first responders and could play a major role in improving outcome following acute stroke.

Bibliography

Amber R, Watkins W. The community impact of code gray. *Crit Care Nurs Quart* 2003;26(4):316–22.

American Heart Association. Part 3: Adult basic life support. *Circulation* 2000;102 (suppl):I-204.

American Heart Association. Part 7: The era of reperfusion. *Circulation* 2000;102 (suppl):I-204.

Boatright JR. New urgency for rapid transport of patients with stroke to appropriate hospitals. *J Emerg Nurs* 2003;29(4):344–6.

Crocco T, Gullett T, Davis SM, et al. Feasibility of neuroprotective agent administration by prehospital personnel in an urban setting. *Stroke* 2003;34 (8):1918–22.

Dion JE. Management of ischemic stroke in the next decade: Stroke centers of excellence. *J Vasc Interv Radiol* 2004;15(1 Pt 2):S133–41.

Goldstein LB, Simel DL. Is this patient having a stroke? *JAMA* 2005;293 (19):2391–402.

Harbison J, Hossain O, Jenkinson D, Davis J, Louw SJ, Ford GA. Diagnostic accuracy of stroke referrals from primary care, emergency room physicians, and ambulance staff using the face arm speech test. *Stroke* 2003;34(1):71–6.

Hurwitz AS, Brice JH, Overby BA, Evenson KR. Directed use of the Cincinnati Prehospital Stroke Scale by laypersons. *Prehosp Emerg Care* 2005;9(3):292–6.

Kidwell CS, Starkman S, Eckstein M, Weems K, Saver JL. Identifying stroke in the field. Prospective validation of the Los Angeles prehospital stroke screen (LAPSS). *Stroke* 2000;31(1):71–6.

Kothari R, Hall K, Brott T, Broderick J. Early stroke recognition: Developing an out-of-hospital NIH Stroke Scale. *Acad Emerg Med* 1997;4(10):986–90.

Moulin T, Moulin T, Sablot D, Vidry E, Belahsen F, Berger E, Lemounaud P, Tatu L, Vuillier F, Cosson A, Revenco E, Capellier G, Rumbach L., *Impact of emergency room neurologists on patient management and outcome. Eur Neurol* 2003;50 (4):207–14.

Nor AM, Davis J, Sen B et al. The Recognition of Stroke in the Emergency Room (ROSIER) scale: Development and validation of a stroke recognition instrument. *Lancet Neurol* 2005;4(11):727–34.

Nor AM, McAllister C, Louw SJ, et al. Agreement between ambulance paramedic- and physician-recorded neurological signs with Face Arm Speech Test (FAST) in acute stroke patients. *Stroke* 2004;35(6):1355–9.

Pepe PE, Zachariah BS, Sayre MR, Floccare D. Ensuring the chain of recovery for stroke in your community. *Acad Emerg Med* 1998;5(4):352–8.

Saver JL. Time is brain – quantified. *Stroke* 2006;37(1):263–6.

Saver JL, Kidwell C, Eckstein M, Starkman S. FAST–MAG pilot trial investigators. Prehospital neuroprotective therapy for acute stroke: Results of the Field Administration of Stroke Therapy-Magnesium (FAST-MAG) pilot trial. *Stroke* 2004;35(5):e106–8.

Schroeder EB, Rosamond WD, Morris DL, Evenson KR, Hinn AR. Determinants of use of emergency medical services in a population with stroke symptoms: The second delay in Accessing Stroke Healthcare (DASH II) study. *Stroke* 2000;31 (11):2591–6.

Tirschwell DL, Longstreth WT Jr, Becker KJ, et al. Shortening the NIH stroke scale for use in the prehospital setting. *Stroke* 2002;33(12):2801–6.

Wein TH, Staub L, Felberg R, et al. Activation of emergency medical services for acute stroke in a nonurban population: The T.L.L. Temple Foundation Stroke Project. *Stroke* 2000;31(8):1925–1928.

2 Initial assessment of patients with stroke-like symptoms

Rafael H. Llinas

The clinical bedside evaluation of stroke patients is a vital part of the workup. A detailed history and physical exam is necessary, as localization, etiology, and comorbidities need to be quickly assessed. History and physical exam is vital and is the best way to diagnose stroke imitators.

General medical examination

Stroke is primarily a medical disorder. The causes and risk factors of stroke are the same as the risk of atherosclerotic heart and peripheral vascular disease. Hypertension, diabetes, coronary artery disease, and hyperlipidemia are the main risk factors.

➠ Initial examination must include a general medical examination (Table 2.1).

General health and appearance

1. A comment on general health, whether the patient is vomiting or in distress can suggest etiology.
2. In general, patients presenting with coma on arrival, vomiting, severe headache, current warfarin therapy, systolic blood pressure >220 mmHg, or glucose level >170 mg/dl in nondiabetic patients are more likely to have a hemorrhagic stroke but these criteria alone are not sufficient to differentiate between ischemic and hemorrhagic stroke.

Vital signs

Vital signs are important to observe carefully. Stroke patients are often, but not always, hypertensive as the brain attempts to increase its own cerebral perfusion. Blood pressure will also be elevated in subarachnoid hemorrhage and intracerebral hemorrhage as the brain attempts to increase the cerebral

Table 2.1: Medical issues that present with or as strokes

Endocarditis
Acute myocardial infarction
Hyper/hypoglycemia
Malignant cardiac arrhythmias
Acute renal failure
Acute hepatic failure
Acute or chronic intoxications
Neoplasm with hypercoagulable states or metastasis
Hypoxia

perfusion pressure by increasing systemic blood pressure. Very high systemic blood pressure may suggest an intracerebral hemorrhage.

1. The presence of hypertension can sometimes help differentiate stroke from stroke imitators.
2. A diastolic blood pressure of >90 and/or SBP>150 is predictive of stroke over other imitators.

Elevated temperature is unusual in acute stroke. A significantly elevated core temperature with acute stroke should raise the possibility of endocarditis or generalized sepsis. It is unlikely that acute aspiration will lead to fever within hours.

1. High fevers with acute neurological deficits should raise the suspicion of sepsis, central nervous system, or cardiac infection as a cause of acute neurological deterioration.

Last and most importantly, pulse evaluation can lead to clues about the primary cardiac source of emboli.

1. Irregularly irregular rhythm of atrial fibrillation.
2. Aortic dissection: absent right-sided pulses seen with dissection of the ascending aorta as well as significant systolic blood pressure difference on the right side compared to the left of 20 mmHg or greater.
3. Diffuse large vessel vasculitis as in Takayasu's arteritis "pulseless disease" will present with absent pulses throughout. Abnormal peripheral pulses are a sign more often found in strokes than in stroke imitators.

Fundiscopic examination

1. A fundiscopic examination is probably most helpful when Hollenhorst plaques are seen in one or both retina.
   a) These are bright, highly retractile, atheromatous materials usually found at the bifurcation of retinal blood vessels.

b) This can suggest unilateral or bilateral cholesterol embolization especially from symptomatic carotid stenosis.
2. "Copper wire" changes seen on fundiscopic examination with long-standing hypertension and can suggest diffuse atherosclerotic disease.
3. Chronic ocular ischemia can cause iris atrophy, pallor of the optic disk, and central venous retinopathy.

Carotid/vertebral artery examination

1. Listening for carotid or vertebral bruits in asymptomatic patients may not be indicated.
2. In acute symptomatic patient listening, and carotid palpating arteries are very important for initial plans concerning treatment and imaging evaluation of acute stroke patients.
3. In general the presence or absence of bruits should not dissuade the clinician from vascular imaging studies.

Palpation of the facial arteries can be sometimes used to suggest carotid occlusion or high-grade stenosis. The arteries of the face originate from the external carotid artery (ECA) and can usually be palpated

➠ in front of the ear (superficial temporal artery)
➠ in the nasolabial area (the facial artery)
➠ on each side of the nose (angular artery)
➠ from the internal carotid medial orbit pulse (supraorbital artery).

If there is an internal carotid occlusion, one may be able to detect pounding external carotid pulses ipsilateral to the carotid occlusion. One can palpate enhanced flow through the ECA branches by finding pounding pulses at medial canthus and ipsilateral eyebrow region (Figure 2.1). Easily felt angular pulse and brow pulses suggest ipislateral carotid occlusion.

In some patients, the internal carotid artery (ICA) supplies the supra-orbitalartery through the ophthalmic artery. When the internal carotid is occluded, there is an attempt to increase collateral flow to the brain through the ECA.

1. This reversal of flow can sometimes be detected clinically by the loss of the supraorbital pulse with compression of the superficial temporal artery.
2. In ICA occlusion, the ECA, instead of the ICA, supplies blood flow to the supraorbital artery through the superficial temporal artery. By compressing the superficial temporal artery, the supraorbital artery pulse may be diminished suggesting that the supraorbital artery is receiving most of its blood flow from the ECA and that there may be an ICA stenosis or occlusion. The specificity and sensitivity of this test have not been formally studied.

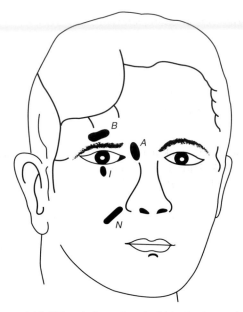

A. Angular pulse easy felt in ICA occlusion and can be felt in 1in 10 normal adults without occlusion;
B. brow pulse rarely easily palpated without ICA occlusion;
N. nasolabial pulse may be increased but is less reliable than A and B pulses;
I. infraorbital pulse may indicate maxillary to ophthalmic artery collateralization. Less helpful
Adapted from Fisher CM. Facial pulses in internal carotid artery occlusion. *Neurology* 1970:20(5); 476–78.

Figure 2.1 Facial pulses in internal carotid artery occlusion. A: Angular pulse easy felt in ICA occlusion and can be felt in 1 in 10 normal adults without occlusion; B: brow pulse rarely easily palpated without ICA occlusion; N: nasolabial pulse may be increased but is less reliable than A and B pulses; I: infraorbital pulse may indicate maxillary to ophthalmic artery collateralization. Less helpful. Adapted from Fisher CM. Facial pulses in internal carotid artery occlusion. *Neurology* 1970; 20(5): 476–78.

Carotid bruits are best heard with the diaphragm, as most bruits are high pitched. The difficulty of a carotid examination is that a bruit of the ECA or transmitted cardiac murmurs may make diagnosis difficult. The pitch and volume of the carotid bruit will change as the stethoscope is placed closer to the bifurcation and stenosis whereas transmitted cardiac murmurs will be louder closer to the heart.

Listening for orbital bruits when listening for carotid bruit can also be helpful.

1. Orbital bruit may suggest either enhanced flow through the ECA system or increased flow due to high grade stenosis.
2. The bruit may occur ipsilateral or contralateral to the affected ICA. For the most part murmurs are not transmitted to the orbital area.

3. Orbital bruits often reflect contralateral ICA stenosis or occlusion due to enhanced flow through the ECA system ipsilaterally, secondary to high flow through the anterior communicating artery as collateral flow moves from unaffected to affected side.

It is useful to listen to cervical bruits in an acute stroke patient to begin to formulate a hypothesis for the etiology of the stroke. Imaging is necessary to confirm carotid stenosis.

1. The carotid pulse in the neck arises from the common carotid artery and not from the ICA. Thus, only occlusion of the common carotid will diminish the cervical carotid pulse. The internal carotid pulse can be felt in the posterior pharynx only.
2. Vertebral bruits are best heard in the posterior neck. Often bruits heard in the vertebral artery position actually represent enhanced flow through a normal artery due to occlusion, stenosis, or congenital hypoplasia of the contralateral vertebral artery. In general, this is a difficult maneuver to perform and imaging is probably the best choice.

Cardiac examination

1. A careful cardiac examination should be performed.
   a) New murmur should raise the possibility of concomitant myocardial with secondary embolization although in the acute setting it can be difficult to confirm whether a murmur of mitral or aortic regurgitation is new or old.
   b) On rare occasions large atrial myxomas can present with mitral regurgitation, as the mitral valve is forced open by the myxoma and by a "tumor plop" that can be mistaken for an S3.
2. Valvular heart disease and atrial fibrillation, in the presence of neurological deficits, can suggest stroke over stroke mimic.

Neurological examination

➠ The neurological examination remains the best test to determine localization of stroke.
➠ A detailed neurological examination is important in differentiating true stroke from stroke imitators.
➠ The National Institute of Health Stroke Scale (NIHSS) is a scale of stroke severity. It does not confirm etiology, localization, or rule out neurological disorders that may imitate stroke.
➠ The Folstein Mini-Mental Status examination is a good test to follow for severity of dementia or delirium. It is inappropriate in the evaluation of acute stroke.

Mental status

ALERT

Comment on how awake the patient is.

1. Reduced consciousness is seen with damage to the bifrontal or bithalamic regions, or brainstem reticular activating system.
2. If the patient is hyperalert, think alcohol/barbiturate withdrawal or psychiatric disease.

ORIENTATION

Should be done in terms of ascending difficulty. (a) Where are you? (b) What is the date (day, month, year)? (c) Orientation to person (who they think they are), and (d) Why are you here, or what's going on?

1. Disorientation is usually seen in delirium or memory impairment.
2. If a patient does not know who he/she is or thinks he/she is Julius Caesar, consider psychiatric cause.

ATTENTION

Can the patient attend to concentration tasks? For example, doing the days of the week forward and backward, months of the year forward and backward. Difficulty with concentration is poorly localizing, as it can be seen with metabolic disturbances, pain, and anxiety.

MEMORY

Long-term memory (questions like Where did you go to high school? When's your birthday? and Where do you live? is usually preserved in most people with memory deficits.

LANGUAGE

Examine the following items:

⟹ Speech output and flow
⟹ Comprehension
⟹ Repetition
⟹ Writing
⟹ Reading
⟹ Prosody.

In *fluent aphasia*, speech flows but has phonemic paraphasic errors (flotch for watch). In *nonfluent aphasia*, speech is sparse, nongrammatical, but with meaningful words haltingly spoken, and patients are often frustrated (Table 2.2).

1. Every patient should *write* and *read*. This is the *minimum* required language testing for aphasia.

Table 2.2: Basic aphasia testing

Aphasia	Fluency	Comprehension	Repetition
Broca's	Poor	Adequate	Poor
Wernicke's	Adequate	Poor	Poor
Conduction	Adequate	Adequate	Poor
Global	Poor	Poor	Poor
Transcortical motor	Poor	Adequate	Adequate
Transcortical sensory	Adequate	Poor	Adequate
Transcortical global	Poor	Poor	Adequate

Source: Adapted from Damasio AR. Aphasia *NJEM* 1992;326(8):531–39.

2. *Prosody* is best tested by having patients interpret a sentence like "I didn't say she stole my money" by placing the accent on different words, which can drastically alter the meaning of the sentence. Expressive prosody problems localize to nondominant frontal and receptive prosody problems to nondominant temporal regions.
3. Finger agnosia is the inability to name individual fingers. Care should be taken in interpreting this sign, as many languages do not name each individual finger. Finger agnosia is part of the Gerstman's syndrome.

All aphasia localize to the dominant hemisphere.

1. Wernicke's aphasia = superior temporal gyrus.
2. Broca's aphasia = frontal lobe.
3. Conduction = parietal and frontal lobes (arcuate fasciculus).
4. Global aphasias = large hemispheric strokes or tumors.
5. Transcortical motor aphasia = anterior to Broca's area in frontal lobe or thalamus.
6. Transcortical sensory = dominant posterior, temporal-occipital area, think of watershed strokes.
7. Transcortical global = poorly localizing; can also occur with watershed strokes.
8. Alexia without agraphia = dominant occipital lobe and/or splenium of the corpus callosum lesion.

CALCULATION

➡ Acalculia occurs primarily as part Gerstmann's syndrome (acalculia, agraphia, right left confusion, finger agnosia) affecting angular gyrus of the dominat parietal lobe.

NEGLECTS

More common with right hemipshere lesions.

1. *Sensory neglect* is extinction to double simultaneous stimulation and localizes to the occipital-parietal region.
2. *Spatial neglect* is best tested with line bisection task and clock drawing (have them draw it large).
3. *Motor neglect* where people have good strength but are still weak. It localizes to the right frontal lobe.
4. *Anosagnosia* is being unaware of deficits.

APRAXIAS

Patients are unable to perform tasks like finger snapping, clapping, sticking out the tongue, waving goodbye, light a match then blow it out. There can be gait apraxias, dressing apraxia, or apraxia of eye opening.

➠ Often localize to prefrontal cortex or parietal lobe.

Frontal lobe dysfunction

1. Orbital frontal lesions present with emotional disinhibition (grasping, crying, inappropriate sexual comments).
2. Dorsolateral prefrontal lesions present with working memory problems. This is probably best tested by giving the patient three objects and having them repeat all three at 30 s and 5 min with distraction.
3. Mesiofrontal lesions lead to abulia (patients lie like a bump on a log, saying nothing, and doing little).

Dermatological examination

A careful skin examination in atypical stroke patients is important and can provide clues to the diagnosis of several stroke syndromes.

1. Malar rash can be seen in systemic lupus erythematosus (SLE). SLE can cause stroke due to hypercoagulable states as well as from Libman–Sacks endocarditis.
2. Levido reticularis is a skin pattern found in Sneddon's syndrome, which is an uncommon antiphospholipid antibody syndrome variant. It can present with strokes and is also associated with SLE. The rash is often found on the trunk and extremities.
3. Splinter hemorrhages and Janeway lesions can be seen with subacute and occasionally acute bacterial endocarditis. Endocarditis not only causes embolic stroke but also mycotic cerebral aneurysms.
4. A reddish purplish rash in the buttocks, groin, and upper thighs can be found in Fabry's disease. It is an X-linked disease found in males in which the rate of incidence of stroke is 10–24 percent . Most common strokes are posterior circulation, penetrating artery disease, and intracerebral hemorrhages.

Cranial nerves

I-Olfactory

Test each nostril separately. Don't use anything noxious like alcohol or peppermint.

1. Reduction can occur after head trauma suggesting a fracture of the cribiform plate.
2. Patients with orbital groove meningiomas and people with Alzheimer's often have decreased smell.
3. Olfaction is rarely tested in the setting of acute stroke-like symptoms.

II-Optic

Test visual acuity in each eye, look for field loss in both eyes, look at optic fundus for papilledema and at vessels.

III-Oculomotor, IV-Trochlear, and VI-Abducens

Is there a ptosis? Look at each pupil separately and note the size and amount of contraction to light. Does the contralateral pupil constrict when you shine light? Does one eye constrict to direct light but less/more to consensual light? If there is a significant pupillary size difference, is it worse with the lights on (III palsy) or worse with the lights off (Horner's syndrome)? Is the difference the same either way (physiologic anisocoria)?

1. Always describe what you see, no jargon.
2. Have patients follow your finger in the six cardinal directions, observe voluntarily eye movements, and if comatose with head movements, do the eyes move normally? Is there nystagmus? Which direction is the fast phase and which is the slow phase? Is the nystagmus worse in one direction? Does the nystagmus change direction as they follow your finger? Do the eyes move together or is one eye unable to make a specific movement? Is there double vision? Does it get better when they close one eye, if so, is it worse when looking at close objects or when they are far away? Is the double vision worse in one of the six cardinal directions?
   a) Worsening horizontal diplopia when looking at close objects suggests CN III nerve problem.
   b) Worsening horizontal diplopia when looking at far objects suggests CN VI nerve problem.
3. Examining pupillary function is very important especially in the sleep or comatose patient.
   a) Very small pin point but symmetric pupils can be due to opiate use and can also be a sign of bilateral pontine injury from stroke or increased intracranial pressure.

b) Anisocoria can be due to a large and poorly constrictive pupil or a small and poorly dilating pupil. Pupils should be examined in the light and again in the dark. In general, if an anisocoria is more pronounced with lights on, this raises a concern for pupillary constriction deficit as in a third nerve palsy. An anisocoria that is more pronounced in the dark is probably due to a deficit of pupillary dilatation as in Horner's syndrome.

4. Cortical visual changes can be seen with strokes involving the occipital parietal areas.

a) A Balint's syndrome can occur with bilateral parieto-occipital damage. Such patients will appear blind or have reduced vision but will have normal pupillary function.

i) They have a triad of findings on visual examination.
- optic ataxia, which is the inability to accurately reach objects with their hands because of poor visual cues. Without vision there is no ataxia or sensory loss.
- optic apraxia, which is the inability to move their eyes to a new area of fixation. The request "Can you move your eyes to the right?" typically results in the patient's eyes moving in various directions.
- simutanagnosia, which is the inability to perceive more than one object at a time. Drawing a house with doors, windows, and smoke stack best tests this. The patient will identify each object separately but will not put the whole picture together as a house.

V-Trigeminal

Test fine touch and pin sensation of the face (both sides). Vertex of head to just under the eye is V1, under eye to above jaw is V2, and mandible is V3. Motor component of V is jaw opening and jaw closing. Consider testing vibration on the forehead if you suspect the sensory loss to be factitious.

VII-Facial

Does the face look symmetric? Can they raise their eyebrows? Can they close their eyes against resistance? Is there an equal nasolabial fold on both sides, or is one gone? When they smile do the corners of both sides turn up? Sometimes both sides end up normal but one side moves slower. These are signs of subtle facial weaknesses.

1. Classically if the whole face is paralyzed, then it is a peripheral seventh, and if it's just the mouth, it is a central seventh. However, both types of palsy can present either way.

2. A branch associated with the seventh nerve mediates taste and so is volume pitch control of hearing. Ask whether things have a funny taste, whether taste has gone on one side of the tongue, and whether everything sounds tinny on one side. These are peripheral seventh cranial nerve signs.

3. The rule of upper and lower face being lower motor neuron versus lower face being just upper motor neuron can lead one astray. There are plenty of examples of their type presenting with just lower face or upper and lower face. One useful way to differentiate is the volitional versus the emotional smile.

   a) With peripheral palsy, the smile should be asymmetric regardless of whether it is emotional or volitional. The axons to the muscles are damaged so no movement occurs.

   b) With upper motor neuron lesion, sometimes the patient will have an intact emotional smile but an absent volitional smile.

VIII-Auditory/vestibular

Hearing is tested grossly with finger rubbing or ticking of a watch.

1. Weber test is done with a 512-Hz tuning fork placed on the forehead or front teeth. The sound should be heard in both ears. If it is louder in the one ear, this can suggest nerve damage in the contralateral ear or conduction deafness in the ipsilateral ear.

2. Rhinne uses the 512-Hz fork. Place fork in front of ear then place on mastoid process. Ask which is louder, air or bone. If air is greater than bone, then it is normal or a neural hearing loss. If bone is greater than air, then there's a conduction (nonnerve) hearing loss.

3. In general, this is not an issue with most stroke patients. Except with strokes involving the anterior inferior cerebellar artery (AICA). The labyrinthine artery comes off the AICA and occlusion of this artery can result in unilateral hearing loss, which resembles sensory neural hearing loss type. Occasionally bilateral acute hearing loss can be the presenting symptom of a basilar artery occlusion as both AICAs are occluded.

IX-Glossopharyngeal–X-vagus complex

1. Do both sides of the palate elevate symmetrically or does one side rise and the other side not move? If the right side does not elevate, it is a right palate weakness.

2. Touching the posterior pharynx with a pin or cotton swab tests sensation.

3. Putting a swab on the tonsillar pillars tests gag. Absence of a gag is not abnormal by itself; almost all people with dentures have little or no gag.

IX-Spinal accessory

Ask the patient to shrug his shoulders and keep them up. Push down on the shoulders; you should not be able to break them even in the elderly. Ask the patient to forcibly turn his head and use your hand to try to resist the movement.

XII-Hypoglossal

I look at the speed of tongue movement and the strength by which a person can indent the cheek with their tongue on either side. I try to push it back in on either side and thus compare the two sides.

1. Care should be taken in evaluating tongue weakness. Simply sticking out the tongue in a patient with a facial droop can resemble a tongue deviation. The above technique is probably better to evaluate tongue weakness.
2. Upper motor neuron weakness of the tongue will present with tongue weakness pointing toward the lesion as the normal side of the tongue pulls the entire tongue away from the side of weakness.
3. Hypoglossal nerve weakness through lesion of the nerve or nucleus presents with atrophy of the tongue and tongue deviation away from the lesion. It is best to think about tongue weakness being weakness on the left or right and then an anatomic localization can be applied.

Motor

Bulk and tone

Increased tone can occur in the acute setting and is not always a late manifestation of stroke. It can occur in the acute setting especially due to deep white matter and basal ganglia strokes. This is likely due to the fact that the descending inhibitory fibers from the motor cortex are affected.

Drift

Have the patient hold hands out, palms up. Ask them to close their eyes. With subtle weakness the hand internally rotates and moves down. Upward motion can be a parietal lobe finding. If the hand starts to move abnormally, this can be a sign of proprioceptive problems.

Strength

Weakness occurs in patterns: single nerve pattern, single root pattern, diffuse-symmetric proximal greater than distal weakness, diffuse-symmetric distal greater than proximal weakness, and upper motor neuron pattern weakness. (Extensors weaker than flexors in arms and extensors stronger than flexors in legs.)

Coordination

(Not called the cerebellar exam. Coordination is also controlled by sensation and strength.)

Rapid alternating movements

Can the patient do rapid finger taps between thumb and forefinger? Look for irregularity of rhythm. Segmentation of motion, thumb to each finger in a row and back is a good test for subtle weakness.

Finger to nose

1. Remember that ataxia on finger to nose can be due to weakness or sensory loss of the limb also.
2. If they do well several times, ask them to do it again with their eyes closed. If they miss consistently even with practice always to the right/ left of target, this is past pointing.
3. Sensory ataxia suggests either a thalamic or parietal lobe lesion.
4. Weakness can occur anywhere in the neuro axis. Ataxia with finger to nose is typically a cerebellar or pontocerebellar lesion.

Heel to shin

This is the finger to nose equivalent in the leg. Ataxia on heel/shin can occur in the absence of abnormal finger to nose testing.The patient should place their heel on their knee and then slide it down the tibia to the ankle. Wavy, shaking, or falling off is considered abnormal. Medial cerebellum damage can lead to normal limb movements with truncal ataxia and abnormal heel to shin.

Rebound/overshoot/mirror test

These are looking for abnormal control of the limb.

➠ Rebound is tested either by holding arms out and tapping on both arms; there should be a single correction then the arms will resume position. Abnormal is if the limb oscillates like a spring, in comparison with the normal limb.
➠ Overshoot is tested by having the arms straight above the head and then bringing them down fast to a sudden stop. Abnormal is when one limb does not stop short but overshoots to halt position more than once.

⇒ Mirror test is done with the patient and you pointing fingers, you move, they move like a mirror. If they overshoot movements more than once or twice, that is abnormal. This is primarily a cerebellar sign.

Sensation

Fine touch

Always ask whether they have numbness and ask them to draw the area out with their finger. This is a fast and efficient way to test in people who know they have numbness. Use a piece of cotton to test fine touch and touch points. Fine touch travels in dorsal columns. Look for focal loss versus distal gradients.

Extinction

This is a cortical/subcortical sign. Hard to test if the primary modalities are gone. Touch the left side, ask where the person felt it, touch the right side ask where they felt it, and then touch both sides and ask where they felt it. People with cortical/subcortical, frontal/parietal lesions will ignore one of the stimuli when two stimuli are given together. Right hemispheric lesions ignore left stimuli when two stimuli are given.

Pin prick/temperature

Use either pin or temperature since they both test spinothalamic sensation. I like temperature for screening and pin for demarcating an abnormality. Look for patterns distal versus proximal or in a spinal cord level.

Vibration

Remember vibration is one of the first modalities to go in peripheral neuropathies. It runs in dorsal columns.

Proprioception

Also runs in dorsal columns.

Cortical sensory loss

The following are sensory loss from cortical lesions, usually parietal lobe dysfunction:

1. Agraphasthesia is when the patient cannot identify a number written traced on the palm of their hand, always do both sides.

2. Astereognosis is the inability to recognize objects just by the feel.
3. Atopographia is the inability to determine where exactly a sensation is located or which direction a sensation is moving. Test by touching a patch of skin with their eyes closed and asking them to touch the same spot. Run a finger up or down a patch of skin and ask which direction the finger is moving.
4. Two-point discrimination is tested with two sharp objects close together, then slowly separate them and note when they realize there are two points, then compare of equivalent area on the other side.

Romberg test

1. A false positive Romberg occurs with cerebellar or eighth nerve dysfunction. In these cases the patient feels unsteady and feels like he or she will fall with eyes open and then does so with eyes closed. This is not a Romberg sign. Patient should be normal with eyes open and very unsteady with eyes closed.
2. Romberg's sign demonstrates loss of propriception in the lower extremities.

Gait

Description

As usual describe what you see. Is the gait wide or narrow based? Is it shuffling? Can they figure how to walk? Does one foot drag? Do they slap their feet when they walk? Most important is, is it wide or narrow based, do they fall to one side over and over?

1. *Tandem gait* Can they walk with one foot in front of the other? If they fall every time to the same side when they tandem, this can be a sign of focal cerebellar dysfunction. It can be the only sign of a cerebellar hemorrhage!!
2. *Forced gait* People will show subtle hemiparesis if you have them walk on the outside of their feet. You can see fisting of the hand if there is a subtle pyramidal weakness.

Reflexes/toes

Reflexes are tested at the ankles, patella, biceps, triceps, and wrist. Reflexes are given a number:
4 = Clonus with reflex,
3 = Abnormal spread (you hit biceps and triceps goes),

2 = normal,
1 = can get with augmentation procedures
0 + unable to elicit even with augmentation,
+ /– to differentiate gradations.

⟶ Babinski reflex (abnormal only) is elicited by scratching to lateral aspect of each foot. Toes are up/down mute or equivocal.

NIH stroke scale

The NIH stroke scale is a useful scale in determining the severity of stroke. It is not a diagnostic scale and there is no localization or etiological subsection to the scale. The NIH stroke scale is a very important skill to master in the acute evaluation of the stroke patient. It is vital to be able to evaluate and follow improvement of worsening of the NIH stroke scale. Remember: (a) Always use first answer. (b) NIH stroke scale underestimates right hemisphere and posterior circulation lesions as it is heavily weighted toward language deficits (Figure 2.2).

1. The NIH stroke scale underestimates severity of stroke especially when the stroke involves the nondominant hemisphere.
2. It does not have detailed cognitive or neglect testing.
3. Patients with delirium may end up having high stroke scales.
4. An NIH stroke scale of zero is more likely to be due to a stroke mimic with the chances of a stroke being a true stroke increasing as the NIH stroke scale increases.

Stroke imitators

Examination of acute stroke patients is an important way to differentiate stroke from stroke imitators. Thirty-one percent of acute stroke evaluation are stroke mimics (Table 2.3). A study found that patients with neurological signs that are consistent with the Oxford Community Stroke Project Classification (OCSP) of neurological deficits were more likely to have a stroke than not.

OCSP classification

The OCSP defines strokes as a cluster of symptoms such as patient with hemiparesis, homonymous hemianopia, and new disorders of higher cerebral dysfunction. For example, dysphasia are classified in the total anterior circulation infarct (TACI) group (Table 2.4).

1. Patients with two of the above features or with isolated cortical dysfunction (e.g., dysphasia) are classified in the PACI group.

Instructions	Definitions	Score
1a LOC	0 = Alert 1 = Arousable by minor stimulation 2 = Obtunded 3 = Unresponsive or reflex response	
1b LOC questions Month and age	0 = Answers both questions correctly 1 = Answers one question correcly 2 = Answers neither question correctly	
1c LOC commands	0 = Performs both tasks correctly 1 = Performs one task correctly 2 = Performs neither task correctly	
2 Best gaze: Horizintal eye movements	0 = Normal 1 = Partial gaze palsy 2 = Total gaxe parasis	
3 Visual fields	0 = No visual loss 1 = Partial hemianopia 2 = Complete hemianopia 3 = Bilateral hemianopia	
4 Fascial palsy	0 = Normal 1 - Minor paralysis 2 = Parial paralysis 3 = Cpmplete paralysis	
5 and 6 Molor arm and leg	0 = No drift 1 = Drift 2 = Some effort against gravity 3 = No effort against gravity 4 = No movement Ampulation = N/A	5a LUE _____ 5b RUE _____ 6a LLE _____ 6b RLE _____
7 Limb ataxia	0 = Absent 1 = Present in one limb 2 = Present in both limbs	
8 Sensory	0 = Normal 1 = Mild to moderate loss 2 = Severe loss	
9 Best language	0 = Normal 1 = Mild to moderate aphasia 2 = Severe aphasia 3 = Mute, global aphasia	
10 Dysarthria	0 = Normal 1 = Mild to moderate 2 = Severe Intubated = N/A	
11 Extinction and inattention	0 = No abnormality 1 = One of the sensory modalities 2 = Profound hemi-inattention	

Figure 2.2 NIH stroke scale.

Table 2.3: Most common stroke imitators

Condition	Total number (%)
Seizure	23 (21.1%)
Sepsis	14 (12.8%)
Toxic/metabolic	12 (11.0%)
Space-occupying lesion	10 (9.2%)
Syncope/presyncope	10 (9.2%)
Acute confusional state	7 (6.4%)
Vestibular dysfunction	7 (6.4%)
Acute mononeuropathy	6 (5.5%)
Functional/medically unexplained symptoms	6 (5.5%)
Dementia	4 (3.7%)
Migraine	3 (2.8%)
Spinal cord lesion	3 (2.8)
Other	3 (3.7%)
Total	109 (100%)

Adapted from Hand PJ, Kwan J, Lindley RI, Dennis MS, Wardlaw JM. Distinguishing between stroke and mimic at the bedside. *Brain Attack Study Stroke* 2006;37:769–75.

Table 2.4: Historical and clinical findings suggestive of stroke over stroke imitators

Variable	OR	95%CIs
Know cognitive impairment	0.33	(0.14–0.76)
An exact onset ould be determined	2.59	(1.30–5.15)
Definite history of focal neurological symptoms	7.21	(2.48–20.93)
Any abnormal vasular findings	2.54	(1.28–5.07)
Abnormal findings in any other system	0.44	(0.23–0.85)
NIHSS $= 0$		
NIHSS 1–4	1.92	(0.70–5.23)
NIHSS 5–10	3.14	(1.03–9.65)
NIHSS > 10	7.23	(2.18–24.05)
The signs could be lateralized to the left or right side of the brain	2.03	(0.92–4.46)
OCSP classification was possible	5.09	(2.42–10.70)

Adapted from Hand PJ, Kwan J, Lindley RI, Dennis MS, Wardlaw JM. Distinguishing between stroke and lmimic at the bedside. *Brain Attack Study Stroke* 2006;37: 769–75.

2. Those patients with isolated motor or sensory deficits, or sensorimotor strokes or ataxic hemiparesis are classified in the lacunar infarct (LACI) group.
3. Patients with brainstem or cerebellar signs in the posterior circulation infarct (POCI) group.
4. Patients who could by physical exam be placed into one of these groups were less likely to have a stroke imitator than a stroke.

Seizures

One of the most common neurological events that may be misinterpreted as acute stroke is seizure with postictal Todd's paralysis.

1. Seizures often have postictal neurological signs. The most common symptom is depressed consciousness. In focal onset seizures, especially if the seizure originates in frontal lobe, there may be a hemiparesis.
2. Seizures involving frontal lobe may present for forced gaze deviation initially and with postictal state gaze deviation away from the hemiparesis just as in stroke patients.
3. Seizures originating from temporal or parietal lobes may also have aphasia similar to that of stroke involving the same vascular territory. The history is probably the most helpful way to differentiate the two.

Toxic/metabolic encephalopathy

Delirium or encephalopathy is a known cause for acute stroke calls. They are particularly difficult as mild encephalopathy can present with confused speech, which may resemble a posterior or Wernicke's aphasia. Patients may develop encephalopathy acutely or over hours or days.

1. Physical exam findings that suggest an encephalopathy over stroke would be (a) inattention and inability to maintain a coherent stream of thought or action, (b) asterixis, (c) fever, and (d) abnormal admission labs particularly elevated WBC, liver function tests, or ammonia.
2. In general, one needs to be careful of the aphasia only stroke without other cortical or subcortical findings such as hemiparesis, neglect, sensory loss, and visual filed cuts.

Space-occupying lesions

Space-occupying lesions of all sorts may present with stroke-like symptoms but they are rarely acute in onset.

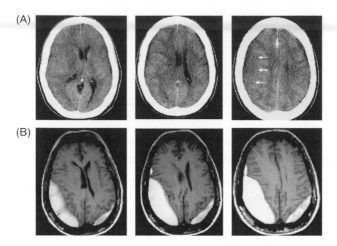

Figure 2.3 Imaging of subdural hematomas. Row A represents a subacute subdural seen on a head CT scan. It is difficult to resolve. Row B shows the same patient after an MRI scan clearly slowing bilateral subacute/chronic subdural hematomas.

1. Typically they occur over weeks to months although families may only notice symptoms late in the presentation.
2. Typically anatomic lesions will present with exam imaging mismatch.
3. The patient will have a trivial weakness or subtle cortical deficits but a large lesion on CT imaging. This is a tell-tale feature of slow-growing tumors and masses.

Subdural hematomas are of particular concern. Whereas acute subdural hematoma after fall is an easy-enough diagnosis to make, subacute subdural hematomas are more complex. Subacute and chronic subdural hematoma may present with recurrent transient ischemic attacks. This can be particularly tricky as subacute subdural hematomas may be isodense to brain after only a few weeks (Figure 2.3).

Syncope

Syncopal spells can be misinterpreted as stroke. Typically an acute syncope can be felt either by lay people or some physicians as a stroke.

1. In general a vast majority of strokes do not present with loss of consciousness. It would require bilateral damage to the frontal lobe, thalamus, or brain stem to accomplish.
2. A top of the basilar embolus may present with coma but will typically present with coma and brain stem findings and are not typically transient spells.

3. Acute onset of coma with abnormal eye and crossed cranial nerve finds are suggestive of diffuse brain stem dysfunction that may be secondary to basilar artery embolus.
4. A vast majority of syncopal spells are secondary to cardiogenic causes.

Vestibular dysfunction

The acute onset of vertigo especially in the elderly may suggest to many a cerebrovascular event. It can be somewhat difficult to differentiate from vestibular nerve dysfunction or labyrthine dysfunction.

1. In general, most posterior circulation strokes can be differentiated from vestibulopathy by the presences of limb weakness, Babinski's reflex, facial weakness, dysphagia, dysarthria, gaze palsies, and intra-nuclear ophthalmoplegia and diplopia, all of which are very uncommon in pure vestibular dysfunction.
2. Cerebellar strokes may present with vertigo and almost no other findings except gait unsteadiness and perhaps some lower extremity ataxia. In these cases a careful look at eye movements can be helpful.
3. In cerebellar or other central lesions the nystagmus may be purely vertical or horizontal. It may also change direction with the direction of gaze and not inhibited with fixation. As opposed to peripheral vestibular dysfunction, which is often combined, horizontal and rotator nystagmus on one direction, inhibited with fixation should not be associated with any other cranial nerve defects.

Migraine

Migraine is typically a disorder of young women although it has been described in older men and women. The migraine aura is caused by a spreading depression that presents with increased activity surrounded by decreased activity. Migraine visual aura will have a bright "leading edge" followed by loss of visions. The same is true of somatosensory auras where there may be a leading edge of paresthesia followed by sensory loss. Perhaps the most important historical aspect of migraine causing focal neurological deficits is that the symptoms usually "match" over 15–50 min. In most TIA and stroke the deficits are maximal at onset with fluctuations but do not tend to start off slight and worsen in a consistent pattern. Otherwise it is very difficult to use the physical examination to differentiate the two.

1. Migraine with aura that may cause, hemianopia, hemiplegia, aphasia, or confusion represents a proportion of cases seen in the emergency room and in any urgent stroke clinic.
2. The historical points that should be obtained are (a) patient history of migraine headaches, (b) frequency of aura associated or unassociated with a vascular headache 30–60 min later, (c) the history of the deficits

and whether they were maximal at onset or spread slowly over 5–20 min, and (d) history of similar spells in the patient or patient's family members. In the heat of acute evaluation, the history is of the utmost importance.

3. Clinical exam is less helpful except that a majority of patient with migraines will have an absence of cerebrovascular risk factors, normal cardiac examination, and will often be normotensive.

Spinal cord lesion

Lesions of the spinal cord may present acutely with asymmetrical examination and may resemble stroke. Spinal cord lesions can resemble a pure motor hemiparesis or a sensory motor stroke. The deficits can be acute and diffuse hyperreflexia may not occur for some time. Assessing the patient with a complete neurological examination is important.

1. Spinal cord injury patients should clearly have no cortical deficits (field cut, aphasia, neglect, gaze deviation) and really should have no facial weakness.
2. High spinal cord injury patients may present with sensory loss of the lower mandible but no sensory loss should exist in the frontal or mandibular branches of cranial nerve V.
3. Patients with new weakness after a fall even if it is a hemiplegia should be considered to have a spinal cord injury first.
4. Tell-tale bruising on the forehead may suggest cervical hyperextension and a central cord injury after a fall. In patients without cranial nerve defects, stroke can still be the diagnosis.

Summary

Imaging plays an important role in stroke care but in the acute setting there are many instances where the physical exam plays a vital role. As rt-PA is most effective from 0 to 90 min from onset, there is increasing pressure to evaluate patients quickly. A history and physical is probably the most effective way to ascertain etiology and localization for stroke evaluation. There are a number of stroke mimics that can confuse the picture and the clinician should be wary of these. Experience and understanding of the limitations of the stroke scale and possible mimics are vital to the appropriate care of the acute stroke patient.

Bibliography

Adams, Jr HP, Adams RJ, Brott T, et al. Guidelines for the early management of patients with ischemic stroke. *Stroke* 2003;34:1056–83.

Baloh RW. Differentiating between peripheral and central causes of vertigo. *Otolaryngol Head Neck Surg* 1998;119:55–9.

Bamford J, Sandercock P, Dennis M, Burn J, Warlow C. Classification and natural history of clinically identifiable subtypes of cerebral infarction. *Lancet* 1991;337:1521–6.

Buttner U, Helmchen C, Brant T. Diagnostic criteria for central versus peripheral positioning nystagmus and vertigo: A review. *Acta Otolaryngol* 1999;119:1–5.

Caplan LR. The frontal-artery sign – a bedside indicator of internal carotid artery disease. *N Engl J Med* 1973;288:1008–9.

Christou I, Felberg RA, Demchuk AM, et al. A broad diagnostic battery for bedside transcranial Doppler to detect flow changes with internal carotid artery stenosis or occlusion. *J Neuroimaging* 2001 July;11(3):236–42.

Fink JN, Selim MH, Kumar S, et al. and the association of National Institutes of Health. Stroke Scale scores and acute magnetic resonance imaging stroke volume equal for patients with right- and left-hemisphere ischemic stroke? *Stroke* 2002 Apr;33(4):954–8.

Fisher CM. Facial pulses in internal carotid artery occlusion. *Neurology* 1970 May;20 (5):476–8.

Hand PJ, Kwan J, Lindley RI, Dennis MS, Wardlaw JM. Distinguishing between stroke and mimic at the bedside. *The brain attack study Stroke*. 2006;37:769–75.

Lauritzen M, Aling J, Pailson BO. Orbital bruits and retinal artery pressure in internal carotid artery occlusion. *Clin Neurol Neurosurg* 1981;83(1):7–10.

Libman RB, Wirkowski E, Alvir J, Rao TH. Conditions that mimic stroke in the emergency department. Implications for acute stroke trials. *Arch Neurol* 1995;52:1119–22.

Linfante I, Llinas RH, Schalug G, Chaves C, Warach S, Caplan LR. Diffusion-weighted imaging and National Institutes of Health Stroke Scale in the acute phase of posterior-circulation stroke. *Arch Neurol* 2001 Apr;58(4):621–8.

Panzer RJ, Feibel JH, Barker WH, Griner PF. Predicting the likelihood of hemorrhage in patients with stroke. *Arch Intern Med* 1985;145:1800–3.

Pessin MS, Panis W, Prager RJ, Millan VG, Scott RM. Auscultation of cervical and ocular bruits in extracranial carotid occlusive disease: A clinical and angiographic study. *Stroke*, 1983;14(2): 246–9.

Ropper AH, Fisher CM, Kleiman GM. Pyramidal infarction in the medulla: A cause of pure motor hemiplegia sparing the face. *Neurology* 1979 Jan;29(1):91–5.

Savitz S, Caplan LR. Vertebrobasilar disease. *NEJM* 2005 352:2618–26.

3 Clinical stroke syndromes and localization

Sean I. Savitz

Specific stroke syndromes are caused by occlusion or hemorrhage of a cerebral blood vessel supplying a specific vascular territory in the brain. Accurate diagnosis of the specific type of stroke and vascular brain lesions requires matching the patient's symptoms and signs to known patterns of ischemia and hemorrhage.

Ischemic stroke syndromes

Stroke syndromes caused by vessel occlusions can be categorized based upon whether the vascular lesion is in the anterior or posterior circulation.

Syndromes of occlusive disease and brain ischemia in the anterior circulation

The main supply of the anterior circulation derives from the carotid arteries, which course through the neck into the brain and give off the ophthalmic artery to the eye, the middle and anterior cerebral arteries feeding the medial and anterior segments of the cerebral hemispheres, the anterior choroidal and posterior communicating arteries.

INTERNAL CAROTID ARTERY (ICA) STENOSIS AND OCCLUSION
Features of retinal ischemia
One of the most localizing clues to an ICA lesion is transient monocular blindness (amaurosis fugax). This is caused by occlusion of the retinal artery, which comes off the ophthalmic artery.

1. A shade falls from above but may move from the sides. After a few seconds or minutes, the shade recedes.
2. The upper or lower visual field may only be affected if a branch vessel off the retinal artery is selectively blocked.

3. Fundoscopy should assess for retinal infarcts, cholesterol crystals, and platelet plugs.

Hemispheral features

Infarction in the cerebral hemisphere occurs most commonly in the Middle cerebral artery (MCA) territory and causes weakness of the contralateral hand and face more than the leg, contralateral cortical sensory loss, aphasia (if left hemisphere), and neglect of the left side (if right hemisphere).

1. Some patients with tight ICA stenosis present with brief, multiple Transient ischemic attack (TIAs) over several weeks.
2. Sudden, brief episodes of limb shaking can occur and are called limb shaking TIAs.

THE MCA SYNDROMES

Main stem ischemia

Occlusion at the main stem of the MCA causes infarction of the basal ganglia and internal capsule before the take-off of the lenticulostriate branches (Figure 3.1). Striatocapsular damage causes hemiparesis of the face, arm, and leg, dysarthria, and usually minimal sensory loss. Cortical findings are variable depending on the collateral circulation of the convexity.

Superior division MCA ischemia

The superior branch of the MCA supplies the frontal and superior parietal lobes. Patients have hemiplegia more severe in the face, hand, and arm, hemisensory loss, conjugate eye deviation to the ipsilateral side, and neglect of the contralateral side of space if the nondominant hemisphere is affected.

➧ Left hemisphere lesions cause aphasia which evolves over time to a Broca's type (sparse effortful and telegraphic speech, preserved comprehension).
➧ Right hemisphere lesions cause anosognosia and aprososida.

Inferior division MCA ischemia

The inferior branch of the MCA supplies the inferior parietal and temporal lobes. In contrast to superior division MCA stroke, there are no elementary motor or sensory signs. The clinical spectrum of include:

➧ contralateral visual field defects
➧ Wernick-type aphasia (if left hemisphere)
➧ agitation (right hemisphere)
➧ poor visual-spatial constructions (right hemisphere).

ANTERIOR CEREBRAL ARTERY SYNDROME

This artery supplies the medial frontal lobe (Figure 3.2). Occlusive lesions cause a pattern of weakness affecting the leg and foot more so than the arm

Lesion		Artery/occluded	Infarct, surface	Infarct, coronal section	Clinical manifestations
Middle cerebral artery	Entire territory	Anterior cerebral — Superior division, Lenticulostriate (Medial, Lateral); Internal carotid — Middle cerebral — Inferior division			Contralateral gaze palsy, hemiplegia, hemisensory loss, spatial neglect, hemianopsia Global aphasia (if on left side) May lead to coma secondary to edema
	Deep				Contralateral hemiplegia, hemisensory loss Transcortical motor and/or sensory aphasia (it on left side)
	Parasylvian				Contralateral weakness and sensory loss of face and hand Conduction aphasia, apraxia and Gerstmann's syndrome (if on left side) Constructional dyspraxia (if on right side)
	Superior division				Contralateral hemiplegia, hemisensory loss, gaze palsy, spatial neglect Broca's aphasia (if on left side)
	Inferior division				Contralateral hemianopsia or upper quadrant anopsia Wernicke's aphasia (if on left side) Constructional dyspraxia (if on right side)

Figure 3.1 Patterns of MCA occlusion. (Reprinted from Ciba Collection of Medical Illustrations, Volume I, Part II: *The Nervous System,* Frank Netter, 1986, with permission from Elsevier.)

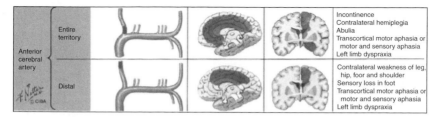

				Incontinence Contralateral hemiplegia Abulia Transcortical motor aphasia or motor and sensory aphasia Left limb dyspraxia
Anterior cerebral artery	Entire territory			
	Distal			Contralateral weakness of leg, hip, foor and shoulder Sensory loss in foot Transcortical motor aphasia or motor and sensory aphasia Left limb dyspraxia

Figure 3.2 Patterns of ACA occlusion. (Reprinted from Ciba Collection of Medical Illustrations, Volume I, Part II: *The Nervous System*, Frank Netter, 1986, with permission from Elsevier.)

or face; the deltoid muscle can also be weak. A grasp reflex of the contralateral hand may be present. Sometimes, aphasia can develop if the supplementary motor cortex is infarcted.

➠ Bilateral frontal lobe infarctions can occur if there is only one anterior choroidal artery (ACA) syndrome supplying both sides of the brain and cause abulia, urinary incontinence, and paraparesis.

ACA SYNDROME

This artery supplies the globus pallidus, lateral geniculate body, posterior limb of the internal capsule. The classic syndrome consists of

➠ hemipareis and hemisensory loss of the face, arm, and leg
➠ homonymous hemianopsia
➠ absence of cortical findings

Often, some features are not present but hemiparesis is the most common finding.

Syndromes of occlusive disease and brain ischemia in the posterior circulation

Anatomy Figure 3.3 shows the blood supply of the posterior circulation.

Typical symptoms Dizziness, vertigo, headache, vomiting, double vision, loss of vision, ataxia, weakness, or numbness involving both sides of the body are frequent symptoms in patients with vertebrobasilar ischemic disease. Clinical signs suggestive of posterior circulation ischemia include

➠ bilateral or crossed motor or sensory signs
➠ ataxia
➠ decreased level of consciousness
➠ oculomotor and lower cranial nerve deficits

BRAIN STEM SYNDROMES
Lateral medullary infarction (Wallenberg syndrome)

This condition is most often caused by a vascular occlusive lesion within the intracranial vertebral artery. The clinical features depend upon the extent of

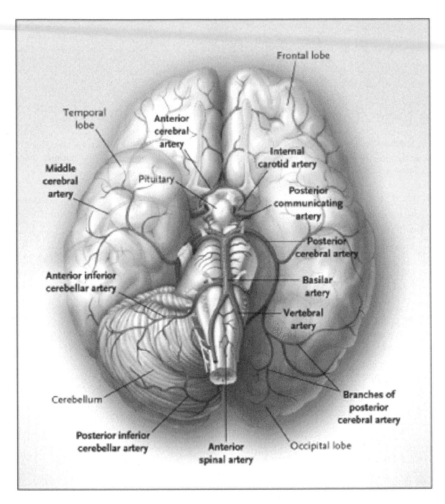

Figure 3.3 Posterior circulation. The posterior circulation nourishes the brain stem (medulla, pons, midbrain), cerebellum, occipital lobes, posterior temporal lobe, and thalamus. The arterial supply consists of the vertebral arteries feeding the medulla and joining together to form the basilar artery, which nourishes the pons with deep arterial penetrators before merging with the Circle of Willis at the base of the brain to give off the posterior cerebral arteries. (Reprinted from Savitz SI, Caplan LR. Vertebrobasilar Disease. *N Engl J Med. 2005;* 352:2618–2626 with permission from the publishing division of the Massachusetts Medical Society).

the damage within the lateral tegmentum of the medulla and consist of the following (Figure 3.4):

- vertigo or feeling off balance (vestibular nuclei)
- nystagmus (vestibular nuclei)
- pulling sensation or leaning to one side (inferior cerebellar peduncle)
- facial sensory changes ipsilateral (trigeminal nucleus)
- contralateral loss of pain/temperature in body/limbs (spinothalamic tract)

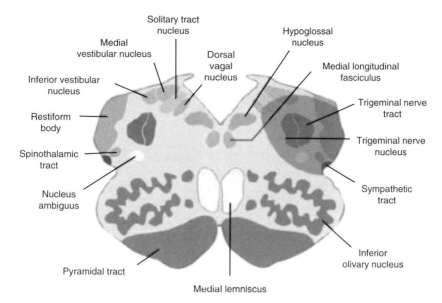

Figure 3.4 Lateral medullary infarction. (Reprinted from Savitz SI, Caplan LR. *Vertebrobasilar Disease. N Engl J Med. 2005;* 352:2618–2626 with permission from the publishing division of the Massachusetts Medical Society).

➤ Horner's of the ipsilateral eye (sympathetic tract)
➤ autonomic changes (sympathetic tract)
➤ oropharyngeal paresis ipsilateral (nucleus ambiguus)

Medial medullary infarction

The most common finding is contralateral hemiparesis, due to involvement of the corticospinal tracts, and posterior column sensory loss (such as proprioception), due to involvement of the medial lemniscus. Although most localizing, ipsilateral tongue paresis can occur but is least common.

Pontine syndromes due to basilar artery occlusions

Bilateral symptoms and signs or crossed findings (involving one side of the face and the contralateral side of the trunk and limbs) are most common. Here are the typically features:

1. hemiparesis on one side and some motor or reflex abnormality on the other;
2. ataxia or limb incoordination combined with hemiparesis;
3. bulbar weakness (face, pharynx, larynx, and tongue): dysarthria, dysphonia, dysphagia;
4. oculomotor: gaze palsies, INO, nystagmus, diplopia;
5. exaggerated crying and laughing;
6. palatal myoclonus;
7. sensory loss not typically prominent.

When the ventral pons is severely infarcted bilaterally, the patient may develop a locked-in syndrome causing quadriplegia, aphonia, and impaired horizontal gaze but consciousness and vertical eye movements are preserved.

Midbrain strokes

1. Resulting from occlusion of basilar branches:
   a) *Dorsal midbrain* Supranuclear upgaze paralysis, light-near dissociation, and convergence retraction nystagmus.
   b) *Ventral midbrain* Decreased level of consciousness, bilateral downgaze paralysis.
2. Resulting from occlusion of branches from the PCA: Many syndromes have been described depending on the area of the midbrain affected. One syndrome, called Weber syndrome, includes an ipsilateral third nerve palsy, and a contralateral hemiparesis. Involvement of the red nucleus causes a tremor.

TOP OF THE BASILAR SYNDROME

This syndrome is typically due to embolic infarction of the rostral midbrain and thalamus and consists of the following:

➧ Small, poorly reactive pupils
➧ Defective vertical gaze
➧ Hypersomnolence
➧ Hallucinations
➧ Memory deficits
➧ Decreased level of consciousness
➧ Involuntary seizure-like or posturing movements of extremities

PCA SYNDROMES

The most common finding is a hemianopia that the patient may or may not recognize depending on whether the injury extends into the parietal lobe which controls awareness of deficits. The lateral thalamus is supplied by a small branch of the PCA (thalamogeniculate) and ischemia in this territory causes sensory symptoms and signs of the contralateral hemibody. Additional features include the following.

Left posterior cerebral artery (PCA) ischemia

Alexia without agraphia, Gerstmann's syndrome, and visual agnosia.

Right PCA ischemia

Prosopagnosia (inability to recognize faces), visual neglect, disorientation to place. Inability to form new memories can occur if the medial temporal lobes are involved on either side.

Bilateral PCA stroke

Cortical blindness in which patients cannot see or identify objects correctly but have normal papillary responses (Anton's syndrome). Agitated confusion can occur and resembles delirium but any right hemisphere infarct may cause confusion.

CEREBELLAR SYNDROMES
Posterior inferior cerebellar artery (PICA) distribution

PICA territory ischemia causes vertigo similar to peripheral vestibulopathies, lateral pulsion or veering to the ipsilateral side, ipsilateral limb ataxia, headache, and vomiting. This condition often coexists with the lateral medullary syndrome because the PICA originates from the intracranial vertebral artery.

Anterior inferior cerebellar artery (AICA) distribution

Lesions within this territory can not only simulate some features of the lateral medullary syndrome but also affect cranial nerves VII and VIII.

1. AICA ischemia is typically associated with aural symptoms because it gives off the internal auditory artery, supplying the inner ear.
2. Episodes of tinnitus, hearing loss, and vertigo may represent inner ear ischemia and herald an AICA stroke.

Superior cerebellar artery (SCA) distribution

Very rare to occur in the absence of other infarcts in regions supplied by other arteries arising from the rostral basilar artery. By itself, SCA ischemia involves the pontine and midbrain tegmentum and superior cerebellar surface.

1. The classic syndrome is ipsilateral limb ataxia and Horner's syndrome, contralateral loss of pain and temperature of the face, arm, and leg, and contralateral fourth nerve palsy.
2. Limb ataxia and intention tremor are more prominent than PICA or AICA strokes.

Small vessel syndromes (penetrating artery disease)

These syndromes result from changes within small arteries that arise from the major basal cerebral arteries (see Table 3.1). Degeneration or occlusion of these arteries causes small deep infarcts called lacunae in the basal ganglia, thalami, brain stem (pons, cerebral peduncles, pyramids), and white matter within the corona radiata. They do not typically occur in the cortex or cerebellum.

1. Symptoms are primarily motor or sensory.
2. There are no headaches, no changes in alertness or behavior, and no seizures.

Table 3.1: Vascular distribution of small vessel disease

Artery	Origin	Areas affected
Lenticulostriate	MCA stem	Internal capsule
Thalamogeniculate	PCA	Thalamus
Anterior choroidal	ICA	Corona radiata, internal capsule, LGN
Deep perforators	Basilar	Pons, midbrain

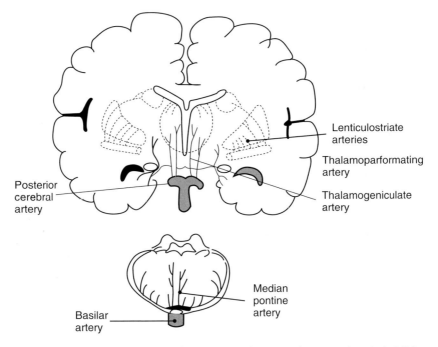

Figure 3.5 Small artery strokes. (Reprinted from *Caplan's Stroke, 3rd Edition: A Clinical Approach*, Louis Caplan, Copyright (2000), with permission of Elsevier.)

3. Typical arteries affected are depicted in Figure 3.5.

The most common syndromes are

1. *Pure motor weakness* Face, arm, and leg without cognitive, sensory, or visual abnormalities.
   a. *Location* Anywhere in the corticospinal tract from the corona radiata to the medulla but most commonly → internal capsule or pons.
2. *Pure sensory loss* Numbness or paresthesias in face, arm, and leg without cognitive, motor, or visual abnormalities.

   a. *Location* Ventrolateral thalamus (most common), lateral tegmental pons (less common).
3. *Ataxic hemiparesis* Weakness and ataxia on one side of the body without sensory, visual, or cognitive abnormalities.
   a. *Location* Anywhere from where the corticospinal and pontocerebellar tracts travel together (typically, the pons or posterior limb of internal capsule).
4. *Sensorimotor symptoms* Weakness and tingling variably affects face, arm, and leg (often leg is more affected than arm) on one side.
   a. *Location* Corona radiata affecting both corticospinal and sensory tracts.
5. *Dysarthria-clumsy hand syndrome* Slurred speech, facial and tongue weakness, clumsiness of the hand.
   a. *Location* Pons.

Watershed syndromes

These infarcts occur at the border zone between two arterial territories either between MCA and ACA or MCA and PCA. Global hypoperfusion is a common cause of watershed syndromes.

1. MCA-ACA
   a) Weakness primarily involves the shoulder and hip, sparing the hand and foot and causing a "man-in-a-barrel" pattern.
   b) Sometimes, saccadic eye movements are impaired due to damage of the frontal eye fields. Transcortical motor aphasias may also occur.
2. MCA-PCA
   a) These infarcts involve the parietal-occipital and parieto-temporal areas and cause transcortical sensory aphasia and Balint's syndrome (optic ataxia, ocular apraxia, and simultagnosia).

Intracerebral hemorrhage syndromes

Hemorrhage causes specific symptoms referable to the area affected and general symptoms referable to raised intracranial pressure such as headache, vomiting, and depressed level of consciousness.

General symptoms

1. Onset of symptoms can be sudden similar to vascular occlusions but a distinguishing feature is progression of clinical deficits over minutes to hours because of hematoma expansion.
2. Headache is common but not invariable.
3. Focal signs appear first depending on the location and extent of the bleed.

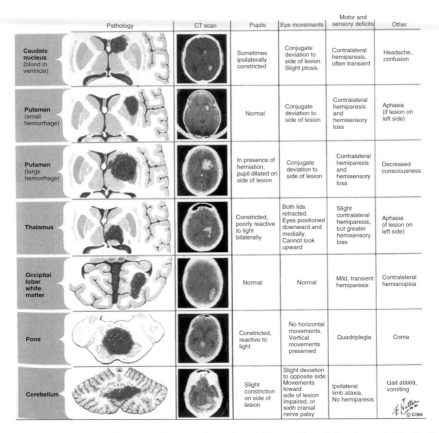

Pathology	CT scan	Pupils	Eye movements	Motor and sensory deficits	Other
Caudate nucleus (blood in ventricle)		Sometimes ipsilaterally constricted	Conjugate deviation to side of lesion. Slight ptosis	Contralateral hemiparesis, often transient	Headache, confusion
Putamen (small hemorrhage)		Normal	Conjugate deviation to side of lesion	Contralateral hemiparesis and hemisensory loss	Aphasia (if lesion on left side)
Putamen (large hemorrhage)		In presence of herniation, pupil dilated on side of lesion	Conjugate deviation to side of lesion	Contralateral hemiparesis and hemisensory loss	Decreased consciousness
Thalamus		Constricted, poorly reactive to light bilaterally	Both lids retracted. Eyes positioned downward and medially. Cannot look upward	Slight contralateral hemiparesis, but greater hemisensory loss	Aphasia (if lesion on left side)
Occipital lobar white matter		Normal	Normal	Mild, transient hemiparesis	Contralateral hemianopsia
Pons		Constricted, reactive to light	No horizontal movements. Vertical movements preserved	Quadriplegia	Coma
Cerebellum		Slight constriction on side of lesion	Slight deviation to opposite side. Movements toward side of lesion impaired, or sixth cranial nerve palsy	Ipsilateral limb ataxia. No hemiparesis	Gait ataxia, vomiting

Figure 3.6 Hemorrhage syndromes. (Reprinted from Ciba Collection of Medical Illustrations, Volume I, Part II: *The Nervous System*, Frank Netter, 1986, with permission from Elsevier.)

4. Vomiting occurs from ventricular blood irritating the fourth ventricle or downward displacement on the brain stem from raised pressure or brain stem compression.
5. Decreased level of consciousness may indicate a cerebral hematoma causing shift and damage to the other hemisphere, bilateral thalamic damage, or brain stem compression.
6. The most common locations can be found in Figure 3.6.

PUTAMINAL HEMORRHAGE

The usual findings of a large hematoma are

1. Contralateral hemiparesis (involving the internal capsule)
2. Hemisensory loss (involving the sensory tracts)
3. Conjugate eye deviation toward ipsilateral side
4. Other findings may include nonfluent aphasia (if left sided), left-sided neglect (if right sided).

THALAMIC HEMORRHAGES

Neurological features differ depending on the size, location, and pressure effects on the third ventricle. The posterior hematomas in the distribution of the thalamogeniculate artery cause primarily contralateral sensory changes but can cause concurrent hemiplegia depending on whether the internal capsule is involved.

1. There are many characteristic occulomotor findings:
   a) Paralysis of upward gaze.
   b) Hyperconvergence of one or both eyes. Patients may appear as if they are peering downward and inward at the top of their noses.
   c) Ocular skew is also possible in which one eye rests below the other.
   d) Wrong way eyes. Eyes rest toward the opposite side of each other.
   e) Disconjugate gaze. Impaired abduction of both eyes (pseuosixth).
2. There may also be pupillary abnormalities:
   a) Small and poorly reactive to light.
3 Many different cortical signs:
   a) Aphasia (if left sided).
   b) Neglect and anosognosia (if right sided).
4 Arousal may also be affected:
   a) Decreased alertness.
   b) Hypersomnolence.

PONTINE HEMORRHAGES

These hemorrhages typically start in the penetrating vessels supplying the tegementum and base of the pons.
 The typical signs of medial pontine hematomas include

1. quadraparesis
2. limb stiffness
3. coma
4. no horizontal eye movements
5. rapid or irregular respirations
6. headache and vomiting may occur if bleeding dissects into the fourth ventricle
7. some cases start with hemiparesis and then progress to deafness, dysarthria, facial numbness, limb weakness followed by coma.

The typical signs of lateral hematomas include:

1. pure motor or ataxic hemiparesis
2. unilateral cranial nerve abnormalities
3. oculomotor (if affecting the lateral tegmentum): ipsilateral gaze paresis, INO, one and a half syndrome, contralateral sensory loss, and ipsilateral ataxia.

LOBAR HEMORRHAGES

Hematomas develop at the gray-white junction and dissect into the white matter. Symptoms and signs depend on the location.

1. *Frontal* Patients may have contralateral hemiparesis, conjugate ipsilateral eye deviation, aphasia (if left sided), and abulia.
2. *Parietal* Patients may have contralateral hemisensory loss with neglect of the affected side, a contralateral field cut, aphasia (if left sided), visua-spatial disorders (if right sided).
3. *Temporal* Agitation and delirium if right sided, aphasia (if left sided), visual field cuts. These hematomas can cause uncal herniation and brain stem compression leading to stupor and coma and an ipsilateral dilated pupil.
4. *Occipital* Contralateral hemianopia is most common.

CEREBELLAR HEMORRHAGES

Clinical features may mimic a gastrointestinal disorder including nausea and vomiting but typically there is no diarrhea.

1. A distinguishing sign is difficulty walking or maintaining a sitting or standing position.
2. Headache is common.
3. Progression to coma can be rapid and is life threatening.
4. Brain stem compression can be diagnosed by finding ipsilateral abducens or gaze palsy and bilateral pyramidal signs such as extensor plantar responses.

Bibliography

Caplan LR. Top of the basilar syndrome: Selected clinical aspects. *Neurology* 1980;30:72–9.

Fisher CM. Occlusion of the internal carotid artery. *Arch Neurol Psychiatry* 1951;65:346–77.

Fisher CM. Lacunes, small deep cerebral infarcts. *Neurology* 1965;15:774–84.

Hollenhorst R. Ocular manifestations of insufficiency or thrombosis of the internal carotid artery. *Am J Ophthalmol* 1959;47:753–67.

Savitz SI, Caplan LR. Vertebrobasilar disease. *N Engl J Med* 2005;352:2618–26.

Schmidley J, Messing R. Agitated confusional states in patients with right hemisphere infarctions. *Stroke* 1984;15:883–5.

The Hunt for a Stroke Etiology

4 Ischemic stroke

Thomas J. Wolfe and Osama O. Zaidat

Establishing the etiology of ischemic stroke is important for determining the most appropriate management of each patient. A complete history and physical, including a comprehensive neurological examination, is pivotal in guiding the workup of ischemic stroke etiology. Early neuroimaging helps in differentiating ischemic from hemorrhagic infarction, as clinical signs have proven to be less reliable. Thorough and directed evaluation for potential causes in various age groups would lead to timely diagnosis and treatment.

Pertinent information from the history and physical

1. Natural history of symptoms can help define etiology
   a) Transient ischemic attack (TIA)
      i) Typically, symptoms resolve within 30 minutes
      ii) Traditionally, defined by resolution of neurologic symptoms within 24 hours from onset
      iii) Practically, symptoms persisting longer than 1–2 hours are often associated with infarction
      iv) Transient monocular blindness (TMB) or amaurosis fugax can be associated with ipsilateral carotid disease
   b) Completed infarction
      i) Symptoms typically maximal at onset and persistent
      ii) Commonly seen with embolic etiology
   c) Stuttering symptoms
      i) More often associated with small vessel–related infarction
   d) Crescendo +/− decrescendo
      i) Suggestive of thrombotic process
   e) Other review of symptoms
      i) Loss of consciousness, headache, nausea and vomiting, and seizures are often seen with hemorrhagic stroke, although altered mental status can be seen with acute basilar artery occlusion

      ii) Seizure may be the presenting symptom of stroke in the elderly

      iii) Neck pain and headache are associated with dissection and vasculitis

  f) Comorbid conditions associated with increased stroke risk include the following (details regarding individual items are discussed in the other sections):

Modifiable risk factors

    i)   Prior stroke

    ii)   HTN

    iii) Coronary artery disease and myocardial infarction (MI)

    iv) Congestive heart failure (CHF)

    v)   Diabetes mellitus

    vi) Hyperlipidemia

    vii) Sickle cell disease

    viii) Autoimmune diseases

    ix) Malignancy

    x)   Elevated body mass index

    xi) Recent cardiac or cerebral angiography

    xii) Tobacco use

    xiii) Stimulants (cocaine, methamphetamine)

    xiv) Intravenous drug use

2. Medications

  a) Vasopressors can contribute to small vessel arteriopathy

    i)   Pseudoephedrine

    ii)   Midodrine

  b) Antihypertensives can contribute to hypoperfusion

  c) Direct prothrombotic effects

    i)   Contraceptives, especially with smoking

    ii)   Estrogen-receptor modulators

    iii) Estrogen replacement

  d) "Antiplatelet failure"/"antiplatelet resistant"

    i)   Inadequate platelet inhibition despite intended benefit

    ii)   Inadequate platelet inhibition despite increasing the antiplatelet dosing

Mechanisms of ischemic stroke

Ischemic stroke typically results from embolism to the cerebral arteries, arterial thrombosis and dissection, cerebral hypoperfusion, or states of impaired cerebral oxygenation. Vasospasm (subarachnoid hemorrhage related, toxin related – cocaine, sympathomimetic, angiography related) can also contribute to an ischemic event, especially with the presence of a distal arterial stenosis. Based on the mechanism of injury, acute management and secondary prevention are tailored.

Cardiac embolism

The following list of conditions has been associated with an increased risk of ischemic stroke from cardioembolism.

1. Acute myocardial infarction (AMI)
    e) One in forty chance of stroke after AMI with 6 months, up to 20 percent incidence in patients age >75 years
    f) Anterior wall involvement increases risk
    g) Reduced ejection fraction also independent risk factor
2. CHF
    a) Relative risk of 1.8 with ejection fraction < 28 percent compared to > 35 percent.
    b) Increased left atrial size has also been associated with increased risk
3. Atrial fibrillation (a fib)
    a) Common with AMI, CHF, postcardiac surgery
    b) In the community, actual stroke rates of 0.9–2.3 per 100 person-years
    c) Increased risk of stroke in those older than 65 years of age, prior stroke, history of coronary artery disease (12 percent annual stroke risk and 18 percent with history of mitral valve stenosis). Lone a fib in young patients is associated with 1 percent annual stroke risk
4. Patent foramen ovale (PFO) and paradoxical emboli
    a) The presence of PFO in medically treated patients under 55 years of age with cryptogenic stroke does not impart increased risk of stroke recurrence without concurrent atrial septal aneurysm (ASA)
    b) Transcranial Doppler (TCD) with agitated saline exam may be as sensitive as transesophageal echocardiography (TEE) at detecting PFO
    c) TCD is not capable of assessing for ASA
5. Valvular disease contributing to embolic material (thrombotic, fibrinic, calcific)
    a) Rheumatic heart disease
    b) Prosthetic mitral and aortic valves
        i) Mechanical valves are more prone to thrombus formation than bioprosthetic valves
        ii) Mechanical valves invariably require therapeutic anticoagulation
    c) Mitral valvuloplasty frequently leads to emboli
    d) Mitral valve prolapse
        i) Lifetime relative risk 2.2 of stroke
        ii) Especially seen with older age and thickened leaflets
    e) Mitral annular calcification
    f) Aortic calcifications, particularly after percutaneous cardiac procedures

    g) Aortic atheroma; particularly complex one with > 4 mm thickness, mobile and ulcerated

    h) Bacterial endocarditis

    i) Marantic vegetations in systemic lupus erythematosus

    j) Anticardiolipin antibody syndrome – possibly increases risk of left-sided cardiac valve abnormalities

Artery-to-artery embolism

Embolic material is derived from sources distal to the aortic valve in artery-to-artery embolism. This material subsequently mobilizes distal to its site of origin.

1. Atheroemboli in large and medium artery atherosclerotic disease
    a) Mechanisms of atherosclerosis
        i) "Response to injury" hypothesis suggests that endothelial damage occurs and results in a fibroproliferative response
        ii) Lipid deposition, lipid oxidation, and calcification make a plaque more prone to contribute to increased risk
    b) Metabolic and physiologic stressors to endothelial cells contributing to atherosclerosis
        i) Hypertension
        ii) Hyperlipidemia
        iii) Hyperglycemia
        iv) Sickle cell disease
        v) Hyperhomocysteinemia
        vi) Free radicals
        vii) Tobacco smoke
        viii) Cocaine
        ix) Antibodies toward heat shock proteins, oxidized low-density lipoprotein, and beta-2 glycoprotein1
    c) Characteristics of unstable or ruptured atherosclerotic plaques
        i) Unstable plaques typically have the following characteristics:

        (1) Large extracellular lipid-rich core
        (2) Thin fibrous cap due to reduced collagen content and smooth muscle density
        (3) Increased numbers of activated macrophages and mast cells

        ii) Plaque disruption occurs at points of maximal stress resulting from mechanical and hemodynamic forces
2. Aortic arch atheromatous disease
    a) Highest risk is associated with plaques > 4 mm in thickness
    b) Coronary and cerebral catheter angiography may disrupt aortic plaques

   c) Typically investigated by TEE, but CT angiography may be an
      alternative and less invasive investigation
3. Arterial dissection
   a) Traumatic causes
      i)   Motor vehicle accidents
      ii) Cervical spine manipulation, specifically vertebral artery trauma
           (i.e., chiropractic, beauty shop sink)
      iii) Arterial catheterization and angiography
   b) Increase risk associated with the following:
      i)   Hypertension and atherosclerotic disease
      ii) Fibromuscular dysplasia
      iii) Hyperhomocysteinemia and methylenetetrahydrofolate reduc-
           tase (MTHFR) mutations
4. Arterial thrombus formation in hypercoagulable states with distal
   embolization or complete occlusion due to in situ arterial thrombosis
5. Large vessel arteriopathy associated with sickle cell disease
6. Cardiothoracic surgery
   a) "On-pump" microembolic phenomenon
   b) Aortic manipulation during the procedure
   c) Postoperative atrial fibrillation

Small artery occlusive disease, lacunar infarction

The concept of lacunar syndrome in evaluating ischemic stroke has
been found to be 95 percent sensitive and 93 percent specific in determining
small vessel etiology. Lacunar syndrome utilization had a positive predictive
value of 90 percent and negative predictive value of 97 percent in diagnosing
lacunar infarction. Symptoms related to the lacunar syndromes were
outlined above. Pathophysiologic mechanisms of lacunar infarction follow:

1. Hyaline arteriosclerosis: related to comorbid diabetes and HTN
2. Microatheromatous emboli: from large and medium vessel plaque
3. Lipohyalinosis – typically as a consequence of uncontrolled HTN
4. Fibrinoid necrosis – seen in chronic HTN and vasculitis
5. Atherosclerotic plaque side branch disease; by the plaque extending
   into the ostium of small perforator and occluding it
6. Cerebral autosomal dominant arteriopathy with subcortical infarcts
   and leukoencephalopathy (CADASIL)
   a) Small granular arteriopathy
   b) Chromosome 19q123, Notch 3 gene
   c) Diagnosed with genetic testing or skin biopsy, testing should be
      reserved for situations with high clinical suspicion based on family
      history, infarct distribution, and recurrence without other sig-
      nificant risk
7. Vaso-occlusive crisis in sickle cell disease

Hypoperfusion and hypoxemia

"Watershed" infarction typically occurs in response to a global decrease in cerebral perfusion. Watershed ischemia results from lack of perfusion to the zones between primary cerebral arterial territories. Hemispheric hypoperfusion can also contribute to watershed infarction, especially in the setting of ipsilateral carotid stenosis. Intracranial stenosis arteries can lead to recurrent TIA with the same symptomatology. Tandem stenotic lesions further increase this chance of focal perfusion abnormalities. Hypoxemia results in a generalized reduction of cerebral oxygenation, leading to less focal ischemic injury.

1. Some causes of decreased systemic perfusion and hypoxic states include the following:
   a) Sepsis, SIRS
   b) Intraoperative hypotension
   c) Cardiopulmonary arrest
   d) Cardiac arrhythmia
   e) Volume depletion
   f) Antihypertensive medication
   g) Pulmonary embolus
   h) Pneumonia
   i) Carbon monoxide toxicity

Thrombotic stroke and hypercoagulable states

Evaluating for a hypercoagulable state as the etiology of ischemic stroke is indicated most in patients with a history of unexplained thrombotic events. Younger patients (<50 years of age), those with "cryptogenic" stroke, previous thrombotic event, late gestational or recurrent pregnancy loss, and those with a family history of thrombosis are more likely to have a positive hypercoagulable evaluation. These select patients should undergo a full hypercoagulable workup due to its implication on treatment and secondary prevention. The relationship between venous thromboembolism (VTE) and ischemic stroke is particularly important in the setting of PFO and paradoxical emboli. Hereditary abnormalities more commonly increase risk of venous thrombosis, especially in the setting of a concurrent acquired risk factor.

The timing of hypercoagulable evaluation is important. During the acute phase of thrombosis, several clotting factors are consumed, potentially contributing to falsely low levels in acute testing. Because of this, factor testing should be delayed for 1–2 weeks from onset of thrombosis. Warfarin, by inhibiting vitamin K–dependent clotting protein synthesis, also confounds interpretation of factor levels. Heparin may reduce antithrombin III levels and interfere with aPTT testing. Since aPTT is a screening test for antiphospholipid (APL) antibodies, heparinization may complicate establishing an etiology. Blood sampling for coagulation factors and APL antibodies should be performed prior to initiation of anticoagulation. If anticoagulation is initiated prior to lab evaluation, coagulation factor testing should be deferred until 1–2 weeks after therapy is discontinued, as an outpatient. The PT and a PTT assays may help rule out either single or multiple factor deficiencies from liver disease or inherited defects. Specific tests for inherited mutations are not affected by anticoagulation.

1. Acquired risk for thrombosis has been associated with the following:
   a) age
   b) obesity
   c) recent surgery or trauma
   d) immobility
   e) facility confinement (hospitals and nursing homes)
   f) malignancy
   g) contraceptive and estrogen replacement
   h) pregnancy/postpartum
   i) thrombocytosis
   j) increased lipoprotein a
2. Hereditary gene abnormalities:
   a) antithrombin III (ATIII)[1]
   b) protein C (PC) deficiency[2]
   c) protein S (PS) deficiency[3]
   d) factor V Leiden (FVL) and activated PC resistance
   e) prothrombin G20210A
   f) MTHFR and hyperhomocysteinemia
3. Autoimmunity:
   a) Vasculitis
      i) Small vessel (microscopic polyangiitis, leukocytoclastic, Henoch-Schönlein purpura, Cryoglobulinemia)
      ii) Medium vessel (ANCA associated, PAN, Churg-Strauss)
      iii) Large vessel (Giant cell arteritis, Takayasu's arteritis)
   b) APL antibody syndrome
   c) Lupus anticoagulant (LA) and anticardiolipin antibodies (ACAs)
   d) Hypocomplementemia
   e) Sjögren's
   f) TTP/ITP
   g) Other antibodies:

---

[1] Consumed during acute thrombosis and may be decreased postoperatively and in DIC or severe liver disease; reduced by heparin.

[2] Consumed during acute thrombosis and may be decreased postoperatively and in DIC or severe liver disease; reduced by warfarin.

[3] See note 2.

    i) Anti-β2 glycoprotein 1 (facilitates APL and increases risk alone)

    ii) Antiphosphatidylethanolamine (Henoch-Schönlein purpura)

    iii) Antiphosphotidylserine

When should I order certain tests to evaluate ischemic stroke etiology?

Every patient will need an individual assessment for determining the etiology of their stroke. It is difficult to establish a firm protocol for this evaluation, but by understanding the mechanism of ischemic stroke, a practical approach can be taken when ordering diagnostic tests. Simply, each patient requires a comprehensive history and physical, monitoring of cardiovascular function, neuroanatomic and neurovascular imaging, laboratory analysis, and other imaging to complete the review of systems (see Figure 4.1).

1. Cardiac evaluation
   a) A *12-lead electrocardiogram* and *telemetry monitoring* aid in ruling out MI and atrial fibrillation
   b) *Echocardiogram with bubble study* to assess ejection fraction, wall motion and structural abnormalities, and PFO
      i) Transthoracic echocardiogram (TTE)
         (1) Noninvasive screening exam
         (2) Technically inferior to TEE at evaluating atrial anatomy
      ii) Transesophageal echocardiogram (TEE)
         (1) Better first choice in younger patients due to higher incidence of PFO-related stroke
         (2) Allows for aortic imaging
         (3) Considered the "gold standard" for evaluating atrial anatomy
   c) *Transcranial Doppler*
      i) May detect PFO with greater sensitivity than TEE
      ii) Use in association with either TTE or TEE due to the lack of ability to assess atrial anatomy
2. Vascular anatomy and physiologic evaluation
   a) Carotid ultrasound
      i) Excellent screening exam in anterior infarction
      ii) Limited to examining extracranial vessels
   b) Transcranial Doppler
      i) Evaluation of flow velocities can identify vessel stenosis
      ii) Unable to localize stenosis beyond major cerebral branches
   c) Magnetic resonance angiography (MRA)
      i) Allows for concurrent vascular imaging of the neck, which will be essential if posterior infarction is suspected
      ii) Highly sensitive for dissection

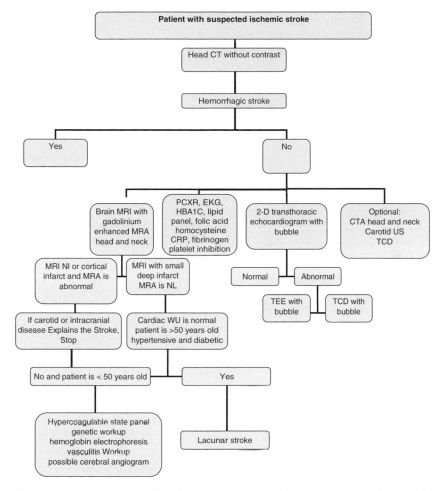

Figure 4.1 Suggested algorithm for diagnostic evaluation for patients with ischemic stroke.

    d) Computerized tomographic angiography (CTA)
        i)   Allows for imaging down to aortic arch
        ii) Anterior and posterior evaluation
        iii) Possibly as sensitive as MRA, but typically easier to obtain
    e) Digital subtraction angiography (DSA)
        i)   Considered the "gold standard" for vascular imaging
        ii) May be essential in evaluating vasculitis
        iii) Procedural stroke risk ~1 percent
  3. Neuroimaging
    a) Computerized tomography (CT)
        i)   Excellent at ruling out hemorrhagic infarction, but not highly
            sensitive at localizing acute infarction

ii) Signs of acute infarction
   (1) Loss of gray-white differentiation
   (2) Loss of insular ribbon
   (3) Focal sulcal effacement
   (4) "Hyperdense MCA" sign
iii) Subacute to chronic infarction
   (1) Hypodense vascular territory or lacune

b) Magnetic resonance imaging (MRI)
  i) Diffusion-weighted imaging helps in localizing an acute infarction
  ii) MRI is superior to CT at illustrating the extent of premorbid cerebrovascular disease and characterizes the lesion better

c) Perfusion-weighted imaging
  i) Indicated when there is suspicion of hypoperfusion syndrome
  ii) Helpful in the absence of diffusion abnormality on MRI

4. Laboratory evaluation
  a) Initial screening tests
    i) CBC
    ii) Electrolytes and hepatic function
    iii) Coagulation studies (PT/INR, PTT, or aPTT)
    iv) Cardiac enzymes (CK, CK-MB, troponin I)
    v) Fasting cholesterol panel (total, HDL, LDL, triglycerides)
    vi) High sensitivity C reactive protein
    vii) ESR
    viii) Homocysteine
    ix) Hemoglobin A1C, glycosylated hemoglobin
    x) Platelet inhibition testing (PFA-100, PGY212, Verify now …)

  b) Specific testing
    i) Hypercoagulability testing
      (1) Timing of testing is imperative for diagnostic accuracy (details discussed earlier)
      (2) Initial screening panel: PC, PS, ATIII, APCR, prothrombin gene mutation, MTHFR, APL antibodies (LA, ACA, β-2 glycoprotein), ANA
    ii) CADASIL testing (see above in lacunar infarct section)

5. General systems evaluation
  a) Chest x-ray
    i) Pulmonary disease can contribute to cardiac arrhythmia
    ii) Evaluation for aortic tortuosity or calcification, which suggests vascular disease
  b) Swallowing study

Bibliography

American Academy of Neurology Practice Guidelines. 2005–6 edition.

Avierinos JF, Brown RD, Foley DA, Nkoma V, et al. Celebral ischemic events after diagnosis of mitral valve prolapse: a community-based study of incidence and predictive factors. *Storke* 2003; 34(6):1339–44.

Eber B. Anticardiolipin antibody and stroke: Possible relation of valvular heart disease and embolic events. *Cardiology* 1992;80(2):156–8.

Bauer K. Hypercoagulable states. *Hematology* 2005 Sep–Oct;10:S1–39.

Boiten J, Lodder J. Lacunar infarcts. Pathogenesis and validity of the clinical syndromes. *Stroke* 1991;22(11):1374–8.

Gorelick PB, Alter M. *The prevention of stroke*. New York: Parthenon Publishing, 2002.

Klein LW. Clinical implications and mechanisms of plaque rupture in the acute coronary syndromes. *Am Heart Hosp J* 2005 Fall;3(4):249–55.

Lee SJ, Kavanaugh A. Autoimmunity, vasculitis, and autoantibodies. *J Allergy Clin Immunol* 2006 Feb;117(2):S445–50.

Levine SR. Hypercoagulable states and stroke: A selective review. *CNS Spectr* 2005 Jul;10(7):567–78.

Lichtman JH, Krumholz HM, Wang Y, Radford MJ, Brass LM. Risk and predictors of stroke after myocardial infarction among the elderly: Results from the cooperative cardiovascular project. *Circulation* 2002;105:1082–7.

Loh E, Loh E., Sutton M. Wun CC et al. Ventricular dysfunction and the risk of stroke after myocardial infarction. *NEJM* 1997 Jan;336:251–7.

Mandal K, Mandal K, Jahangiri M, Xu Q. Autoimmune mechanisms of atherosclerosis. *Handb Exp Pharmacol* 2005;170:723–43.

McKenzie SB, Clare CN, Smith LA, Lee Sang JE. Laboratory test utilization in the diagnosis of hypercoagulability. *Clin Lab Sci* 2000;13(4):215–21.

Mohr JP, Albers GW, Amarenco P, et al. American Heart Association Prevention Conference IV. Prevention and Rehabilitation of Stroke. Etiology of stroke. *Stroke* 1997;28:1501–6.

Ross, R. The pathogenesis of atherosclerosis. *Mech Ageing Dev* 1979 Mar;9(5–6):435–40.

van Laar PJ, van der Grond, J.; Mali, WP, Hendrikse, J. Magnetic resonance evaluation of the cerebral circulation in obstructive arterial disease. *Cerebrovasc Dis* 2006;21:297–306.

Wang TJ, Massaro JM, Levy DL, et al. A risk score for individuals with new-onset atrial fibrillation in the community, the Framingham study. *JAMA* 2003;290:1049–56.

Witt BJ, Ballman KV, Brown RD Jr, Meverden RA, Jacobsen SJ, Roger VL. The incidence of stroke after myocardial infarction: A meta-analysis. *Am J Med.* 2006 Apr;119(4):354.e1–9.

5 Hemorrhagic stroke

Angelos Katramados and Panayiotis Varelas

Introduction

Although a hemorrhagic stroke typically presents with a catastrophic onset, it is frequently a manifestation of a long-standing process that may have been unidentified. Several conditions may result in a "spontaneous" hemorrhage. Table 5.1 shows the most common etiologies of intracranial hemorrhages.

1. Primary hemorrhages are considered as those that are associated with arterial hypertension or amyloid angiopathy.
2. Chronic hypertension usually results in deep-seated or subcortical hemorrhages. These are located in the basal ganglia, thalamus, pons, and cerebellum. They are attributed to long-standing small vessel disease.
3. Many of the superficial or lobar hemorrhages are, likewise, associated with cerebral amyloid angiopathy in the elderly population.

It might be a mistake, however, to make etiologic assumptions based only on the presence of risk factors or the location of the hematoma. The advent of modern imaging techniques has revealed an increasing number of structural lesions that would otherwise remain undiagnosed. An adequate workup for secondary causes is always warranted to ensure optimal management and secondary prevention. In all cases, clinical and radiologic data should be taken into account before we reach a safe diagnostic conclusion.

History and clinical examination

It is very common for an intracerebral hemorrhage to present with an acutely decreased level of consciousness. Nausea, vomiting, and a severe headache can be noted even without increased intracranial pressure. All the above features occur much more often in hemorrhagic than in ischemic strokes.

➠ History can give valuable diagnostic insight into the etiology of a specific hemorrhage.

60

Table 5.1: Causes of intracerebral hemorrhage

Traumatic (cerebral contusion)
Spontaneous (nontraumatic)
  Hypertension
  Amyloid angiopathy
  Vascular malformations
    Arteriovenous malformations
    Cavernous angiomas
    Venous angiomas
Intracranial aneurysms
Arterial thrombosis (hemorrhagic transformation)
Venous thrombosis (dural sinuses or deep venous system)
Coagulopathy
    Systemic (thrombocytopenia, disseminated intravascular
    coagulation, polycythemia, hemophilia, von Willenbrand
    disease, sickle cell anemia, coagulation factor deficiencies.)
    Drug related (thrombolytic therapy, heparin, warfarin,
    antiplatelets)
Neoplastic
    Solid tumors (primary or metastatic)
    Leukemia
Vasculitis
Drug abuse (cocaine, amphetamines, phenylpropanolamine,
phenylcyclidine, MAOIs)
Miscellaneous (heat stroke, fat embolism, protracted migraines)

Table 5.2 summarizes the most important diagnostic clues that can be obtained. Recent concurrent trauma can be ascertained by direct witnesses or suspected by the setting that the patient was found in. However, we should not automatically assume that this will always be the direct etiology of the hemorrhage. Many times, trauma may result from loss of consciousness or a seizure after a hemorrhage has developed.

➡ Concomitant medical conditions such as malignancies, coagulopathies, known vascular lesions can provide accurate directions for timely subsequent workup.

Significant risk factors such as age, chronic hypertension, and alcohol use can also be documented from the patient or from his or her environment. History of recent anticoagulant or thrombolytic use may provide a specific diagnosis even if laboratory values have normalized in the interim. Recent pregnancy, hypercoagulability, or dehydration may precipitate the development of cerebral venous thrombosis and hemorrhagic venous infarcts.

Table 5.2: History

Trauma
Recent use of anticoagulants, thrombolytics, antiplatelets
Over the counter medications, recreational drugs
Alcohol use
History of malignancy, hematologic disorders
Recent pregnancy
Prior ischemic stroke or hemorrhage or family history of such
Known vascular malformations or family history of such
Known coagulopathy

Table 5.3: Clinical examination

Signs of recent trauma
Bleeding tendency
Hepatic or renal disease
Skin marks of recent intravenous drug use
Clinically evident mass lesions

Clinical examination (Table 5.3) can reveal stigmata of coagulopathy or hepatic disease. Recent trauma, especially in the head, may be difficult to identify. Skin marks or recent intravenous drug use may alert to the possibility of vasculitis or endocarditis.

➠ Acute hypertension is seen very commonly in the setting of recent intracranial hemorrhage and is not necessarily a marker of long-standing hypertension.

Laboratory test

Initial diagnostic tests are outlined in Table 5.4. A complete blood count and coagulation parameter testing will assist in the diagnosis of hematologic disorders or coagulopathies. The effect of warfarin and unfractionated heparin is usually evident in the thrombin and thromboplastin times, respectively. Evaluation of a biochemical profile may reveal the presence of hepatic or renal failure. A urine drug screen will provide rapid information about recent use of cocaine, amphetamines, or other drugs that have been associated with intracranial hemorrhages.

➠ Further testing should be guided by the relevant clinical presentation.

An elevated sedimentation rate, or positive antinuclear antibodies, in the correct clinical setting may provide further support of an underlying

---

Table 5.4: Laboratory testing

Routine tests
  Complete blood count.
  Biochemical profile
  Coagulation parameters
  Liver function tests
  Drug screen

Selected patients
  Blood cultures
  Clotting factors levels
  Antinuclear antibodies
  Erythrocyte sedimentation rate
  Hemoglobin electrophoresis
  HIV ELISA

---

vasculitis or autoimmune disorder. Hemoglobin electrophoresis, testing of clotting factors, or tumor markers can be performed if necessary. Blood cultures will be required if there is a documented or suspected history of endocarditis.

Computed tomography (CT)

CT without contrast is universally required in any patient with a clinical diagnosis of acute stroke.

➠ Several attempts have been made to predict the presence of bleeding on clinical grounds only; however, the distinction between ischemia and hemorrhage can be made only by radiologic criteria.

Radiological signs on CT that can assist in making a diagnosis are shown in Table 5.5. Acute hemorrhage typically appears as an area of increased density in the cerebral parenchyma.

➠ A possible exception is that in extremely anemic patients, intracerebral blood will have lower density or may even be isodense to the adjacent parenchyma.

Multiple areas of hemorrhage can be present. The presence of concurrent subarachnoid, intraventricular hemorrhage or extraaxial hematomas can be documented.

1. Intracranial calcifications, unexpected vascular structures or a peri-sylvian location of the hemorrhage may all point to a secondary cause.
2. Edema that is out of proportion to the hemorrhage may be suggestive of underlying ischemia or malignancy and requires further investigation.

Table 5.5: Useful diagnostic clues that can be revealed by computed tomography

Intraparenchymal hemorrhage (deep or lobar)
Concurrent intraventricular, subarachnoid hemorrhage,
epidural or subdural hematomas
Infarction of arterial territories
Signs of dural sinus thrombosis
Edema surrounding the area of hemorrhage
Calcifications suggestive of vascular lesions
Perisylvian hemorrhage
Cord sign (thrombosed vein)
Delta sign (contrast enhancement around thrombosed sagittal sinus)

The addition of iodinated contrast may be necessary if the patient is too unstable or has other contraindications for magnetic resonance imaging (MRI). It can reveal areas of impaired blood-brain barrier suggestive of neoplasia or inflammation. Underlying arteriovenous malformations or vascular tumors will also be picked up although with less sensitivity than with MRI.

⮡ Most primary hemorrhages, however, in the subacute phase will demonstrate peripheral enhancement on CT and pose further diagnostic problems.

MRI

In the hyperacute phase, CT remains the test of choice although MRI techniques with comparable sensitivity have been developed.

⮡ The role of the MRI is invaluable in identifying underlying vascular lesions that might be responsible for the hemorrhagic event (Table 5.6). Small intracranial aneurysms or arteriovenous malformations may be evident.

Mass lesions will be easily shown although, again, the presence of perilesional edema or enhancement may be related to the impairment of the blood-brain barrier by the acute process.

⮡ Serial imaging in the subacute phase may be necessary to make the distinction between intratumoral and primary hemorrhage.

Acute ischemia in relation to hemorrhage (hemorrhagic transformation) can be easily identified by MRI. In this case, the hemorrhage is usually a secondary phenomenon and there can be significant temporal delay compared to the initial ischemia. Ischemia may respect arterial territories and represent a true arterial infarct, often embolic.

> **Table 5.6:** Lesions identified by magnetic resonance imaging
>
> Small vascular lesions (aneurysms, angiomas, AVMs)
> Tumors
> Ischemic lesions (arterial, venous)
> Areas of previous hemorrhage

⇒ Venous thrombosis may also be present either in the dural sinuses (cortical edema hemorrhage) or in the deep venous system of the brain, in which case, it may masquerade as a deep-seated hemorrhage.

Multiple areas of previous hemorrhage can be demonstrated. Those, especially if small (microbleeds), are suggestive of small vessel disease caused by long-standing hypertension or amyloid angiopathy. This finding, depending on the topographic distribution, can help make a noninvasive diagnosis and may have significant implication for recurrence or future use of anticoagulants. However, it may be very difficult to exclude prior history of trauma or multiple cavernous angiomas.

⇒ Venous ischemia should be suspected with bilateral hemorrhagic lesions associated with the major dural sinuses, with gyriform hemorrhagic transformation, or if the area of infarction does not respect arterial territories. MRI may demonstrate the absence of flow void in the sinuses, although gradient-echo, T2-weighted sequences are usually required to demonstrate the actual thrombus.

CT and MR angiography

Noninvasive techniques are continuously gaining acceptance in the imaging of the intracranial vasculature. They are employed when previous studies have suggested an aneurysm, AVM, or other vascular lesion.

1. CT requires administration of potentially nephrotoxic contrast but overall it is safer compared to conventional digital subtraction angiography (DSA). In experienced hands it can identify aneurysms with a sensitivity comparable to that of DSA. Inferior results have been reported in arteriovenous malformations.
2. MR angiography can also help delineate vascular anatomy in suspected underlying lesions.

Cerebral angiography

Currently, the main role of intraarterial DSA is in identifying macroscopic vascular lesions. Obviously, this is an invasive technique and procedural risks should be weighted carefully against potential benefits, especially in critically ill patients.

1. Intra- and extracranial aneurysms can be identified. Intricate details of the aneurysm, including the size, projection, neck, perforating branches, flow dynamics, can be studied in depth.
2. Vasospasm may be seen if there is a component of subarachnoid hemorrhage.
3. Vascular malformations are also optimally seen by DSA. It can easily distinguish the arterial, capillary, and venous phases of blood flow. The arterial feeders, the nidus, any intranidal aneurysms, and the draining veins are delineated.
4. DSA also remains the gold standard technique for evaluation of vasculitis.
5. Amyloid angiopathy usually does not have distinctive angiographic features. Angiography should be performed, however, as underlying lesions are frequently encountered in lobar hemorrhages.
6. Vasculitis has also been described in patients with amyloid angiopathy, and may have a radiographic appearance of multiple stenotic areas alternating with areas of dilatation.

Histopathology

Usually, cases with pure vascular involvement (ischemia, aneurysmal rupture) can be diagnosed by imaging modalities only. If there is a suspicion of parenchymatous involvement, only pathologic examination can provide a definitive diagnosis. This is typically the case in malignant neoplasms, central nervous system (CNS) vasculitis, encephalitis, or amyloid angiopathy. Again, the benefit of the diagnosis depends on the availability of specific treatment and should be balanced against the significant morbidity of a brain biopsy.

Cerebrospinal fluid (CSF) analysis

CSF analysis is rarely performed in the acute phase as an inflammatory reaction to the hemorrhage is very commonly present. It may be rarely indicated later on, if other tests have not been able to identify a responsible process, especially if vasculitis or other CNS inflammation is suspected. The presence of xanthochromia in the CSF during the hyperactive phase (less than 10 hours) is indicative of a sentinel hemorrhage, usually from a previously ruptured cerebral aneurysm.

General protocol

Figure 5.1 summarizes a proposed protocol for the diagnostic workup of intracerebral hemorrhage. After an initial history and clinical examination,

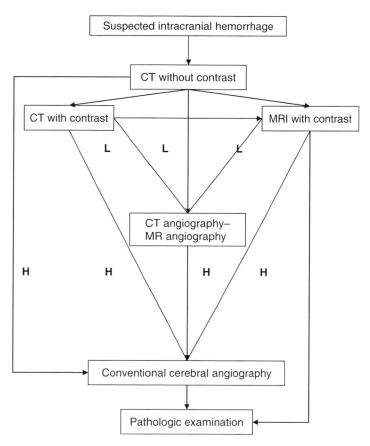

Figure 5.1 Protocol. L: Low suspicion of underlying vascular lesion, H: High suspicion of underlying vascular lesion (see text for specific criteria).

every patient with a suspected clinical diagnosis of acute stroke should undergo an emergent CT scan of the head without contrast.

1. If an intracranial hemorrhage is identified in the CT of the head, an MRI with contrast can be performed if the patient is stable and does not have relevant contraindications. Otherwise, a CT of the head with contrast may identify many of the responsible or concurrent structural lesions.

2. At this point, an assessment should be made whether there is a high suspicion for an underlying vascular lesion. This will be the case in young, normotensive patients with characteristics of hemorrhage that do not fit a typical hypertensive etiology. Such characteristics may be the presence of extraaxial hematomas, temporal or perisylvian location of primary hemorrhage, a subarachnoid hemorrhage, an intraventricular component, or history of cocaine use.

3. Clinical judgment will be necessary as many deep-seated hemorrhages may harbor underlying lesions and not be of hypertensive etiology as previously thought.
4. The next step should be a DSA if the presence of a macroscopic vascular lesion (AVM, aneurysm, vasculitis, moya-moya), as determined above, is very likely and its diagnosis will affect further management.
    i)   This means that it may be performed, even in patients who would not be surgical candidates, as direct embolization or stenting can be performed at the time of the exam.
    ii) Despite the advent of noninvasive angiographic techniques, conventional DSA remains the optimal diagnostic test. The timing of the exam will be determined by the treating physicians based on the patient's condition and available resources.
5. CT and MR angiography have now evolved to be useful noninvasive screening tests for the assessment of the intracranial vasculature. They can be employed when there is a low suspicion for a responsible vascular lesion or if circumstances do not allow for a timely DSA. Positive findings may need to be confirmed by DSA. Individual institutions should develop their own algorithms based on patient volume and their particular experience with each procedure.
6. Obviously, if a patient is deteriorating rapidly and requires decompressive surgery, appropriate surgical management will take precedence over diagnostic studies.
7. False-negative imaging results are possible as pressure from the expanding hematoma may obliterate an AVM and blood-brain barrier impairment may prevent identification of a tumor. If a lesion is still suspected despite negative examinations, serial imaging in 2–3 months may be necessary after the edema has subsided and the blood-brain barrier has been restored.
8. Finally, if a mass lesion is evident, biopsy and pathologic examination may be necessary. Additional information can be provided when tissue fragments are included in specimens of evacuated hematomas.
    i)   When cerebral amyloid angiopathy is the primary diagnosis, diagnostic biopsy is usually discouraged, as there is no therapeutic benefit and the risk of bleeding complications is very high.
    ii) Other therapeutic surgical procedures, such as decompression or evacuation of the hematoma, can be performed relatively safely, if necessary.

Conclusion

With the refinement of imaging techniques, many intracerebral hemorrhages that were previously ascribed to hypertension or amyloid angiopathy are now attributed to various underlying pathophysiologic processes. At the same time, the therapeutic armamentarium has been significantly expanded, to the point that most lesions are approachable by interventional or surgical techniques. Clinical judgment is required, in order to correctly identify the relevant conditions and guide therapeutic interventions and secondary prevention. Hopefully, as more diagnostic modalities become available, noninvasive imaging will gain more acceptance and obviate the low but still significant procedural risk of conventional angiography.

Bibliography

Broderick JP, Adams HP, Jr, Barsan W, et al. Guidelines for the management of spontaneous intracerebral hemorrhage: A statement for healthcare professionals from a special writing group of the Stroke Council, American Heart Association. *Stroke* 1999 Apr;30(4):905–15.

Fewel ME, Thompson BG, Jr, Hoff JT. Spontaneous intracerebral hemorrhage: A review. *Neurosurg Focus* 2003 Oct;15(4):E1.

Halpin SF, Britton JA, Byrne JV, Clifton A, Hart G, Moore A. Prospective evaluation of cerebral angiography and computed tomography in cerebral haematoma. *J Neurol Neurosurg Psychiatry* 1994 Oct;57(10):1180–6.

Hino A, Fujimoto M, Yamaki T, Iwamoto Y, Katsumori T. Value of repeat angiography in patients with spontaneous subcortical hemorrhage. *Stroke* 1998 Dec;29(12):2517–21.

Imaizumi T, Horita Y, Hashimoto Y, Niwa J. Dotlike hemosiderin spots on T2*-weighted magnetic resonance imaging as a predictor of stroke recurrence: A prospective study. *J Neurosurg* 2004 Dec;101(6):915–20.

Izumihara A, Ishihara T, Iwamoto N, Yamashita K, Ito H. Postoperative outcome of 37 patients with lobar intracerebral hemorrhage related to cerebral amyloid angiopathy. *Stroke* 1999 Jan;30(1):29–33.

Jayaraman MV, Mayo-Smith WW, Tung GA, et al. Detection of intracranial aneurysms: Multi-detector row CT angiography compared with DSA. *Radiology* 2004 Feb;230(2):510–18.

Kidwell CS, Chalela JA, Saver JL, et al. Comparison of MRI and CT for detection of acute intracerebral hemorrhage. *JAMA* 2004 Oct;292(15):1823–30.

Matsumoto M, Kodama N, Sakuma J, et al. 3D–CT arteriography and 3D-CT venography: The separate demonstration of arterial-phase and venous-phase on 3D-CT angiography in a single procedure. *AJNR Am J Neuroradiol* 2005 Mar;26 (3):635–41.

Osborn AG. *Diagnostic cerebral angiography.* Philadelphia, PA: Lippincott Williams & Wilkins, 1998.

Sanelli PC, Mifsud MJ, Stieg PE. Role of CT angiography in guiding management decisions of newly diagnosed and residual arteriovenous malformations. *Am J Roentgenol* 2004 Oct;183(4):1123–6.

Shah MV, Biller J. Medical and surgical management of intracerebral hemorrhage. *Semin Neurol* 1998;18(4):513–19.

Tung GA, Julius BD, Rogg JM. MRI of intracerebral hematoma: Value of vasogenic edema ratio for predicting the cause. *Neuroradiology* 2003 Jun;45(6):357–62.

Wasay M, Azeemuddin M. Neuroimaging of cerebral venous thrombosis. *J Neuroimaging* 2005 Apr;15(2):118–28.

Weir CJ, Murray GD, Adams FG, Muir KW, Grosset DG, Lees KR. Poor accuracy of stroke scoring systems for differential clinical diagnosis of intracranial haemorrhage and infarction. *Lancet* 1994 Oct 8;344(8928):999–1002.

Wong AA, Henderson RD, O' Sullivan JD, Read SJ, Rajah T. Ring enhancement after hemorrhagic stroke. *Arch Neurol* 2004 Nov;61(11):1790.

Zhu XL, Chan MS, Poon WS. Spontaneous intracranial hemorrhage: Which patients need diagnostic cerebral angiography? A prospective study of 206 cases and review of the literature. *Stroke* 1997 Jul;28(7):1406–9.

Zwimpfer TJ, Brown J, Sullivan I, Moulton RJ. Head injuries due to falls caused by seizures: A group at high risk for traumatic intracranial hematomas. *J Neurosurg* 1997 Mar;86(3):433–7.

6 Other causes of stroke

Andrew W. Tarulli

Although the majority of cerebral infarctions are related to atherosclerotic disease, hypertension, and emboli, uncommon causes of stroke should be kept in mind, especially in younger patients. Stroke is the classical apoplectic neurological disease, but stroke mimicry by other neurological and nonneurological conditions also deserves careful consideration. Table 6.1 lists uncommon causes of stroke by pathogenesis, whereas Table 6.2 separates them by involvement of associated organ systems.

Vasculitis

Primary angiitis of the central nervous system (CNS)

This necrotizing arteritis is characterized by granulomatous giant cell and epithelioid cell infiltrates of all cerebral vessels, especially those of small- and medium caliber. Neurologic presentations include ischemic stroke, hemorrhage (mostly lobar), headache, movement disorders, and demyelinating disease.

1. Patients with ischemic strokes typically have evidence of other CNS disease.
2. Brain biopsy is the gold standard for diagnosis. Angiography is of low specificity and sensitivity.

The combination of corticosteroids (prednisone 1 mg/kg/day) and cyclophosphamide (1–2 mg/kg/day) is superior to corticosteroids alone.

Temporal arteritis

This systemic arteritis has a predilection for medium and large vessels. Presenting features include headache, visual loss, jaw claudication, scalp tenderness, diaphoresis, weight loss, anorexia, and malaise. Polymyalgia rheumatica commonly accompanies temporal arteritis.

Table 6.1: Uncommon causes of stroke

Vasculitis
    Primary angiitis of the CNS
    Temporal arteritis
    Behcet's disease
    Polyarteritis nodosa
    Churg-Strauss syndrome
    Takayasu's arteritis

Connective tissue disorders
    Systemic lupus erythematosus
    Marfan syndrome
    Ehlers-Danlos syndrome
    Fibromuscular dysplasia

Angiopathies
    Moyamoya syndrome
    Susac's syndrome
    HERNS
    Osler-Weber-Rendu disease
    Arterial dissections
    Sneddon's syndrome

Metabolic disorders
    CADASIL
    Fabry's disease
    MELAS

Hematologic and oncologic causes
    Hyperviscosity syndromes
    Cancer-related strokes

Pregnancy-related strokes
    Postpartum cerebral angiopathy
    Peripartum cardiomyopathy
    Metastatic choriocarcinoma
    Amniotic fluid emboli
    Pituitary apoplexy

Substance abuse
    Heroin
    Cocaine
    Amphetamines
    PCP
    Complications of an addictive lifestyle

(continued)

Table 6.1: *(continued)*
Infections
  Bacterial
    Listeria
    Syphilis
    Tuberculosis
    Bartonella
  Viral
    Herpes zoster
    Cytomegalovirus
    Human immunodeficiency virus
    Herpes simplex
  Fungal
    Aspergillosis
    Candidiasis
    Mucormycosis
    Cryptococcosis
    Histoplasmosis
  Parasitic
    Cysticercosis
Migrainous infarctions

▸ Visual loss is a neurologic emergency caused by anterior ischemic optic neuropathy.

Strokes from temporal arteritis most commonly involve the posterior circulation. Elevated C-reactive peptide (CRP) is a more sensitive diagnostic test than erythrocyte sedimentation rate (ESR).

▸ The combination of a CRP greater than 2.45 mg/dl and an ESR greater than 47 mm/hr has a 97% specificity for temporal arteritis, although rare patients with temporal arteritis have ESR less than 20 mm/hr.

Superficial temporal artery biopsy establishes the diagnosis. Skip lesions necessitate sampling of several centimeters to ensure maximal sensitivity.

▸ If temporal arteritis is strongly suspected, prednisone 60 mg should be administered immediately, especially in patients with anterior ischemic optic neuropathy.

Prednisone 60–80 mg/day should be prescribed for 4–6 weeks followed by gradual reduction so that the patient is asymptomatic and the ESR is normal. Treatment should be continued for at least 1 year.

Table 6.2: Causes of stroke with sites of involvement outside of CNS

Heart/great vessels
Takayasu's arteritis
Systemic lupus erythematosus
Marfan syndrome

Lungs/airways
Churg-Strauss
Systemic lupus erythematosus
Osler-Weber-Rendu disease

Kidneys
Systemic lupus erythematosus
Fibromuscular dysplasia
HERNS

Joints
Marfan syndrome
Ehlers-Danlos syndrome

Eyes
Temporal arteritis
Behcet's disease
Marfan syndrome
Susac's syndrome
HERNS

Auditory/vestibular system
Susac's syndrome

Skin
Polyarteritis nodosa
Systemic lupus erythematosus
Marfan syndrome
Osler-Weber-Rendu disease
Sneddon's syndrome
Fabry's disease

Behcet's disease

The clinical triad of recurrent oral and genital ulcerations, uveitis, and vasculitis is referred to as Behcet's disease. Its most common neurologic presentation is meningoencephalitis, but strokes also occur.

⟶ Venous sinus thrombosis is the most common cause of stroke. Other causes include aneurysms, arteriovenous malformations (AVMs), arterial dissections, large artery occlusions, and intracranial or spinal hemorrhages.

Immunosuppression and possibly anticoagulation may prevent stroke recurrence.

Other vasculitides

Polyarteritis nodosa (PAN) is a necrotizing vasculitis that affects the peripheral nerves, muscles, joints, skin, kidney, and gastrointestinal tract. Strokes are uncommon and are usually lacunar. The best prevention of strokes related to PAN is not clear. Corticosteroids may produce more strokes whereas antiplatelet agents appear to prevent recurrence.

Churg-Strauss syndrome is a necrotizing vasculitis that causes asthma, eosinophilia, and multisystem vascular involvement. Like PAN, strokes are usually lacunar.

Takayasu's arteritis is an arteritis of unknown origin involving the aortic arch and proximal portion of the major branches. It occurs predominantly in young women. Strokes are usually related to hypertension or obstruction of the carotid or brachiocephalic arteries. Stroke prevention involves blood pressure control and antiplatelet agents.

Connective tissue disorders

Systemic lupus erythematosus (SLE)

This connective tissue disorder causes stroke by several mechanisms including

➠ hypercoagulable states
➠ cardiogenic emboli (from Libman-Sacks endocarditis)
➠ atherosclerosis
➠ vasculitis
➠ thrombogenic cytokine formation
➠ intracranial hemorrhage

Laboratory evaluation for SLE (ANA, anti-dsDNA Ab, anti-Sm Ab) can be reserved for those patients with other evidence of SLE by history or physical exam. Warfarin may help prevent recurrent emboli. The role of steroids in stroke prophylaxis is less clear and not universally recommended.

Marfan syndrome

This is an autosomal dominant disorder caused by mutations of the protein fibrillin. Clinical features include pectus excavatum, joint hypermobility, ectopia lentis, and dilatation or dissection of the ascending aorta. Mechanisms of stroke include arterial dissection, valvular dysfunction, and aneurysmal rupture. Beta blockers and valve reconstruction reduce the likelihood of stroke.

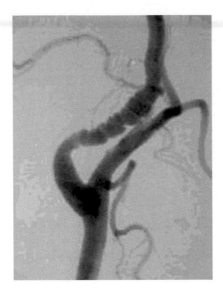

Figure 6.1 Angiogram demonstrating the beading on a string consistent with fibromuscular dysplasia.

Ehlers-Danlos syndrome

This group of connective tissue disorders is characterized by fragile or hyperelastic skin, hyperextensible joints, and vascular lesions. Mechanisms of stroke in Ehlers-Danlos syndrome include aneurysmal rupture, carotid-cavernous fistulae, and arterial dissection. Specific treatment depends on stroke mechanism.

Fibromuscular dysplasia (FMD)

This connective tissue disorder most commonly affects middle-aged women.

⇛ It classically involves the internal carotid and renal arteries, but can affect almost any artery.

Stroke mechanisms include arterial dissection, aneurysmal rupture, and stasis with thrombus formation and distal embolization.

⇛ Angiography demonstrates a sausage-like string-of-beads appearance of the internal carotid artery (ICA). These changes can also be demonstrated on CT angiogram (CTA) or magnetic resonance angiogram (MRA) (Figure 6.1).

The best prevention of FMD-related stroke is not known. Options include antiplatelet agents, anticoagulants, thromboendarterectomy, and endovascular intervention.

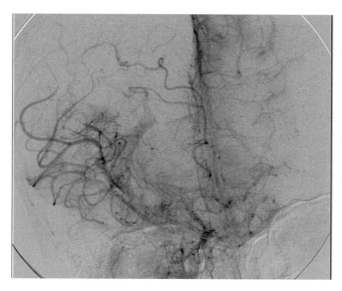

Figure 6.2 An angiogram demonstrating the changes seen in Moyamoya disease.

Angiopathies

Moyamoya syndrome

The name of this syndrome is derived from Japanese for "something hazy like a puff of cigarette smoke drifting in the air."

➠ Progressive occlusion of the intracranial ICAs at their intracranial bifurcations (the T-portions) results in prominent anastomosing channels that appear as angiographic clouds of smoke (Figure 6.2).

Etiologies include sickle cell disease, neurofibromatosis, Takayasu's arteritis, Down syndrome, atherosclerosis, and FMD. It is more common in women and has a bimodal distribution.

➠ Children younger than 15 years present with transient episodes of hemiparesis precipitated by physical exertion or hyperventilation whereas adults are most commonly affected by subcortical hemorrhages.

Surgical revascularization improves collateral blood flow, decreases moyamoya vessels, and reduces the risk for further stroke.

Susac's syndrome

The clinical triad of Susac's syndrome consists of

➠ acute and subacute multifocal and diffuse encephalopathy
➠ hearing loss
➠ visual loss

It affects mainly adult women. The etiology is unknown, but is thought to be microangiopathy of the arterioles of the brain, retina, and cochlea. Treatments are usually unsuccessful, but include corticosteroids, cyclophosphamide, azathioprine, antiplatelets, calcium channel blockers, IVIg, and plasmapheresis.

Hereditary endotheliopathy with retinopathy, nephropathy, and stroke (HERNS)

This autosomal dominant vasculopathy causes progressive visual loss beginning in the third or fourth decades, followed by focal neurological deficits in 5–10 years.

➧ Stroke-like episodes occur in most patients and may be the presenting symptoms.

These strokes may progress over several days before reaching completion. Later in the disease, signs of multifocal cortical and subcortical involvement occur.

➧ More than half of patients have migraines and about half have evidence of renal dysfunction.

Multiple T2 hyperintensities can be seen on magnetic resonance imaging (MRI) in the deep white matter, often before neurologic symptoms develop. The best treatment for stroke related to HERNS is unclear. Aspirin is often prescribed. Corticosteroids can help reduce edema.

Osler-Weber-Rendu disease

This autosomal dominant disorder is characterized by cutaneous, mucosal, and visceral vascular malformations that may hemorrhage spontaneously.

➧ Facial telangiectasias are the most common sign. The lungs and digestive tract are also commonly affected.

Neurological complications include brain abscesses, meningitis, and rupture of AVMs. Cerebral vascular malformations are most commonly telangiectasias or cavernous angiomas. AVMs, aneurysms, and carotid-cavernous fistulas are less common.

➧ The most common cause of ischemic strokes in Osler-Weber-Rendu is paradoxical emboli from pulmonary AVM.

Hyperviscosity syndromes and gaseous emboli from pulmonary vessel-respiratory pathway fistulae can also occur.

➧ Patients with Osler-Weber-Rendu disease and stroke should undergo chest CT angiography to look for evidence of pulmonary AVM .

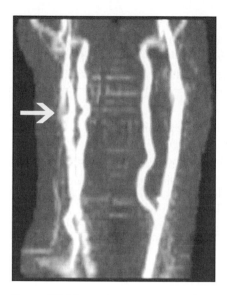

Figure 6.3 Magnetic resonance angiogram demonstrating dissection of the right internal carotid artery.

Resection or embolization of pulmonary AVMs is recommended to prevent stroke recurrence. Treatment of cerebrovascular malformations depends on type and location.

Arterial dissections

A tear within an arterial wall leads to bleeding and dissection within the media along the longitudinal course of the artery.

▸ This is the second leading cause of stroke in patients younger than 45.

The main precipitant of arterial dissection is trauma including motor vehicle accidents, chiropractic manipulation, and even mild mechanical stress caused by simply looking over the shoulder. Often, the trauma is trivial and the patient does not remember the precipitating event. Connective tissue disorders are a risk factor for dissection. Stroke may result in blood flow stasis and intraluminal thrombosis.

Carotid artery dissection (Figure 6.3) most commonly involves the extracranial ICA in its pharyngeal and distal intracranial segments. Signs include those related to the ipsilateral eye and cerebral hemisphere.

▸ The proximity of the carotid artery to the oculosympathetic pathways may produce an ipsilateral Horner's syndrome. Because the ICA passes through the retropharyngeal space, dysfunction of the lower cranial nerves may be present.

Dissections of the extracranial vertebral artery (VA) usually affect the vessel between its emergence from the vertebral column and its dural penetration, or in the first segment of the artery above the VA origin but before entrance into the transverse foramina. Pain often precedes neurologic symptoms by hours or days. Symptoms include dizziness, diplopia, dysarthria, clumsiness, and imbalance.

1. Transient ischemic attacks (TIAs) are less common in VA dissections than in ICA dissections.
2. MRA with fat saturation or CTA of the neck confirms the presence of dissection.
3. Extracranial VA dissection should also be evaluated with MRA of the chest to study the takeoff from the subclavian arteries.

Ultrasonography and conventional angiography are now used less often to establish the diagnosis.

Treatment of arterial dissection is controversial, but short-term anticoagulation is often used to reduce the risk of embolization of thrombus. For extracranial ICA dissection, there are no randomized trials to compare anticoagulants or antiplatelet drugs with control or to each other. The reported nonrandomized trials did not show a difference between anticoagulant and antiplatelet drugs. Extracranial dissections may produce only headache, pain, and TIAs without lasting neurologic deficits. Most extracranial dissections heal spontaneously with time. Intracranial dissections are less common but usually cause severe deficits or even death.

Sneddon's syndrome

Sneddon's syndrome is the combination of ischemic strokes and livedo reticularis, a purplish mottling of the skin distributed over the lower trunk, buttocks, and proximal thighs. Women are affected more often than men. The etiology is not clear, but may be related to a hypercoagulable state, such as the antiphospholipid antibody state, or small vessel vasculopathy.

➠ Livedo reticularis is usually the first manifestation of the disease, preceding the neurological symptoms by an average of 10 years.

Migrainous symptoms usually occur synchronously with the onset of livedo reticularis. TIAs and strokes are multiple and recur in the same or different vascular territories. Mild to severe cognitive impairment may occur in later stages. Subarachnoid hemorrhage and seizures are also reported.

1. Extensive laboratory evaluation to exclude hypercoagulable states should be performed.
2. Skin biopsy of the normal flesh-colored area within the bordering livedo is of the highest diagnostic yield.

The optimal treatment of Sneddon's syndrome is not clear. Many clinicians prefer anticoagulation because of the presumed relationship between Sneddon's syndrome and antiphospholipid antibody syndrome. Others use antiplatelet agents. There is no clear benefit for immunosuppression.

Metabolic diseases

Cerebral autosomal dominant arteriopathy with subcortical infarcts and leukoencephalopathy (CADASIL)

This autosomal dominant disorder is caused by a mutation of the notch3 gene on chromosome 19. The mean age of onset is between 45 and 50 years.

⇒ Although recurrent ischemic strokes are the most common presentation, approximately half of patients develop cognitive deficits.

In the earlier stages of CADASIL, there are typically T2 hyperintensities in the basal ganglia and periventricular white matter. As the disease progresses, white matter lesions can involve the whole of the cortex including the subcortical U fibers.

⇒ The diagnosis can be made by skin biopsy or genetic analysis.

The best treatment for CADASIL is not clear, and involves addressing other modifiable stroke risk factors.

Fabry's disease

Fabry's disease is an X-linked recessive disorder caused by deficiency of α-galactosidase with resulting lysosomal accumulation of glycosphingolipids.

1. Episodic pain crises of the hands and feet are the most common early symptoms.
2. Angiokeratomas appear in clusters in the superficial layers of the skin, usually in the periumbilical area, the extensor surfaces of the elbows and knees, and the hip and genital areas.
3. Ophthalmological exam discloses whirl-like corneal opacities, dilatation and tortuosity of the conjunctival vessels, and abnormalities of retinal vessels.

Ischemic strokes typically occur in middle age and are more common than hemorrhagic strokes. Mechanisms of cerebral ischemia include

⇒ intracranial arterial dolichoectasia
⇒ progressive occlusion of small arteries or arterioles secondary to glycosphingolipid accumulation
⇒ cardiogenic embolism

⟶ impaired autonomic function
⟶ prothrombotic states

Alpha-galactosidase supplementation may improve renal function and peripheral neuropathy symptoms, but there is little data on its efficacy for stroke prevention. Patients have about a 75 percent chance of recurrent events.

Mitochondrial encephalomyopathy, lactic acidosis, and stroke-like episodes (MELAS)

This maternally inherited disorder is secondary to mitochondrial respiratory chain dysfunction. Patients usually present before age 40.

⟶ Diagnostic features include migraine-like headaches in the setting of stroke-like episodes and prolonged focal or generalized seizures.

Strokes usually occur in the posterior half of the brain and do not follow single arterial territories. Chronic progressive external ophthalmoplegia, pigmentary retinopathy, optic atrophy, cardiac conduction defects, diabetes, and hypothyroidism may also occur.

⟶ Diagnosis is established by muscle biopsy that demonstrates ragged red fibers.

Treatments are largely supportive and consist of antioxidant vitamin supplements and respiratory chain cofactors including

⟶ coenzyme Q10 (50–300 mg/day)
⟶ creatine (up to 10 g/day)
⟶ L-carnitine (3 g/day)
⟶ vitamin E (200–400 IU/day)
⟶ ascorbic acid (2 g/day)

Newer studies suggest a benefit of L-arginine infusions and oral L-arginine supplementation.

Hematologic and oncologic causes

Hyperviscosity syndromes

High blood viscosity increases the risk of ischemic strokes. Hyperviscosity syndromes can result from one of three mechanisms:

⟶ plasma protein abnormalities (e.g., Waldenstrom's macroglobulinemia)
⟶ increased cellularity (e.g., polycythemia vera and leukemia)
⟶ decreased red cell deformability (e.g., sickle cell anemia)

Frequent phlebotomy and plasma exchange may prevent recurrent strokes.

Strokes in the setting of cancer

In patients with cancer, stroke is second only to metastasis as a cause of CNS pathology. There are multiple mechanisms by which cancer causes stroke.

1. Tumor may activate the coagulation system and produce a hypercoagulable state.
2. Nonbacterial thrombotic endocarditis (NBTE) is seen most commonly in adenocarcinomas and generally affects left-sided valves.
3. Tumor emboli occur most commonly with tumors of the heart or lung.
4. Venous sinus thrombosis usually occurs with hematological malignancies.
5. Strokes may also occur as a result of cerebrovascular compression and infiltration, intracranial hemorrhage, chemotherapy, and radiotherapy.

Treatment largely depends on stroke etiology. Stroke is overall a poor prognostic factor in cancer.

Substance abuse

A variety of substances abuse can produce either ischemic or hemorrhagic strokes.

1. Strokes related to heroin frequently follow the reintroduction of intravenous heroin after a period of abstinence.
2. Amphetamines may cause a necrotizing angiitis that resembles PAN.
3. Cocaine produces ischemic strokes by multiple mechanisms including
   a) hypertension and emboli of impurities. Particles of drugs and fillers are trapped in lung arterioles and small arteries, causing an obliterative arteritis or development of pulmonary arteriovenous shunts.
   b) Hemorrhagic strokes from cocaine are most commonly lobar hemorrhages.
   c) Subarachnoid hemorrhage from rupture of AVMs and aneurysms is also a frequently recognized stroke subtype with cocaine use.
4. Phencyclidine (PCP) rarely causes intracranial hemorrhage secondary to hypertension.

Infective endocarditis, hepatitis, AIDS, and fungal infections are common complications of an addictive lifestyle and may also produce strokes.

Infections

Bacterial infections

Acute bacterial meningitis may cause strokes by occluding pial arteries and veins.

➠ *Listeria monocytogenes* produces an inflammatory disorder involving predominantly the pontine and medullary tegmentum (*Listeria rhombencephalitis*). Multiple lower cranial nerve palsies, oculomotor palsies, and vestibular symptoms may result.

Meningovascular syphilis is now uncommon. It is characterized by an inflammatory infiltration of the adventitia of medium- to large-caliber arteries that cause progressive stenosis. Most often, meningovascular syphilis-related strokes involve the middle cerebral artery.

Tuberculosis may cause obstruction of capillaries from small tuberculous emboli leading to microinfarcts. The anterior and middle cerebral arteries are most commonly involved.

Bartonella henselae, the cause of cat-scratch disease, is an uncommon cause of stroke related to localized intracranial stenosis and arteritis.

Viral infections

Most virus-related strokes are secondary to vasculitis.

➠ Herpes zoster most commonly causes delayed hemispheric infarction ipsilateral to the site of herpes zoster ophthalmicus.

Symptoms begin days to weeks after onset of rash. Controversy exists as to the mechanism, but the leading theory is that herpes virus is transported to the walls of the ipsilateral proximal basal cerebral vessels along nerve fibers originating in the ophthalmic portion of the Gasserian ganglion. Smooth muscle fibers in these vessels are affected by arteritis and thrombosis in situ.

Cytomegalovirus, HIV, and herpes simplex may also be associated with stroke.

Fungal infections

Aspergillus causes CNS disease by direct extension or embolization. In immunosuppressed patients, strokes are caused by dissemination from a pulmonary source, whereas in immunocompetent patients, strokes are related to vasculitis. Only about 25 percent of patients respond to amphotericin B, voriconazole, or caspofungin.

Candida produces strokes from cerebral abscesses, small vessel thromboses formed by pseudohyphae, and vasculitic microinfarcts. This fungus has a predilection for the middle cerebral artery and should be treated with a combination of amphotericin B and flucytosine.

Mucormycosis may cause an acute necrotizing tissue reaction and thrombosis of the neighboring vessels. Diabetes, acidosis, and immunosuppression predispose to mucor infection. Thrombosis of the cavernous sinus and ICA are common. Debridement, discontinuation of immunosuppression, and amphotericin B are required to effectively treat mucor.

Cryptococcosis and histoplasmosis rarely cause large vessel cerebral vasculitis.

Parasitic infections

Cysticercosis most commonly produces stroke by inflammatory occlusion of arteries at the base of the brain. Lacunar infarctions are more common than large artery occlusions. Patients with cerebral infarction secondary to cysticercosis should receive anticysticercal agents such as praziquantel or albendazole and corticosteroids.

Migrainous infarction

Migraine aura symptoms that persist for longer than an hour can be accompanied by neuroimaging evidence of ischemic stroke. Women under 45 with migraine are at increased risk for stroke, especially those who smoke and use estrogen-containing oral contraceptives. Strokes generally occur in the posterior cerebral and vertebrobasilar artery territories. Intracranial hemorrhage secondary to migraine is less common.

Stroke mimics

Common conditions that can be confused with stroke are listed in Table 6.3.

Intracranial mass lesion

The duration of symptoms with brain tumors is usually weeks to months, but a small percentage of patients with brain tumors may have symptoms for less than one day prior to presentation. Hemorrhage into the tumor, edema, or hydrocephalus may be responsible for apoplectic presentations.

Subdural hematoma

Subdural hematomas are the result of torn intracranial bridging veins. Presentations are protean and can imitate ischemic stroke, seizure, encephalopathy, or dementia. Chronic subdural hematomas may present weeks to months after mild head trauma. Expanding subdural hematomas with progressive neurologic deficits require neurosurgical evaluation and consideration of drainage.

Seizures

The neurologic deficits of seizure can usually be distinguished from those of stroke by a march of symptoms over a period of seconds. Todd's paralysis is

---

Table 6.3: Stroke mimics

Intracranial mass lesions

Subdural hematoma

Seizures
  Todd's paralysis

Migraine
  Migraine aura
  Familial hemiplegic migraine
  Sporadic hemiplegic migraine
  Call's syndrome
  Bartleson's syndrome

Alternating hemiplegia

Posterior leukoencephalopathy

Metabolic disturbances
  Hypoglycemia
  Nonketotic hyperglycemia
  Hyponatremia
  Hypoxia
  Hepatic encephalopathy

Peripheral nervous system disorders

Metabolic insult causing re-expression of old stroke (MICROS)

Psychiatric disorders
  Conversion disorder
  Malingering

---

a postictal paralysis that not only usually follows a partial motor seizure, but may also follow a generalized seizure. The presence of "negative" symptoms may cause Todd's paralysis to be misdiagnosed as a seizure, frequently if the seizure has not been observed or renders the patient unable to communicate. The pathophysiology of Todd's paralysis is unclear and likely represents a combination of neuronal exhaustion and active neuronal inhibition. Spontaneous recovery is the rule. Unexpectedly prolonged Todd's paralysis suggests either a progressive structural lesion or subtle, continuing seizures.

Migraine

Migraine aura can produce neurologic symptoms of sudden onset that resemble ischemic stroke. The clinical picture is often obscured by the lack of headache.

Familial hemiplegic migraine (FHM) is characterized by migraine with aura including motor weakness. Disturbances of consciousness, fever, and CSF pleocytosis can occur.

➤ FHM1 is caused by mutations in the CACNA1A gene on chromosome 19 whereas FHM2 is caused by mutations in the ATP1A2 gene on chromosome 1.

Sporadic hemiplegic migraine has a similar clinical presentation to FHM but lacks a history of similarly affected first- or second-degree relatives. It occurs with approximately the same prevalence as FHM, is more common in men, and is often associated with aphasia.

Call's syndrome is a disorder characterized by headache and fluctuating or recurring motor or sensory deficits. Cerebral angiography shows segmental narrowing of intracranial arteries.

Bartleson's syndrome occurs mainly in young people and is characterized by episodic, severe headaches preceded and accompanied by sensory, motor, speech, and visual disturbances. The CSF shows an elevated opening pressure, lymphocytic pleocytosis, and elevated protein. Recovery is usually complete.

Alternating hemiplegia

Alternating hemiplegia of childhood is a disorder of recurrent hemiplegia beginning before age 18 months. It is associated with dystonia, nystagmus, and progressive cognitive and motor impairment. Benign familial nocturnal alternating hemiplegia also features alternating hemiplegia, but there is no progression to neurologic or intellectual impairment. The etiologies of these conditions are not known, but may be related to migraines or channelopathies.

Posterior leukoencephalopathy

This is an acute-onset condition characterized by headache, nausea, vomiting, seizures, visual disturbances, altered sensorium, and occasionally, focal neurologic deficits. It is usually associated with hypertension. Common causes include

➤ hypertensive encephalopathy
➤ eclampsia
➤ immunosuppressive agents and cytotoxic drugs
➤ renal failure with hypertension

MRI shows edematous lesions of the posterior parietal and occipital lobes. This edema may spread to the basal ganglia, brain stem, and cerebellum. If the condition is recognized promptly, the blood pressure controlled, and offending agents removed, it is completely reversible.

Hypoglycemia

Transient hypoglycemia, usually with a blood glucose level less than 45 mg/dl may produce stroke-like syndromes.

⇒ Patients with hypoglycemia are usually confused or have a diminished level of consciousness, but in some patients, focal neurologic deficits may occur without these findings.

Predisposing conditions included diabetes, alcoholism, and sepsis. Stroke-like symptoms may resolve immediately with glucose administration or resolution may take hours to days.

Nonketotic hyperglycemia

Hyperglycemia can mimic stroke. Although focal deficits often occur after a seizure, a glucose concentration greater than 400 mg/dl may mimic stroke in the absence of a seizure. It is reversible with correction of the hyperglycemia. The mean duration of the symptoms is approximately 5 days.

Other metabolic disorders that may mimic stroke include hyponatremia, hypoxia, and hepatic encephalopathy.

Radial neuropathy

Patients often awaken with radial neuropathies after deep sleep while intoxicated or after surgery, and may not recognize the time of onset of their symptoms.

⇒ Stroke can be clinically differentiated from radial neuropathy by weakness in muscles outside of a radial distribution and alteration in muscle tone and deep tendon reflexes.

In cases that are still unclear, MRI or electromyography/nerve conduction studies can help differentiate the two conditions. Improvement depends on the nature of the injury. Some patients may require surgical intervention whereas others repair spontaneously over 6–8 weeks.

Metabolic insult causing re-expression of old stroke (MICROS)

Patients with prior ischemic stroke are susceptible to reappearance of their old symptoms and signs without a new ischemic stroke.

⇒ Although MICROS has never been formally studied, insults such as urinary tract infections, pneumonia, and medication overdoses appear to be the most common provocative agents.

The precise mechanism of MICROS is unclear, but because the tissue from the initial stroke is infarcted, the pathways that form during the reorganization of the brain during stroke recovery may be disrupted, as they are more susceptible to metabolic fluctuations. Alternatively, MICROS may affect tissue that once belonged to the ischemic penumbra; this tissue may be prone to changes in the metabolic environment that do not affect healthy tissue.

⮕ A negative diffusion-weighted MRI is required to exclude the possibility of stroke recurrence.

This entity is poorly studied, but most cases respond to correction of the causative metabolic abnormality.

Conversion disorder

Conversion disorder is the unintentional production of neurological symptoms that cannot be explained by a known neurological or medical disorder. The most common symptoms of conversion disorder include paralysis, blindness, and language disturbances, often of sudden onset. Patients have secondary gains, and the symptoms of the conversion disorder allow them to be excused from obligations, receive support and assistance from other people, and control other people's behavior.

⮕ This is a diagnosis of exclusion that can only be entertained after extensive medical evaluation proves negative.

Resolution is usually spontaneous, but may be prolonged and helped by psychotherapy.

Malingering

Malingering is the intentional production of false or grossly exaggerated physical or psychological symptoms. Patients have external motivations such as avoiding responsibilities, monetary compensation, and retaliation. Most patients express subjective, vague, ill-defined features, but they may also demonstrate very specific, stroke-like symptoms. The symptoms and signs are inconsistent, but extensive medical evaluation should be performed prior to making the diagnosis. Treatment is challenging and direct confrontation is not recommended.

Bibliography

Bartleson JD, Swanson JW, Whisnant JP. A migrainous syndrome with cerebrospinal fluid pleocytosis. *Neurology* 1981;31:1257–62.
Berkovic SF, Bladin PF, Darby DG. Metabolic disorders presenting as stroke. *Med J Aust* 1984;140:421–4.

Bessen H. Intracranial hemorrhage associated with phencyclidine abuse. *JAMA* 1982;248:585–6.

Bogousslavsky J, Caplan L, eds. *Uncommon causes of stroke*. Cambridge: Cambridge University Press, 2001.

Call GK Fleming MC Sealfon S et al. Reversible cerebral segmental vasoconstriction. *Stroke* 1988;19:1159–70.

Caplan LR. *Posterior circulation disease. Clinical findings, diagnosis, and management*. Cambridge, UK: Blackwell Science, 1996.

Caplan LR, Thomas C, Banks G. Central nervous system complications of "T's and Blues" addiction. *Neurology* 1982;32:623–8.

Caplan LR, Zarins C, Hemmatti M. Spontaneous dissection of the extracranial vertebral artery. *Stroke* 1985;16:1030–8.

Dichgans M, Mayer M, Uttner I, et al. The phenotypic spectrum of CADASIL: Clinical findings in 102 cases. *Ann Neurol* 1998;44:731–9.

Flint AC, Liberato BB, Anziska Y, et al. Meningovascular syphilis as a cause of basilar artery stenosis. *Neurology* 2005;64:391–2.

Frayne J, Gates P. Listeria rhombencephalitis. *Clin Exp Neurol* 1987;24:175–9.

Garg RK. Posterior leukoencephalopathy syndrome. *Postgrad Med J* 2001;77:24–8.

Hayreh SS, Podhajsky PA, Raman R, et al. Giant cell arteritis: Validity and reliability of various diagnostic criteria. *Am J Ophthalmol* 1997;123:285–96.

Houkin K, Kamiyama H, Abe H, et al. Surgical therapy for adult Moyamoya disease. Can surgical revascularization prevent the recurrence of intracerebral hemorrhage? *Stroke* 1996;27:1342–6.

Huff JS. Stroke mimics and chameleons. *Emerg Med Clin N Am* 2002;20:583–95.

Jen J, Cohen AH, Yue Q, et al. Hereditary endotheliopathy with retinopathy, nephropathy, and stroke (HERNS). *Neurology* 1997;49:1322–30.

Kavanaugh M, Myers GJ. Benign alternating hemiplegia of childhood: New features and associations. *Neurology* 2004;62:672.

Koga Y, Akita Y, Nishioka J, et al. L-arginine improves the symptoms of strokelike episodes in MELAS. *Neurology* 2005;64:710–12.

Maccario M. Neurological dysfunction associated with nonketotic hyperglycemia. *Arch Neurol* 1968;19:525–34.

Mitsias P, Levine SR. Cerebrovascular complications of Fabry's disease. *Ann Neurol* 1996;40:8–17.

Rogers LR. Cerebrovascular complications in patients with cancer. *Semin Neurol* 2004;24:453–60.

Roman G, Fisher M, Perl DP, et al. Neurological manifestations of hereditary hemorrhagic telangiectasia (Rendu-Osler-Weber disease): Report of 2 cases and review of the literature. *Ann Neurol* 1978;4:130–44.

Salaki JS, Louria DB, Chmel H. Fungal and yeast infections of the central nervous system. A clinical review. *Medicine* 1984;63:108–32.

Schmidley JW. *Central nervous system angiitis*. Boston: Butterworth Heinemann, 2000.

Selby G, Walker GL. Cerebral arteritis in cat-scratch disease. *Neurology* 1979;29:1413–18.

Slovut DP, Olin JW. Fibromuscular dysplasia. *N Engl J Med* 2004;350:1862–71.

Snyder H, Robinson K, Shah D, et al. Signs and symptoms of patients with brain tumors presenting to the emergency department. *J Emerg Med* 1993;11:253–8.

Wallis WE, Donaldson I, Scott RS, et al. Hypoglycemia masquerading as cerebrovascular disease (hypoglycemic hemiplegia). *Ann Neurol* 1985;18:510–12.

Wong RL, Korn JH. Temporal arteritis without an elevated erythrocyte sedimentation rate. Case report and review of the literature. *Am J Med* 1986;80:959–64.

Zelger B, Sepp N, Stockhammer G, et al. Sneddon's syndrome. A long-term follow-up of 21 patients. *Arch Dermatol* 1993;129:437–47.

Acute Stroke Imaging

Computed tomography in acute stroke

Sanjay K. Shetty and Michael H. Lev

The goal of this chapter is to familiarize the reader with the use of computed tomography (CT) in the setting of suspected acute stroke and to develop an understanding of the role, strengths, and weaknesses of each application of CT. Key points that are necessary to understand the implications on image interpretation and triage will be highlighted.

CT: Considerations

CT offers an increasing array of tools to aid in the detection and characterization of acute stroke. Rapid ongoing improvements in scanner technology continue to expand the role of this modality (Table 7.1).

1. In the acute setting, unenhanced CT, the traditional initial screening modality in the setting of suspected stroke, can reveal the presence of an infarct and/or intracranial hemorrhage.
2. CT angiography (CTA) and CT venography (CTV) evaluate the major intracranial vessels for the presence of intravascular thrombus.
3. CT perfusion (CTP) extends the traditional anatomic role of imaging to evaluate capillary level hemodynamics, attempting to predict whether ischemic tissue is destined to infarct ("infarct core") or is potentially salvageable after prompt recanalization ("penumbra").
4. CTA source images (CTA-SIs), the axial images acquired after bolus administration of contrast, can offer an additional view of perfusion hemodynamics in the detection of infarct.

The potential advantages and disadvantages of CT are summarized below.

Advantages

The major advantages of CT are widespread availability, relatively low cost, and rapid acquisition. CT is also the only available modality in patients with contraindications to magnetic resonance (MR) scanning or in patients who cannot be adequately screened for MR safety.

Table 7.1: Role of CT in the detection and triage of acute stroke: the four key questions

The role of CT in acute stroke

	Unenhanced CT	CTA	CTP (CBV)	CTP (CBF)	CTP (CTA-SI)	CTV
Is there hemorrhage?	+					
Is there intravascular thrombus?		+				+
Is there a "core" of critically ischemic, irreversibly infarcted tissue?	+		+			

Disadvantages

One of the technical disadvantages of CT is the use of ionizing radiation. It is important to remember that acquisitions added to a conventional unenhanced CT scan will increase radiation dose. A second consideration is iodinated contrast, which is required for CTA, CTP, and CTV. Also, postprocessing of CTA and CTP images is more labor intensive than that of MR angiography (MRA) and MR perfusion (MRP) images, although with training and quality control, 3D reconstructions of CTA datasets, as well as quantitative CTP maps, can be constructed rapidly and reliably.

1. Clinically, the risks of contrast-induced nephropathy or anaphylactic reaction are important to consider, particularly in older patients.
   a) Screening patients for renal disease and previous allergy can be difficult in the acute setting.
   b) The use of nonionic iodinated contrast has been shown not to worsen stroke outcome.
   c) Optimized CTA protocols can also reduce the contrast load while improving arterial opacification, including saline bolus following contrast administration.

Unenhanced CT

Unenhanced CT remains a first-line diagnostic test in the evaluation of acute stroke. A checklist for the interpretation of unenhanced CT is presented in Table 7.2.

1. The primary role of CT in the acute setting is the detection of *intracranial hemorrhage*, which can guide subsequent therapy (Table 7.2 and Figure 7.1).

Table 7.2: Checklist for interpretation of unenhanced CT

⇒ Exclude intracranial hemorrhage (Hyperdense or Bright)
    Evaluate parenchyma
    Evaluate subarachnoid space
        Interpeduncular cistern
        Sylvian fissures
        Convexities
   Evaluate ventricles
        Occipital horns of the lateral ventricles
   Evaluated epidural and subdural spaces

⇒ Parenchymal changes of stroke
    Loss of Gray/white Differentiation
        Insular ribbon sign
        Obscured lentiform nucleus
    Cortical and parenchymal swelling
        Focally effaced sulci
        Mass effect on the sylvian fissure or ventricles

⇒ Indirect signs of stroke
    Hyperdense middle cerebral artery sign
    MCA dot sign
    Venous Thrombus: dense cord, dense triangle, dense lateral sinus

---

2. In addition, unenhanced CT scan may detect infarcted brain parenchyma within 6 hr of stroke onset.

   a) The overall sensitivity of unenhanced CT for the detection of acute stroke is difficult to gauge, since published studies vary in scanner parameters and vascular territory. A prospective study of patients imaged in the emergency room (mean interval from onset of symptoms to imaging of 2.3 hr) demonstrated that a neuroradiologist blinded to history had a sensitivity of 38 percent, which increased to 52 percent when the history of suspected stroke was known.

   b) Edema and the resulting decreased attenuation underlie the major parenchymal manifestations of acute stroke: *parenchymal hypodensity, associated loss of gray/white differentiation,* and *parenchymal swelling.*

      i) In the MCA territory, loss of gray/white differentiation results in obscuration of the insular ribbon, the basal ganglia, and posterior limb of the internal capsule.

     ii) Parenchymal swelling can result in subtle narrowing of the cortical sulci or the Sylvian fissure or in compression of the ventricles or basal cisterns.

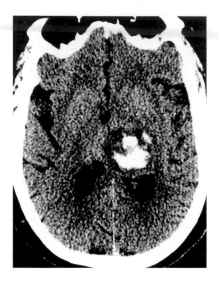

Figure 7.1 Unenhanced CT reveals hyperdense hemorrhage in the left thalamus with surrounding hypodense edema.

iii) Subtle changes require careful attention to these features on every unenhanced CT scan. Infarcts in the posterior fossa are particularly problematic, since beam-hardening artifact from adjacent osseous structures obscures evaluation of the brainstem and cerebellum.

iv) The physical basis of these parenchymal changes offers insight into the subtle changes that are seen on unenhanced CT.

(1) CT scans measure the attenuation of an x-ray beam through a given region of interest, assigning each volume (voxel) an attenuation value, measured in Hounsfield units (HUs), which is proportional to tissue density. Using this scale, on which water is arbitrarily assigned a value of zero, normal gray matter has an attenuation value of 30–35 HU and white matter 20–25 HU.

(2) Gray matter, therefore, appears brighter than white matter when these attenuation values are represented as an image, and subtle changes in attenuation that reduce this contrast between gray and white matter are one of the major parenchymal manifestations of stroke.

(3) In the acute phase (less than 30 min), failure of membrane ion channels caused by inadequate ATP results in *cytotoxic edema*, or movement of water from the extracellular to the intracellular space. This involves a shift in the distribution of water, rather than a change in water content, so the CT appearance will remain essentially unchanged.

(4) In a slightly later phase (greater than 3–6 hr), *vasogenic edema* results from breakdown of tight endothelial junctions in the setting of residual perfusion. Increased water content results in decreased attenuation value or a slightly darker appearance on CT; for every 1 percent increase in water content, there is a corresponding decreased attenuation of 3–5 percent (or 2.5 HU).

v) The significance of these early ischemic changes (EICs) on unenhanced CT is still debated.

(1) Parenchymal hypodensity is considered the most important. Tissue demonstrating severe hypodensity on unenhanced CT is almost invariably destined to infarct, whereas tissue that is only slightly hypodense may not always proceed to infarction.

(2) Parenchymal swelling is relatively less important, with published studies finding no swelling or swelling in only a small percentage of patients in the hyperacute (<3 hr) time frame. In addition, cortical swelling, manifested as effacement of cortical sulci on unenhanced CT scan, may not always represent infarct. In fact, sulcal effacement without associated parenchymal hypodensity has been associated with increased cerebral blood volume (CBV) and reperfusion; these areas do not always proceed to infarct on follow-up imaging.

(3) A possible pitfall is also noted in the subacute phase after stroke (2–6 weeks after stroke onset). The "CT fogging effect," in which infarcted tissue becomes less apparent, is likely due to resolution of low-density edema and infiltration of higher attenuation macrophages and neocapillarity in the infarcted tissue bed.

c) The relatively low sensitivity of unenhanced CT can be improved through optimization of viewing parameters during soft copy review on a PACS workstation. *The contrast between normal and abnormal parenchyma can be emphasized by carefully selecting a nonstandard, narrow viewing range (e.g., window 30 HU and level 36 HU),* which improves sensitivity for stroke detection without loss of specificity or increased interpretation time.

3. Careful review of unenhanced CT may reveal indirect signs of vessel occlusion.

a) An adjunctive sign of infarct is hyperdensity in the proximal middle cerebral artery ("the hyperdense MCA sign") that reflects occlusion of the MCA (Figures 7.2 and 7.9). Because the proximal MCA travels in the axial plane, the vessel appears as an elongated, hyperdense

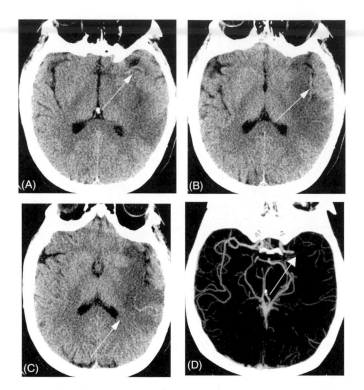

Figure 7.2 (A) Unenhanced CT shows an extreme example of a hyperdense MCA sign: the vessel is visualized from the M1 segment through branch vessels in the Sylvian fissure (M2/M3 segments) (arrows), representing thrombosis. More typically, only the proximal aspect (M1 segment) of the MCA is visualized as hyperdense (see Figure 7.8). (B and C) Note the additional signs of infarct: hypodensity, loss of gray/white differentiation, and mass effect, including effacement of the Sylvian fissure and sulci. (D) CTA confirms occlusion of the MCA proximally (arrow).

structure (80 HU); comparison with the contralateral normal MCA can be valuable in this setting.

   i)   This hyperdensity is most commonly felt to represent hyperdense occlusive thrombus, although some reports suggest that hyperdensity could also result from slow flow.

   ii) This is considered a specific but nonsensitive sign; its incidence is between 1 and 50 percent.

   iii) Differential possibilities for a hyperdense vessel include atherosclerotic calcification and elevated hematocrit.

  b) More distal occlusion (involving the M2 or M3 branches of the MCA) can also be identified in the Sylvian fissure as the vessel crosses perpendicular to the axial plane of section (the "MCA dot sign").

  c) This sign can also be applied in cases of posterior circulation occlusion (Figure 7.3), although hyperdensity in the posterior

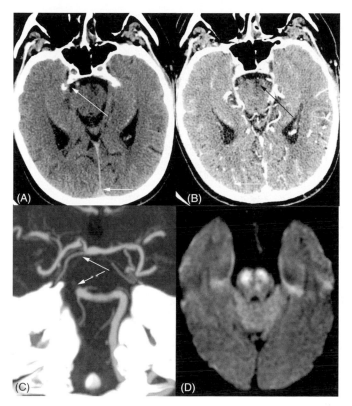

Figure 7.3 A 69-year-old otherwise healthy male presented to the emergency department after a suspected seizure and rapidly deteriorated to stupor and quadriparesis. (A) Unenhanced CT revealed hyperdensity in the basilar artery (arrow), which raised the possibility of basilar thrombosis. (B) CTA source images showed hypodensity in the anterior pons, consistent with infarct, and (C) CTA showed a basilar thrombosis (thrombosed segment is demarcated by arrows).

circulation should be interpreted with caution since beam-hardening effects in the posterior fossa can create an artifactually hyperdense appearance.

In addition to the detection of infarct, the unenhanced CT plays an important part in stroke triage, helping to exclude patients with intracranial hemorrhage or who are at increased risk for development of hemorrhage with therapy.

➠ An infarct larger than one-third of the MCA distribution territory may pose an increased risk of hemorrhagic transformation. The actual significance of this "rule," however, is still debated.

Initial parenchymal changes on unenhanced CT can also play a role in predicting subsequent clinical outcome.

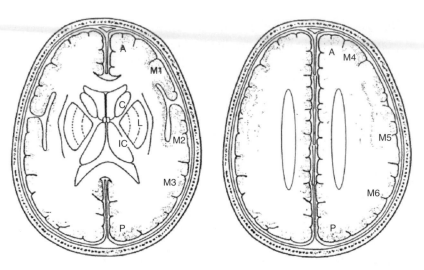

Figure 7.4 The ASPECTS interpretive map, demonstrating the 10 regions within the MCA vascular territory that must be systematically analyzed in the setting of acute stroke. The two standard axial slices are located at the level of the thalamus (left) and just above the level of the basal ganglia (right). The 10 regions include the caudate head (C), lentiform nucleus (L), internal capsule (IC), insula (I), and the six cortical segments (M1–M6). (Reprinted from *THE LANCET*, 355, Barber PA, Demchuk AM, Zhang J, and Buchan AM, Validity and reliability of a quantitative computed tomography score in predicting outcome of hyperacute stroke before thrombolytic therapy, 1670–1674, Copyright (2000), with permission from Elsevier.)

1. Infarct involving greater than 50 percent of the MCA territory is associated with brain herniation.
2. Parenchymal changes in the first 3–6 hr postictus have been found to correlate with stroke severity in some studies.
3. EICs on unenhanced CT have been shown to be a poor predictor of eventual clinical outcome.
4. The Alberta Stroke Programme Early CT Score (ASPECTS) system (discussed below) has been shown to correlate with stroke severity (NIHSS), risk of hemorrhage, and functional outcome.
5. The indirect signs of stroke have also been correlated with outcome: the hyperdense MCA sign has been associated with poor neurological outcome, whereas more distal MCA occlusion (the MCA dot sign) has been correlated with relatively decreased stroke severity and more favorable prognosis.

In the acute setting, reliable and accurate interpretation of the unenhanced CT is clinically important, with consequences for stroke triage and treatment. Improved reliability of infarct detection and characterization may be achieved through the use of ASPECTS, a clinical tool that utilizes a standardized topographic scoring system for MCA territory infarcts, dividing the MCA territory into 10 regions that are systematically analyzed by the reader. This standardized approach can improve reliability of infarct detection. It facilitates a systematic approach and can be taught to relatively inexperienced observers.

Employing the ASPECTS system relies on a systematic evaluation of the noncontrast CT:

1. Two slices are chosen for the analysis: one at the level of the thalami and one just above the level of the basal ganglia.
2. Each of the 10 segments located within the MCA vascular distribution are systematically evaluated. These 10 regions, denoted C, I, L, IC, and M1 through M6, are illustrated in Figure 7.4.
3. Normal segments are scored with one point, whereas any segment with evidence of ischemic change (hypodensity, loss of gray/white differentiation, parenchymal swelling, or sulcal effacement compared with the normal contralateral side) earns zero points.
4. A maximum of 10 points is therefore assigned to normal CT scans, with one point for each of the 10 normal regions. Lower scores correspond to larger regions of MCA infarct.
5. A score of seven has been shown to correlate with infarct involving approximately one-third of the MCA territory, allowing a rapid decision about the appropriate use of thrombolytics in the setting of acute stroke.
6. ASPECTS facilitates accurate interpretation by even relatively inexperienced readers by mandating analysis of the entire MCA distribution for subtle findings of infarct. Importantly, however, the analysis is limited by exclusion of the other vascular distributions and abnormalities that do not fall within the two slices used by ASPECTS.
7. The indirect signs of stroke have also been correlated with outcome: the hyperdense MCA sign has been associated with poor neurological outcome, whereas more distal MCA occlusion (the MCA dot sign) has been correlated with relatively decreased stroke severity and more favorable prognosis.

CTA

CTA expands the role of CT in the acute setting, offering a detailed view of the major vessels following intravenous bolus administration of contrast. This direct visualization of luminal occlusion in the setting of acute stroke offers a direct glimpse at the target of thrombolysis, confirming the clinical suspicion of acute stroke and potentially directing subsequent intraarterial thrombolysis.

The major advantages of CTA include speed of acquisition, generation of accurate anatomic information, and relatively low risk compared to conventional angiography. In addition, CTA provides anatomic information that is not as prone to artifacts as flow-dependent MRA or Doppler US. The principal disadvantages include the inability to provide physiologic data (such as flow rates) and the difficulty of measuring residual luminal diameter in the setting of circumferential atherosclerotic calcification due to beam-hardening artifacts.

Several technical points related to the acquisition of CTA (and CTP, discussed below) deserve mention because of their clinical relevance.

1. *Sufficient intravenous access* is required to deliver injection rates high enough to permit optimal arterial opacification; the high injection rates can lead to extravasation and failed CTA acquisition if the intravenous line is too small or poorly placed.
2. Following bolus administration of contrast, there is a delay before scanning that ensures that the contrast reaches the arteries. Certain clinical factors (such as poor cardiac output or atrial fibrillation) may necessitate alterations in the scan delay.
3. *Reformatted images help to visualize even tortuous vessels in their entirety and are particularly useful for evaluating branch points*. However, reference to the source images is necessary in certain situations, including heavy atherosclerotic calcifications that can obscure true vessel lumen diameter.

The major role of CTA is to identify occlusive thromboembolic disease in the intracranial circulation (Figure 7.5, see also Figures 7.2, 7.3, and 7.6–7.8). Once the occlusion has been localized, the patient can be triaged appropriately and the anatomic information can be used to guide catheter placement for intraarterial intervention. CTA is highly accurate in the detection and characterization of thromboembolic occlusive disease; using conventional catheter angiography as a gold standard, CTA has a sensitivity and specificity of 98.4 and 98.1 percent, respectively, for detection of proximal vessel occlusion. CTA can demonstrate intracranial aneurysms or arteriovenous malformations, which may be contraindications to thrombolytic therapy.

Because it can evaluate the cervical vasculature as part of the same examination, *CTA of the neck is a valuable tool for risk stratification and, in some cases, identifying the underlying etiology of infarction* (Figures 7.5 and 7.7). CTA is comparable and sometimes superior to Doppler US in the evaluation of carotid disease; in evaluating the degree of stenosis using NASCET criteria, CT was accurate in 89 percent of cases compared to 83 percent for sonography, and CTA was more effective in detection of tandem lesions, plaque ulcerations, and vessel anomalies.

1. When evaluating carotid stenosis, for example, *CTA is very accurate in making the crucial distinction between complete occlusion and a residual hairline lumen*; an early study using single-slice helical CT showed accuracy rates between 80 and 95 percent compared to conventional angiography.
2. CTA can also detect vascular dissection, an important differential consideration in younger patients with stroke (Figure 7.5).

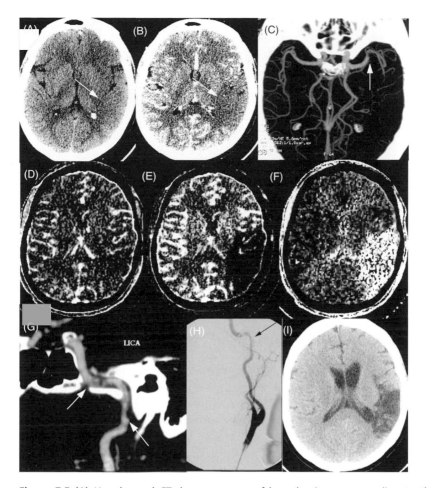

Figure 7.5 (A) Unenhanced CT shows an area of hypodensity corresponding to the inferior division of the left MCA territory (arrow), consistent with infarct. (B) CTA source images improve visualization of this infarct (arrow). Note also the more subtle manifestations of the infarct, including sulcal effacement and mild mass effect on the atrium of the left lateral ventricle. (C) Reformatted CTA image shows occlusion of an M2 branch of the left MCA (arrow). (D–F) CBV, CBF, and MTT maps obtained as through CTP show essentially matched CBV and CBF defects, consistent with an infarct without additional territory at risk. In this region, there is decreased CBV (dark), decreased CBF (dark), and prolonged MTT (bright). (G) Reformatted CTA image shows a carotid dissection (arrow) of the distal left ICA at the skull base, revealing the etiology of the patient's infarct. (F) This was confirmed with conventional angiography (arrow). (G) Unenhanced CT performed 3 months later shows evolution in the appearance of the infarct, with prominent hypodensity and volume loss. Note that the infarct has not changed in size from the initial CBV abnormality, consistent with the initial analysis that showed no additional territory at risk.

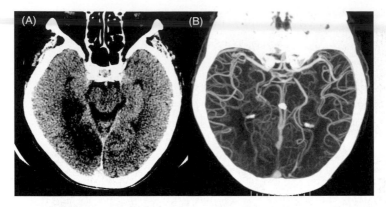

Figure 7.6 (A) Unenhanced CT shows an area of hypodensity in the right occipital and inferior right temporal lobe, consistent with infarct in the right PCA territory. The degree of hypodensity suggests that the infarct is hours-days old. (B) CTA confirms occlusion of the right P2 segment (arrow).

CTP

CTP expands the role of CT by providing insight capillary level hemodynamics and the brain parenchyma. *Perfusion-weighted CT is sensitive to capillary, tissue-level blood flow* and provides insight into the delivery of blood to brain parenchyma. This flow can be described using a variety of parameters, which primarily include cerebral blood flow (CBF), CBV, and mean transit time (MTT).

1. CBV is defined as the total volume of blood in a given unit volume of the brain. This includes blood in the tissues, as well as blood in the large capacitance vessels such as arteries, arterioles, capillaries, venules, and veins. CBV has units of milliliters of blood per 100 g of brain tissue (ml/100 g).
2. CBF is defined as the volume of blood moving through a given unit volume of brain per unit time. CBF has units of milliliters of blood per 100 g of brain tissue per minute (ml/100 g/min).
3. MTT is defined as the *average* of the transit time of blood through a given brain region. The transit time of blood through the brain parenchyma varies depending on the distance traveled between arterial inflow and venous outflow, Mathematically, MTT is related to both CBV and CBF according to the central volume principle, which states that MTT = CBV/CBF.

In simplest terms, CTP relies on direct visualization of the contrast material and images a slab of brain multiple times over a short interval as a bolus of contrast passes through the brain parenchyma. One can calculate the

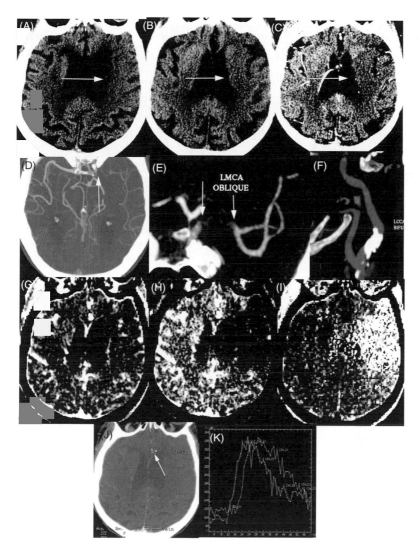

Figure 7.7 (A, B) Unenhanced CT shows hypodensity in the left MCA territory (arrows), consistent with a large MCA territory infarct. (C) CTA source images make the infarct appear more conspicuous (arrow). (D, E) Reformatted images from the CTA show occlusion of the proximal M1 segment (arrows) with evidence of distal collateral flow. (F) CTA of the neck shows severe atherosclerotic narrowing of the proximal left internal carotid artery, the presumed source of the embolus. Note that the axial source images (not shown) are crucial for accurately assessing the degree of narrowing, although evaluation can be obscured by dense atherosclerotic calcification and associated beam-hardening artifact. (G–I) CTP images (CBV, CBF, MTT) show a large area of perfusion abnormality without CBV/CBF mismatch, suggesting no territory at risk. (J) These perfusion images are obtained so that each slab includes a major artery (white arrow) and vein (black arrow) that are perpendicular to the image. (K) The CTP acquisition tracks the bolus of contrast through each voxel of tissue over time, yielding density curves.

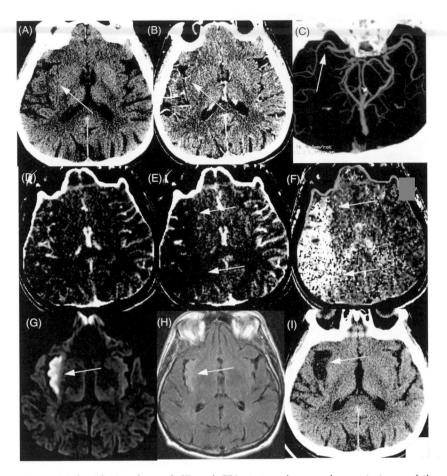

Figure 7.8 (A, B) Unenhanced CT and CTA sources images demonstrate a subtle insular ribbon sign (arrows) and obscuration of the lentiform nucleus, suggesting infarct. Compare with the contralateral normal side to identify subtle changes. (C) CTA shows occlusion of the right MCA. (D–F) CTP images (CBV, CBF, and MTT) show no abnormality on the CBV maps but a large abnormality on the CBF and MTT maps that suggests a large territory at risk. (G–H) DWZ and Flair images 1 day later showing a small impact. (I) Unenhanced CT performed 3 days later again shows no expansion of the infarct (arrow).

kinetics of the contrast bolus through each voxel of tissue and then calculate the above parameters, projecting the values as a map. This allows one to identify the *infarct core* (areas of reduced CBV) and the *ischemic penumbra* of tissue that is in danger of infarction but is not yet irreversibly damaged (areas of reduced CBF that do not correspond to abnormalities on CBV, or the CBF/CBV mismatch). The CTA source images (the axial source images used to reconstruct images of the vessels) are predominantly blood volume (CBV) weighted, so areas that appear hypodense on CTA-SI also correspond to infarct.

Technical considerations

The cine acquisition of CTP forms the final step in the acute stroke imaging evaluation. With dynamic, quantitative CTP, an additional contrast bolus is administered (at a rate of 4–7 ml/s) during continuous, cine imaging over a single brain region. Using the "standard" cine technique, imaging occurs for a total of 45–60 s, to track the "first pass" through the intracranial vasculature. With most scanners, 2 cm of coverage (two 10 mm or four 5-mm thick slices) per bolus is obtained, less than the whole brain coverage afforded by MR-PWI.

1. Certain methods can increase coverage, including performing two separate acquisitions at different levels or toggle table techniques.
2. Because it is important to include a major artery and vein in every acquisition slab and because of the relatively limited coverage of CTP, it is important to select slab locations based on the CTA (Figure 7.7).

Advanced "functional" imaging methods of stroke, like CTP, that accurately distinguish salvageable from nonsalvageable brain tissue are being increasingly promoted as a means to select patients for thrombolysis beyond the 3-hr window for IV therapy. An important goal of advanced stroke imaging is to provide an assessment of ischemic tissue viability that transcends an arbitrary "clock time." With the advent of advanced neuroimaging and modern stroke therapy, a more clinically relevant "operationally defined penumbra" has gained acceptance. *This "operationally defined penumbra" is the volume of tissue contained within the region of CBF/ CBV mismatch on CTP maps, where the region of CBV abnormality represents the "core" of infarcted tissue and the CBF/CBV mismatch represents the surrounding region of tissue that is hypoperfused but salvageable* (Figure 7.8). *CT-CBF/CBV mismatch correlates significantly with lesion enlargement.* Untreated or unsuccessfully treated patients with large CBF/CBV mismatch exhibit substantial lesion growth on follow-up, whereas those patients without significant mismatch – or those with early, complete recanalization – do not exhibit lesion progression. CTP-defined mismatch might, therefore, serve as a marker of salvageable tissue, and thus prove useful in patient triage for thrombolysis.

⇒ Several studies suggest that CBF maps may be more superior to MTT maps for distinguishing viable from nonviable penumbra. This relates to the fact that MTT maps display circulatory derangements that do not necessarily reflect ischemic change, including chronic large vessel occlusions with compensatory collateralization.

CTP interpretation: infarct detection with CTA-SI

As indicated above, theoretical modeling indicates that CTA source images are predominantly blood volume rather than blood flow weighted. *CTA-SI can be used to identify "infarct core" in the acute setting.* CTA-SI subtraction maps, obtained by coregistration and subtraction of the unenhanced head CT from the CTA source images, are appealing for clinical use because they provide whole brain coverage. While both unenhanced CT and CTA-SI can play a role in infarct detection, it is important to remember that they are evaluating different properties of the infarcted tissue: edema and reduced CBV, respectively.

Imaging predictors of clinical outcome

Multiple studies, examining heterogeneous cohorts of patients receiving varied treatments, consistently find that ultimate clinical outcome is strongly correlated with admission "core" lesion volume.

1. In a study of CTP in patients with MCA stem occlusions, patients with admission whole brain CTP lesions volumes >100 ml (equal to approximately one-third the volume of the MCA territory) had poor clinical outcomes, regardless of recanalization status.
2. The degree of early CBF reduction in acute stroke may also help predict hemorrhagic risk. Preliminary results from our group suggest that severe hypoattenuation, relative to normal tissue on whole brain CTP images may also identify ischemic regions more likely to bleed following intraarterial thrombolysis.

Cerebral venous infarcts and CTV

The imaging manifestations of venous thrombosis include regions of edema that do not respect normal arterial distributions (in almost all patients) and intraparenchymal hematoma in 30–40 percent.

Unenhanced CT

Although a number of direct and indirect signs of cerebral venous thrombosis and infarct have been described, it is not uncommon to detect no abnormalities on unenhanced CT (10–26 percent).

1. The direct signs of venous thrombosis are analogous to the hyperdense MCA sign described above, in which hyperdense thrombus is seen within the MCA. In the case of venous thrombosis, this hyperdense clot is seen in a cortical vein (dense cord sign), the transverse sinus (dense lateral sinus sign), the jugular vein (dense jugular sign), or the

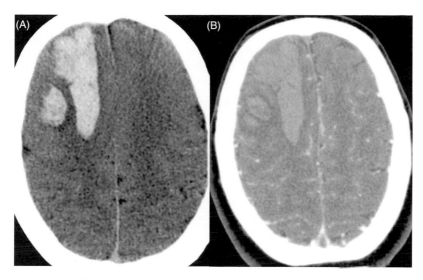

Figure 7 9 (A) Unenhanced CT demonstrates a large right frontal lobe venous hemorrhage with leftward midline shift. (B) Contrast enhanced CT scan shows the "empty delta sign" (arrow) representing superior sagittal sinus thrombosis.

posterior aspect of the superior sagittal sinus (dense triangle sign). These signs should be used with caution, since an elevated hematocrit or hemoconcentration could simulate a hyperdense vessel.

2. Indirect signs are more common and include parenchymal hemorrhage (particularly superficial hemorrhage) or parenchymal edema. Bilateral thalamic infarcts should suggest the possibility of deep venous thrombosis.

Enhanced CT

The classic sign of venous infarct on contrast enhanced CT is the "empty delta" sign, which represents clot in the posterior aspect of the superior sagittal sinus outlined by contrast in surrounding collateral veins (Figure 7.9). Cavernous sinus thrombosis is difficult to diagnose but may be present if there is mon-opacification and expansion of the cavernous sinus.

CTV

This has a high sensitivity compared to conventional angiography and is superior to MRV in identification of cerebral veins and dural sinuses because it directly visualizes the vessels and is not prone to artifacts caused by flow dependence. Potential pitfalls in the interpretation of CTV are the presence of arachnoid granulations, normal structures that can appear as small filling defects, most commonly adjacent to venous entrance sites. Other variants to consider are intrasinus septa and hypoplasia or aplasia of the dural sinuses.

Conclusions

CT offers a growing array of tools in the evaluation of acute stroke. Although the traditional role of CT has been to exclude hemorrhage through an unenhanced CT scan, CT now offers the ability to improve stroke detection, directly visualize vessel occlusion, and evaluate the capillary hemodynamics to identify parenchyma at risk. The wide availability, relatively low cost, and rapid acquisition afforded by CT is particularly appealing. Continued research will continue to expand the potential role of CT and also increase our understanding of its ideal place in the evaluation of acute stroke.

Bibliography

Astrup J, Siesjo BK, Symon L. Thresholds in cerebral ischemia – the ischemic penumbra. *Stroke* 1981;12:723–5.

Barber PA, Demchuk AM, Zhang J, Buchan AM. Validity and reliability of a quantitative computed tomography score in predicting outcome of hyperacute stroke before thrombolytic therapy. ASPECTS Study Group. Alberta Stroke Programme Early CT Score. *Lancet* 2000;355:1670–4.

Gonzalez R, Schaefer P, Buonanno F, et al. Diffusion-weighted MR imaging: Diagnostic accuracy in patients imaged within 6 hours of stroke symptom onset. *Radiology* 1999;210:155–62.

Hacke W, Albers G, Al–Rawi Y, et al. The Desmoteplase in Acute Ischemic Stroke Trial (DIAS): A phase II MRI-based 9-hour window acute stroke thrombolysis trial with intravenous desmoteplase. *Stroke* 2005;36:66–73.

Hamberg LM, Hunter GJ, Kierstead D, et al. Measurement of cerebral blood volume with subtraction three-dimensional functional CT. *AJNR Am J Neuroradiol* 1996;17:1861–9.

Hill MD, Rowley HA, Adler F, et al. Selection of acute ischemic stroke patients for intra–arterial thrombolysis with pro-urokinase by using ASPECTS. *Stroke* 2003;34:1925–31.

Hunter GJ, Hamberg LM, Ponzo JA, et al. Assessment of cerebral perfusion and arterial anatomy in hyperacute stroke with three-dimensional functional CT: Early clinical results. *AJNR Am J Neuroradiol* 1998;19:29–37.

Jovin TG, Yonas H, Gebel JM, et al. The cortical ischemic core and not the consistently present penumbra is a determinant of clinical outcome in acute middle cerebral artery occlusion. *Stroke* 2003;34:2426–33.

Kidwell CS, Saver JL, Mattiello J, et al. Thrombolytic reversal of acute human cerebral ischemic injury shown by diffusion/perfusion magnetic resonance imaging. *Ann Neurol* 2000;47:462–9.

Kucinski T, Vaterlein O, Glauche V, et al. Correlation of apparent diffusion coefficient and computed tomography density in acute ischemic stroke. *Stroke* 2002;33:1786–91.

Lev M, Farkas J, Gemmete J, et al. Acute stroke: Improved nonenhanced CT detection – benefits of soft-copy interpretation by using variable window width and center level settings. *Radiology* 1999;213:150–5.

Lev MH, Farkas J, Rodriguez VR, et al. CT angiography in the rapid triage of patients with hyperacute stroke to intraarterial thrombolysis: Accuracy in the detection of large vessel thrombus. *J Comput Assist Tomogr* 2001;25:520–8.

Lev MH, Gonzalez RG. CT angiography and CT perfusion imaging. In AW Toga, JC Mazziotta (eds), *Brain mapping: The methods*. San Diego: Academic Press, 2002:427–84.

Lev MH, Romero JM, Goodman DN, et al. Total occlusion versus hairline residual lumen of the internal carotid arteries: Accuracy of single section helical CT angiography. *AJNR Am J Neuroradiol* 2003;24:1123–9.

Lev MH, Segal AZ, Farkas J, et al. Utility of perfusion-weighted CT imaging in acute middle cerebral artery stroke treated with intra-arterial thrombolysis: Prediction of final infarct volume and clinical outcome. *Stroke* 2001;32:2021–8.

Nabavi DG, Cenic A, Craen RA, et al. CT assessment of cerebral perfusion: Experimental validation and initial clinical experience. *Radiology* 1999;213:141–9.

Ostergaard L, Chesler DA, Weisskoff RM, Sorensen AG, Rosen BR. Modeling cerebral blood flow and flow heterogeneity from magnetic resonance residue data. *J Cereb Blood Flow Metab* 1999;19:690–9.

Patel SC, Levine SR, Tilley BC, et al. Lack of clinical significance of early ischemic changes on computed tomography in acute stroke. *JAMA* 2001;286:2830–8.

Rohl L, Ostergaard L, Simonsen CZ, et al. Viability thresholds of ischemic penumbra of hyperacute stroke defined by perfusion-weighted MRI and apparent diffusion coefficient. *Stroke* 2001;32:1140–6.

Sanelli PC, Lev MH, Eastwood JD, Gonzalez RG, Lee TY. The effect of varying user–selected input parameters on quantitative values in CT perfusion maps. *Acad Radiol* 2004;11:1085–92.

Schaefer PW, Roccatagliata L, Ledezma C, et al. First-pass quantitative CT perfusion identifies thresholds for salvageable penumbra in acute stroke patients treated with intra–arterial therapy. *AJNR Am J Neuroradiol* 2006 Jan;27(1):20–5.

Schlaug G, Benfield A, Baird AE, et al. The ischemic penumbra: Operationally defined by diffusion and perfusion MRI. *Neurology* 1999;53:1528–37.

Schramm P, Schellinger PD, Fiebach JB, et al. Comparison of CT and CT angiography source images with diffusion-weighted imaging in patients with acute stroke within 6 hours after onset. *Stroke* 2002;33:2426–32.

Schramm P, Schellinger PD, Klotz E, et al. Comparison of perfusion computed tomography and computed tomography angiography source images with perfusion-weighted imaging and diffusion-weighted imaging in patients with acute stroke of less than 6 hours' duration. *Stroke* 2004;35(7): 1652–8.

Schwamm LH, Rosenthal ES, Swap CJ, et al. Hypoattenuation on CT angiographic source images predicts risk of intracerebral hemorrhage and outcome after intra-arterial reperfusion therapy. *AJNR Am J Neuroradiol* 2005 Aug;26(7):1798–803.

Sorensen AG, Buonanno FS, Gonzalez RG, et al. Hyperacute stroke: Evaluation with combined multisection diffusion-weighted and hemodynamically weighted echo-planar MR imaging. *Radiology* 1996;199:391–401.

von Kummer R, Allen KL, Holle R, et al. Acute stroke: Usefulness of early CT findings before thrombolytic therapy. *Radiology* 1997;205:327–33.

von Kummer R, Bourquain H, Bastianello S, et al. Early prediction of irreversible
    brain damage after ischemic stroke at CT. *Radiology* 2001;219:95–100.
Wintermark M, Reichhart M, Cuisenaire O, et al. Comparison of admission
    perfusion computed tomography and qualitative diffusion- and perfusion-
    weighted magnetic resonance imaging in acute stroke patients. *Stroke*
    2002;33:2025–31.
Wintermark M, Reichhart M, Thiran JP, et al. Prognostic accuracy of cerebral blood
    flow measurement by perfusion computed tomography, at the time of emergency
    room admission, in acute stroke patients. *Ann Neurol* 2002;51:417–32.
Wu O, Koroshetz WJ, Ostergaard L, et al. Predicting tissue outcome in acute human
    cerebral ischemia using combined diffusion- and perfusion-weighted MR imaging.
    Stroke 2001;32:933–42.

8 Magnetic resonance imaging in acute stroke

Magdy H. Selim

The use of magnetic resonance imaging (MRI) in the diagnosis and management of acute stroke is rapidly growing. This chapter will highlight the potential applications and limitations of MRI in this setting.

The major limitations of MRI, compared to computed tomography (CT), are

1. decreased availability,
2. higher cost,
3. longer scanning time,
4. contraindications, which limit its utility in some patients such as
   a) clinically unstable patients who require close monitoring and observation;
   b) patients with claustrophobia, pacemakers, metallic implants, or MRI-incompatible prosthetic heart valves; and
   c) morbidly obese patients.

It is necessary to evaluate patients with acute stroke who are considered for MRI for these contraindications.

The advantages of MRI are

1. better image resolution;
2. better anatomical visualization of the brainstem and cerebellum;
3. better visualization of vascular malformations and brain tumors, largely excluding lesions that may mimic stroke;
4. lack of exposure to ionizing radiation;
5. rapid detection of brain ischemia, within minutes of onset, when using diffusion-weighted imaging (DWI);
6. ability to detect petechial hemorrhages and microbleeds, which may impact decision making regarding the use of thrombolytics; and
7. multimodal MRI combining DWI and perfusion-weighted imaging (PWI) can provide rapid, noninvasive information about cerebral hemodynamics and stroke lesion volume.

Pathophysiological principles of MRI

Hydrogen nuclei (protons), which are present in different concentrations in various tissues, become excited when exposed to a magnetic field. They absorb the radio frequency energy of the magnetic field, and then relax by completely releasing it. The energy released over a short period of time (T1 and T2 relaxation time constants) is converted into images. The differences in intensities of the released energy translate into different contrast in the images between various parts of the brain.

The failure of Na^+-K^+ ATP neuronal channels following ischemic injury results in intracellular accumulation of water (i.e., cytotoxic edema) within minutes. Few hours later, plasma proteins and intravacular water leak out of endothelial cells, as the blood-brain barrier (BBB) becomes compromised, into the extracellular space resulting in vasogenic edema and hemorrhagic transformation of the infracted area. The findings seen on MRI reflect these pathophysiological changes.

Technical considerations

The current MRI protocols for stroke imaging include

1. T1-weighted imaging in which the cerebrospinal fluid (CSF) has a lower signal intensity (i.e., darker) than brain tissue.
2. T2-weighted imaging in which CSF has a higher (i.e., brighter) signal intensity than brain tissue.
3. Fluid-attenuated inversion-recovery (FLAIR) imaging in which CSF has the same density of brain tissue.
4. Gradient echo susceptibility-weighted (T2* or GRE) imaging in which blood degradation products such as deoxyhemoglobin produce a susceptibility (dark) effect that can be easily visualized.
5. DWI, which is highly sensitive to diffusion of water molecules and can detect intracellular accumulation of water, which occurs in ischemia, within minutes. This diffusion slowing, that is, cytotoxic edema, results in hyperintense (i.e., bright) signal.
6. PWI, which involves rapid acquisition of T2* images after a bolus injection of gadolinium. This results in T2* shortening (darkening) of the perfused tissue and variable degrees of relative brightening in the hypoperfused tissue.

Clinical applications of MRI in stroke patients

Conventional T1, T2, and FLAIR images

MRI provides an advantage over CT for the detection of cerebral infarction compared with CT, since CT can be negative in a substantial proportion of patients during the early stages of evaluation.

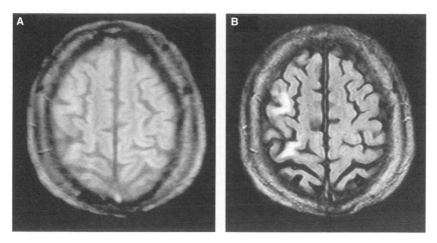

Figure 8.1 (A) T2 image of the high convexity of the brain. (B) FLAIR image at the same level demonstrates unequivocal abnormalities of the cortical surface of the right convexity in two separate gyral regions.

⤳ With conventional sequences, early infarction is best detected on MRI T2 and FLAIR sequences.

However, FLAIR is superior to standard T2 imaging since cortical infarcts, in particular, can be hard to detect on T2 given the similarly high signal of cortical gray matter and adjacent CSF. FLAIR, on the other hand, produces both a strongly T2-weighted image and suppressed CSF signal (Figure 8.1A, B).

⤳ Early signs of vascular occlusions can also be seen on FLAIR images.

Increased intensity (*hyperintense vessel sign*, HVS) can sometimes be seen in cerebral blood vessels of patients with acute ischemic stroke. The FLAIR HVS is often used to describe an increase in intravascular signal intensity of a major brain vessel, and is thought to result from slow flow or stasis, that is, flow-related enhancement, and clot signal intensity, that is, oxyhemoglobin. This sign can be used to assess the status of major cerebral vessels during the hyperacute phase of stroke, if magnetic resonance angiography (MRA) is not available.

1. The sensitivity of FLAIR HVS varies between 40 and 100 percent, within 3 hr of stroke symptom onset.
2. False-positive findings can be seen in the absence of vessel occlusion, likely secondary to slow flow.
3. The diagnostic accuracy of FLAIR HVS is substantially higher than that of hyperdense MCA sign on CT scan.
4. FLAIR images can be used to assess the integrity of BBB after stroke.

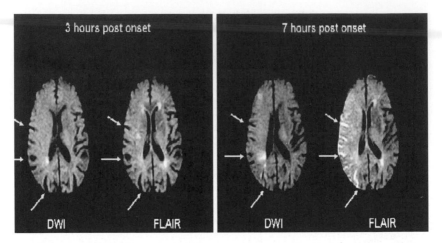

Figure 8.2 An example of HARM. Initial MRI obtained 3 hr after onset of symptoms shows an early evolving lesion adjacent to the posterior horn of the right lateral ventricle on DWI. Precontract FLAIR at 3 hr shows negligible CSF signal. Arrows point to comparable sulci in all images. On the scan at 7 hr after onset (4 hr after gadolinium injection), enhancement is observed in the CSF spaces throughout the right MCA territory, in the sulci and on cortical surface (Warach S, 2004).

FLAIR images, obtained after gadolinium administration, can be used to characterize BBB disruption in acute stroke patients. Disruption of BBB resulting from ischemia and reperfusion is often evident as delayed gadolinium enhancement of the CSF on FLAIR, and is referred to as hyperintense acute reperfusion marker (HARM) (Figure 8.2).

1. In one study, HARM was associated with increased risk for hemorrhagic transformation and worse clinical outcome.
2. Axial, fat-saturation, T1 images are important in patients with suspected arterial dissection.

The so-called crescent moon sign is often seen on these cross-section images in patients with extracranial arterial dissection, where the lumen of the artery appears as a narrow dark flow void surrounded by the high intensity (bright) intraluminal hematoma (Figure 8.3).

➠ T1 and T2 images may provide clues to the diagnosis of venous sinus thrombosis

The thrombosed vein may appear as a hyperintense (bright) signal on standard T1 and T2 images during the subacute phase (days to weeks) due to the presence of methemoglobin within the thrombus. In acute and early subacute stages, a hypointense signal may be seen on T2 images due to the paramagnetic effects of oxyhemoglobin.

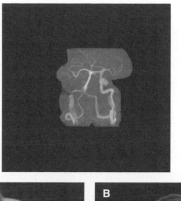

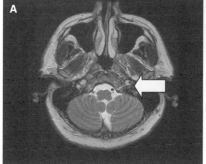
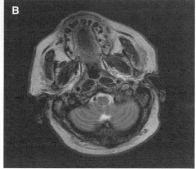

Figure 8.3 (A) Carotid dissection (B,C) Crescent moon sign (arrow) in a patient with carotid dissection.

1. These changes are often subtle and can be easily missed.
2. Gadolinium administration and coronal sections can increase the sensitivity.
3. T1 and T2 images can also be used to diagnose cerebral hemorrhage (Figure 8.4).
4. The MRI picture of hemorrhage depends on the sequence, age of the hemorrhage, and paramagnetic effects of blood degradation products (Figure 8.6).
   a) At the hyperacute phase, oxyhemoglobin may be difficult to distinguish from infarction on T1 images, as the lesion has the same signal as normal tissue (i.e., isointense) with a halo of lower signal (hypointense) because of clot retraction. On T2, the lesion appears hyperintense.
   b) At the acute phase, deoxyhemoglobin may have isointense or hypointense signal on T1, and hypointense signal on T2 images.
   c) During the early subacute phase, methemoglobin appears hyperintense on T1 and hyperintense on T2 images. During the late subacute phase, the lesion appears hyperintense on both T1 and T2 images.

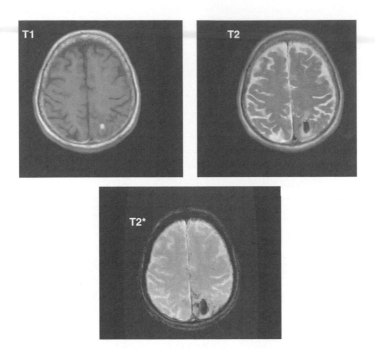

Figure 8.4 T1 and T2 images showing a subacute hemorrhage, approximately 7 days old.

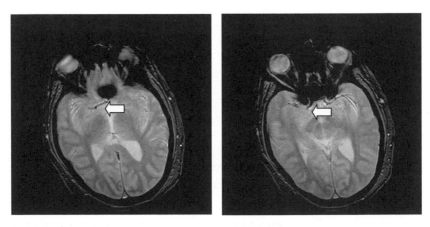

Figure 8.5 Susceptibility (hypodense) MCA sign (arrow).

d) At the chronic phase, the lesion appears isointense on T1 and isointense-to-hyperintense on T2.

Gradient echo susceptibility-weighted (T2*) imaging

⟫ Vessel signs, indicative of thrombosis, can also be seen on GRE/T2* susceptibility images.

The susceptibility vessel sign (SVS) is seen as an area of intravascular signal intensity loss, that is, darkening. The susceptibility or hypodense MCA sign is analogous to the hyperdense MCA sign on CT, where thrombotic occlusion of the MCA/ICA appears as a dark signal within the arterial lumen and the diameter of the signal in the affected vessel appears larger than that of the contralateral side (Figure 8.5). The signal loss (susceptibility effect) is thought to result from deoxyhemoglobin in older clots. Similar susceptibility signs may be seen within the venous sinuses and could provide clues to an underlying venous sinus thrombosis (Figure 8.6).

1. The SVS may be of limited value during the hyperacute phase of stroke.
2. Its diagnostic accuracy improves as time from stroke onset increases due to increased deoxyhemoglobin content with aging of the blood clot.
3. The sensitivity of SVS is lower than the FLAIR HVS, but higher than the hyperdense artery sign on CT scan.
4. T2*/GRE susceptibility-weighted images can reliably diagnose ICH.

Several studies have shown that susceptibility-weighted MRI can reliably show hyperacute hemorrhages soon after their occurrence, petechial microhemorrhages, and old hemorrhages that are not visible on CT scan. Thus, obviating the need to perform CT on every stroke patient. The ability of MRI, but not CT, to detect cerebral microbleeds (Figure 8.7) may have therapeutic implications for the safety on antithrombotic therapy and thrombolysis. Earlier small studies suggested increased risk of hemorrhagic transformation after thrombolysis in patients with ischemic stroke whose MRI showed evidence of "microbleeds." Recent reports, on the other hand, suggests that the presence of microbleeds on GRE images does not increase the risk of thrombolysis-induced hemorrhagic transformation.

1. Like CT, small, isolated SAH can be missed on T2*/GRE MRI.
2. Combining susceptibility-weighted with FLAIR images significantly increases the sensitivity of MRI for detection of SAH.

Diffusion-perfusion MRI and the ischemic penumbra

MR techniques that combine DWI and PWI can identify and separate brain tissue that is irreversibly injured (ischemic core), severely hypoperfused and

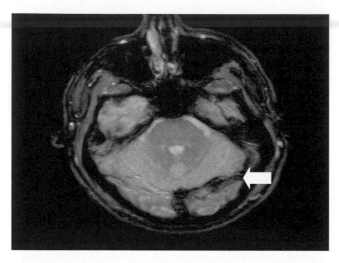

Figure 8.6 Susceptibility abnormality in a patient with sinus thrombosis (arrow).

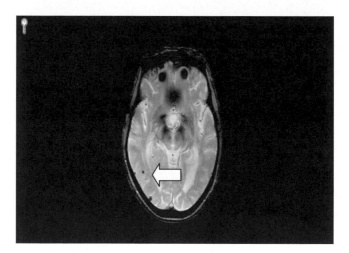

Figure 8.7 T2* MRI showing multiple microbleeds.

at risk of infarction (the penumbra), mildly hypoperfused but not at risk (oligemia) and unaffected (normal).

1. DWI and PWI techniques assess different, but complimentary, aspects of cerebral ischemia.
2. DWI is ideal to detect and qualitatively identify ischemic brain tissue during the hyperacute phase of stroke.
3. PWI can be used to assess regional blood supply and to qualitatively delineate regions of deceased perfusion that may or may not proceed to infarction.

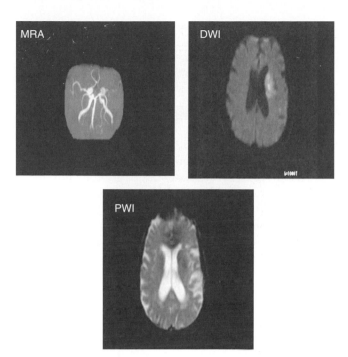

Figure 8.8 MRA, DWI, PWI.

Combining the results of DWI and PWI can provide an estimate of the ischemic penumbra within a few minutes after the onset of cerebral ischemia, where the initial region of DWI abnormality is believed to represent the ischemic core within a larger region of reduced perfusion as defined by PWI.

1. A mismatch in lesion size between DWI and PWI, with a core of restricted diffusion, low ADC and absent perfusion that is surrounded by a zone of variable perfusion deficit, is often seen during the acute phase of cerebral ischemia (Figure 8.8).
2. This PWI-DWI lesion mismatch serves as an approximate MRI marker for the ischemic penumbra and is believed to represent ischemic tissue that is at risk of infarction if reperfusion is not restored in a timely fashion.
3. The ability to determine the existence and extent of potentially salvageable penumbral tissue has important therapeutic implications.
4. There is growing evidence that stroke patients with perfusion greater than diffusion mismatch can benefit from thrombolysis even after 3 hr from stroke onset.

Diffusion-weighted MRI

DWI is by far the most sensitive way to detect ischemic stroke during the hyperacute phase, which is seen as a bright "light bulb" signal within minutes of onset (Figure 8.8a).

1. Although DWI is very sensitive for ischemic changes, it is not highly specific.
   a) DWI abnormalities can be seen in other conditions such as brain tumors, active demyelination, ongoing seizures, infectious or inflammatory lesions, or as artifacts at sites of air-bone interface.
   b) DWI changes due to ischemic stroke follow a vascular territory, which helps to differentiate it from the above conditions.
   c) DWI changes can sometimes be seen in the setting of chronic ischemic lesions. This is often attributed to "T2 shine through" effect, where the old lesion appears bright on both T2 and DWI images.
   d) Although DWI is highly sensitive for stroke diagnosis, there are rare instances where DWI may miss an infarct during the acute phase. This is mostly seen with small brainstem lacunar infarcts.
   e) Some studies suggest that a DWI lesion greater than one-third of MCA territory is associated with increased risk for hemorrhagic transformation after thrombolysis.

DWI provides a qualitative assessment of the movement of water molecules. A quantitative value, called the apparent diffusion coefficient (ADC), can be calculated from DWI images.

1. Brain regions with low ADC values (as seen in ischemia) appear dark on calculated ADC maps.
2. The acute drop in ADC after ischemic insult gradually normalizes to baseline (pseudonormalization) within days. Therefore, it can be used to differentiate between acute/subacute and chronic infarcts (T2 shine through).
3. Volumetric ADC (voxel by voxel) analysis can be used to assess ICH risk after thrombolysis. Several studies have shown that the number of voxels on DWI with ADC $\leq 550 \times 10^{-6}$ mm^2/s is an independent predictor of ICH. However, this analysis is often difficult to perform during the hyperacute phase of stroke evaluation.
4. Diffusion of water molecules is usually imaged in more than one direction to avoid diffusion anisotropy, which may give a false impression of a lesion on DWI and ADC maps.
5. The diffusion motion of all water molecules can be calculated when diffusion/ADC are measured in six or more directions to generate diffusion tensor mapping, which can also be used to examine white matter tracts.

Perfusion-weighted MRI

There are several techniques to perform PWI. Bolus-contrast tracking is the most commonly used technique in the setting of acute stroke. PWI quantifies the amount of contrast that reaches the brain tissue after a fast intravenous bolus injection. Signal intensity (concentration) versus time curves from PWI during bolus transit can be used to calculate physiological parameters of regional blood volume (rCBV), blood flow (rCBF), and mean transit time (rMTT). Comparative evaluation of pre- and postcontrast images for the presence of a mismatch, that is, a perfusion deficit larger than the baseline abnormality, can provide information of the potentially salvageable brain tissue at risk for developing infarction if ischemia is not reversed. Such information may be useful to guide therapeutic interventions, especially in patients presenting after 3 hr from stroke onset.

The use of arterial spin labeling (ALS) to examine brain perfusion after stroke is rising. This methodology uses magnetically labeled arterial blood water as an endogenous tracer to provide CBF measurements.

⇒ ALS-based perfusion may be more sensitive than bolus contract tracking since it can be sampled using a variety of imaging sequences that preserve the signal in regions of high static susceptibility, such as the orbitofrontal cortex.

MRA

MRA can be performed with time-of-flight (TOF) or phase-contrast (PC) techniques. Both are based on the difference in signal between moving blood and surrounding tissue; blood has greater proton density than stationary tissues. Both TOF and PC MRA utilize artifactual signal changes caused by flowing blood to depict the vessel lumen, and do not require contrast administration.

1. TOF is the most widely used technique because of its shorter acquisition time, thinner slices, and larger covering volume.
   a) The three-dimensional (3D) TOF technique is preferred because it provides higher resolution and signal-to-noise ratio than the two-dimensional (2D) technique
   b) TOF MRA, particularly, 2D MRA has poor in-plane flow sensitivity, where saturation of blood flow when the images are parallel to a particular vessel can result in loss of signal intensity and false diagnosis of vascular occlusion.
   c) Similarly, saturation of the scan in low-flow regions can lead to overestimation of the degree of vascular stenosis on 3D images.
   d) 2D TOF MRA provides better images than 3D MRA in slow flow regions.

e) 3D TOF MRA is less sensitive than 2D MRA to turbulent flow artifacts.

f) TOF MRA is flow dependent. Therefore, absence of flow signal does not necessarily mean complete occlusion but rather that flow is below a critical value.

2. PC angiography images blood flow velocity, where the MR signal contains both amplitude and phase information, and is directly proportional to flow velocity.

a) The main advantage of PC MRA is complete suppression of stationary tissue. It is four times slower than TOF MRA, however.

b) 2D PC MRA is particularly helpful in differentiating slow and absent flow from normal flow, that is, it depicts only truly patent vessels.

c) Like 3D TOF MRA, PC MRA has the disadvantage of flow signal dropout due to turbulent flow in tortuous vessels.

3. Contrast-enhanced MRA exploits the gadolinium-induced T1 shortening effects and reduces most of the artifacts of TOF and PC MRA.

4. Magnetic resonance venography (MRV) is recommended when venous sinus thrombosis is suspected. However, it is important to keep in mind that MRV has its limitations and can lead to false-positive, and -negative results.

a) The use of 3D PC or contrast-enhanced MRV can be useful to differentiate slow flow in hypoplastic sinuses from true thrombotic occlusions.

Special considerations

MRI is generally recommended as the imaging modality of choice in the following circumstances:

1. In patients with suspected cerebral vasculitis because it is more sensitive than CT in identifying small ischemic lesions that are more common in vasculitis. Also, MRA can provide screening information on the caliber of large vessels. Conventional angiography is better than MRA in detecting appropriate pathology in medium-sized vessels.

2. In patients with stroke and suspected venous sinus thrombosis as the cause.

3. When arterial dissection is suspected. However, MRI/MRA may not demonstrate a typical abnormality in up to 20 percent of patients with cervical arterial dissection, especially of the vertebral artery. Conventional angiography may be recommended if the MRI/MRA is inconclusive or if there is a strong suspicion for dissection.

4. In patients with suspected spinal cord infarct. MRI may show signal changes and some swelling in the cord, similar to the changes seen in transverse myelitis, a few hours after stroke onset. It may also show

prominent cord vessels suggestive of spinal cord AVM or dural arteriovenous fistula. CT myelography can be reserved to uncertain cases to advance the diagnosis of AVM. Selective angiography of the cord is tedious and in general not recommended in patients with suspected acute spinal cord infarct as it may exacerbate ischemia by occluding a small vessel with catheter manipulations.

Bibliography

Assouline E, Benziane K, Reizine D et al. Intra-arterial thrombus visualized on T2* gradient echo imaging in acute ischemic stroke. *Cerebrovasc Dis* 2005;20(1):6–11.

Brant-Zawadzki M, Atkinson D, Detrick M, Bradley WG, Scidmore G. Fluid-attenuated inversion recovery (FLAIR) for assessment of cerebral infarction. Initial clinical experience in 50 patients. *Stroke* 1996;27(7):1187–91.

Kidwell CS, Chalela JA, Saver JL et al. Comparison of MRI and CT for detection of acute intracerebral hemorrhage. *JAMA* 2004;292(15):182–30.

Noguchi K, Ogawa T, Seto H, et al. Subacute and chronic subarachnoid hemorrhage: Diagnosis with fluid-attenuated inversion-recovery MR imaging. *Radiology* 1997;203(1):257–62.

Schaefer PW, Hunter GJ, He J, et al. Predicting cerebral ischemic infarct volume with diffusion and perfusion MR imaging. *AJNR Am J Neuroradiol* 2002;23 (10):1785–94.

Schellinger PD, Chalela JA, Kang DW, Latour LL, Warach S. Diagnostic and prognostic value of early MR Imaging vessel signs in hyperacute stroke patients imaged <3 hours and treated with recombinant tissue plasminogen activator. *AJNR Am J Neuroradiol* 2005;26(3):618–24.

Schlaug G, Benfield A, Baird AE, et al. The ischemic penumbra: Operationally defined by diffusion and perfusion MRI. *Neurology* 1999;53(7):1528–37.

Selim M, Fink JN, Kumar S, et al. Predictors of hemorrhagic transformation after intravenous recombinant tissue plasminogen activator: Prognostic value of the initial apparent diffusion coefficient and diffusion-weighted lesion volume. *Stroke* 2002;33(8):2047–52.

Selim M, Fink J, Linfante I, Kumar S, Schlaug G, Caplan LR. Diagnosis of cerebral venous thrombosis with echo-planar T2*-weighted magnetic resonance imaging. *Arch Neurol* 2002;59(6):1021–6.

Toyoda K, Ida M, Fukuda K. Fluid-attenuated inversion recovery intraarterial signal: An early sign of hyperacute cerebral ischemia. *AJNR Am J Neuroradiol* 2001;22 (6):1021–9.

Warach S, Latour LL. Evidence of reperfusion injury, exacerbated by thrombolytic therapy, in human focal brain ischemia using a novel imaging marker of early blood-brain barrier disruption.*Stroke* 2004;35(11 Suppl 1):2659–61.

9 Neurosonology in acute stroke

Vijay Sharma, Annabelle Lao,
and Andrei V. Alexandrov

Most patients who suffer from an acute ischemic stroke have arterial thrombi that occlude extra- or intracranial vessels. Fast dissolution of these thrombi often leads to dramatic clinical recovery. This chapter discusses how to diagnose arterial occlusion, monitor recanalization, and potential transcranial Doppler (TCD) applications in the treatment of ischemic stroke.

Fast-track insonation protocol

A fast-track insonation protocol was developed for rapid TCD performance and interpretation in emergency situations.

1. Using such a protocol, urgent TCD studies could be completed and interpreted within minutes at the bedside by the treating clinician, nurse, or technologist.
2. This protocol should be used only by experienced TCD users with knowledge of the clinical status of the patient. The protocol is shown in Table 9.1.
3. The choice of fast-track insonation steps is determined by clinical localization of an ischemic arterial territory.
4. This fast-track TCD examination at bedside results in no time delays to treatment if ultrasound tests are performed simultaneously with other activities such as neurological examination, drawing blood, and vital signs monitoring.

The yield and accuracy of noninvasive vascular ultrasound evaluation (NVUE) in acute cerebral ischemia for lesions amenable to interventional treatment (LAIT), is high both in patients eligible as well as ineligible for thrombolysis (Figure 9.1).

1. The sensitivity, specificity, positive, and negative predictive values for TCD were observed as 96, 75, 96, and 75 percent, respectively.
2. The corresponding values for carotid/vertebral duplex were 94, 90, 94, and 90 percent, respectively.

Table 9.1: Fast-track neurovascular ultrasound examination

Use portable devices with bright display overcoming room light. Stand behind patient headrest. Start with TCD because acute occlusion responsible for the neurological deficit is likely intracranially. Extracranial carotid/vertebral duplex may reveal an additional lesion often responsible for intracranial flow disturbance. Fast-track insonation steps follow clinical localization of patient symptoms.

A. Clinical diagnosis of cerebral ischemia in the anterior circulation

STEP 1: Transcranial Doppler

1. If time permits, begin insonation on the nonaffected side to establish the temporal window, normal MCA waveform (M1 depth 45–65 mm, M2 30–45 mm), and velocity for comparison to the affected side.
2. If short on time, start on the affected side: first assess MCA at 50 mm. If no signals detected, increase the depth to 62 mm. If an antegrade flow signal is found, reduce the depth to trace the MCA stem or identify the worst residual flow signal. Search for possible flow diversion to the ACA, PCA, or M2 MCA. Evaluate and compare waveform shapes and systolic flow acceleration.
3. Continue on the affected side (transorbital window). Check flow direction and pulsatility in the OA at depths 40–50 mm followed by ICA siphon at depths 55–65 mm.
4. If the permits or in patients with pure motor or sensory deficits, evaluate BA (depth 80 – 100 + mm) and terminal VA(40 – 80 mm).

STEP 2: Carotid/vertebral duplex

1. Start on the affected side in transverse B-mode planes followed by color or power-mode sweep from proximal to distal carotid segments. Identify CCA and its bifurcation on B-mode and flow-carrying lumens.
2. Document if ICA (or CCA) has a lesion on B-mode and corresponding disturbances on flow images. In patients with concomitant chest pain, evaluate CCA as close to the origin as possible.
3. Perform angle-corrected spectral velocity measurements in the mid-to-distal CCA, ICA, and external carotid artery.
4. If time permits or in patients with pure motor or sensory deficits, examine cervical portion of the vertebral arteries (longitudinal B-mode, color or power mode, spectral Doppler) on the affected side.
5. If time permits, perform transverse and longitudinal scanning of the arteries on the nonaffected side.

B. Clinical diagnosis of cerebral ischemia in the posterior circulation

STEP 1: Transcranial Doppler

1. Start suboccipital insonation at 75 mm (VA junction) and identify BA flow at 80–100 + mm.
2. If abnormal signals present at 75–100 mm, find the terminal VA (40–80 mm) on the nonaffected side for comparison and evaluate the terminal VA on the affected side at similar depths.

(continued)

Table 9.1: *(continued)*

3. Continue with transtemporal examination to identify PCA (55–75 mm) and possible collateral flow through the posterior communicating artery obstruction.

   STEP 2: Vertebral/carotid duplex ultrasound

1. Start on the affected side by locating CCA using longitudinal B-Mode plane, and turn transducer downward to visualize shadows from transverse processes of midcervical vertebrae.

2. Apply color or power modes and spectral Doppler to identify flow in intratransverse VA segments.

3. Follow VA course to its origin and obtain Doppler spectra. Perform similar examination on another side.

4. If time permits, perform bilateral duplex examination of the CCA, ICA, and external carotid artery as described above.

Notes: ACA indicates anterior cerebral artery; CCA, common carotid artery; ECA, external carotid artery; OA, ophthalmic artery; PCA, posterior cerebral artery; BA basilar artery; and VA, verterbral artery.
Source: Reprinted with permission from Chernyshev et al. (2005).

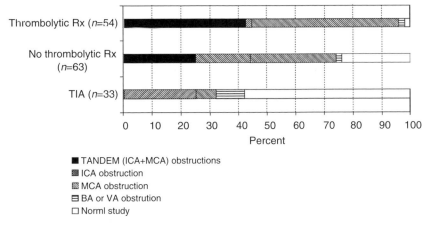

Figure 9.1 Yield of NVUE in acute cerebral ischemia. Ultrasound screening for LAIT was positive in 98 percent of patients eligible for thrombolysis, 76 percent of acute stroke patients ineligible for thrombolysis, and 42 percent in patients with TIAs ($P < 0.001$). From Chernyshev et al. (2005).

Yield and accuracy of TCD and carotid duplex

Invasive angiography shows complete arterial occlusion in 76 percent of acute stroke patients within 6 hr of symptom onset. Although various types of angiographic tests and TCD performed by experienced users show similar results, the scanning protocols and diagnostic criteria used to interpret TCD vary between centers.

1. TCD shows evidence for an acute occlusion in ≥ 70 percent of patients who have significant and fixed neurological deficits and who are candidates for thrombolysis within the first 6 hr.
2. TCD may show signs of an acute occlusion in up to 90 percent of patients who receive intravenous TPA within the first 3 hr after stroke onset particularly if the pretreatment stroke severity is ≥ 10 NIH stroke scale (NIHSS) points.
3. TCD assessment of patients with acute cerebral ischemia can also show intracranial stenotic lesions, spontaneous clot dissolution, and arterial reocclusion.
4. TCD has the highest sensitivity (> 90 percent) for acute arterial obstructions located in the proximal middle cerebral artery (MCA) and ICAs.
5. Spectral TCD has modest sensitivity (55–60 percent) for posterior circulation lesions if performed without transcranial color-coded duplex imaging or contrast enhancement.
6. However, if a nonimage-guided spectral TCD is completely normal, there is less than 5 percent chance that an urgent angiogram will show any acute obstruction (specificity > 96 percent for all proximal arterial systems).
7. After an acute arterial occlusion is found, TCD can determine the beginning, duration, timing, and amount of arterial recanalization. TCD has a sensitivity of 91 percent, and a specificity of 93 percent compared to angiography for MCA occlusion versus complete recanalization in patients receiving thrombolysis for ischemic stroke.
8. TCD can be especially useful at the time of initial clinical assessment of an acute stroke patient. The likelihood of finding an arterial occlusion reduces from 70 to 24 percent when patients are seen later than the first 6 hr after stroke onset.
9. TCD evidence of occlusion helps to identify patients with ischemic nature of acute focal neurological deficits. On the other hand, normal TCD results may be helpful to identify lacunar mechanism or to suspect nonstroke events such as functional deficits or complicated migraine.

In emergency situations, a fast TCD localization of arterial occlusion to such segments as the M2, or M1 MCA, terminal ICA, proximal versus distal basilar artery can help explain the origin of the neurological deficit and indirectly judge collateral blood supply to compensate for an occlusion.

1. This information helps to identify patients with large proximal vessel occlusion and select the next most efficient management step such as

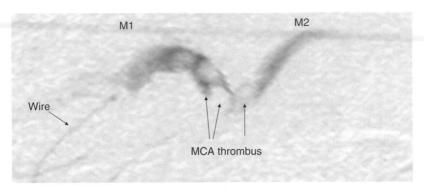

Figure 9.2 Digital subtraction angiography shows TIMI 1 and 2 flow grades at clot location in the distal M1–M2 MCA subdivision after contrast injection with an intraarterial catheter (wire). Note the irregular and sausage-like shape of the thrombus with variable amounts of residual flow at the distal M1 segment and M2 origins.

further diagnostic or interventional procedures despite variable stroke severity.

2. The presence and persistence of a large vessel occlusion or stenosis in patients with acute and spontaneously resolving deficits also point to a greater likelihood for clinical deterioration within the next 24 hr.

3. These TCD findings are also helpful to identify patients with persisting arterial obstructions that will be particularly sensitive to blood pressure changes, head positioning, and inadequate hydration.

TCD and carotid duplex criteria for lesions amenable for intervention

Previously proposed criteria for intracranial occlusions mostly focused on the absence of flow signals at presumed thrombus location and/or velocity asymmetry between homologous segments, that is, MCAs. Although a complete occlusion should produce no detectable flow signals, in reality, some residual flow to or around the thrombus may exist due its irregular shape (Figure 9.2), relatively soft composition, and systolic pressures that cause additional distension of arterial walls. An acute occlusion may therefore produce a variety of waveforms representing this residual flow.

1. The thrombolysis in myocardial infarction (TIMI) flow grading system was developed to assess the residual flow with invasive angiography. We have developed the thrombolysis in brain infarction (TIBI) flow grading system to evaluate residual flow noninvasively and monitor thrombus dissolution in real time.

2. The TIBI system expands previous definitions of acute arterial occlusion by focusing the examiner's attention on relatively weak signals

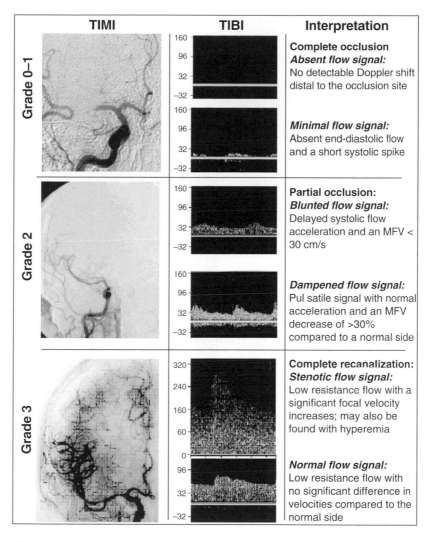

TIMI	TIBI	Interpretation
Grade 0–1	160 / 96 / 32 / –32	**Complete occlusion** *Absent flow signal:* No detectable Doppler shift distal to the occlusion site
	160 / 96 / 32 / –32	*Minimal flow signal:* Absent end-diastolic flow and a short systolic spike
Grade 2	160 / 96 / 32 / –32	**Partial occlusion:** *Blunted flow signal:* Delayed systolic flow acceleration and an MFV < 30 cm/s
	160 / 96 / 32 / –32	*Dampened flow signal:* Pul satile signal with normal acceleration and an MFV decrease of >30% compared to a normal side
Grade 3	320 / 240 / 160 / 60 / 0	**Complete recanalization:** *Stenotic flow signal:* Low resistance flow with a significant focal velocity increases; may also be found with hyperemia
	96 / 32 / –32	*Normal flow signal:* Low resistance flow with no significant difference in velocities compared to the normal side

Figure 9.3 Comparison of TIMI and TIBI flow grading systems and TCD accuracy parameters to determine complete recanalization versus persisting occlusion after thrombolysis in the MCA.

with abnormal flow waveforms that can be found along arterial stems filled with thrombi (Figure 9.3).

3. TIBI flow grades correlate with stroke severity and mortality as well as likelihood of recanalization and clinical improvement.

Acute arterial occlusion is a dynamic process since thrombus can propagate, break up, or rebuild within seconds or minutes thereby changing the degree of arterial obstruction and affecting correlation between TCD and angiography.

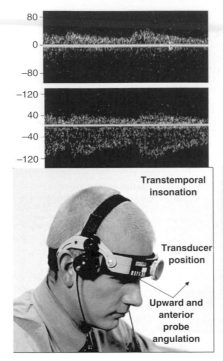
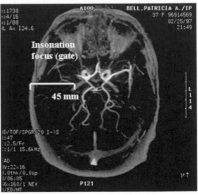

Figure 9.4 The most typical TCD appearance of a proximal M1 MCA occlusion in acute ischemic stroke (left image plate). Magnetic resonance angiogram (right bottom image) shows the relationship of MCA occlusion location to skull structures. Relative TCD transducer position and ultrasound beam are also shown. A typical TCD transducer fixation for continuous monitoring of thrombolysis for MCA stroke is shown in the upper left image (modified with permission from the National Institutes of Neurological Disorders and Stroke rt-PA Stroke Study Group (1955).

1. The occlusion may be a complete occlusion (TIMI grades 0–1) or a partial occlusion corresponding to TIMI grade 2.

2. The presence of a large vessel occlusion on TCD has to be confirmed by other findings such as flow diversion to a branching vessel or a collateral channel (Figure 9.4).

3. Ultrasound may suggest that more than one occlusion is present in the same patient, that is, tandem lesions in the ICA and MCA, or VA and BA. These tandem lesions are detected by combining TIBI flow grading and criteria for collateral flow signals. In other words, if a distal M1 MCA occlusion is present, it should produce antegrade flow diversion to ACA or PCA. If an additional obstruction exists in the proximal ICA, TCD will show either anterior cross-filling via the anterior communicating

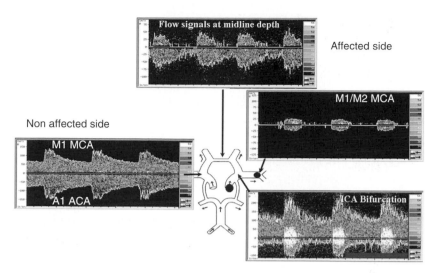

Figure 9.5 An acute tandem M1 MCA and ICA occlusion. TCD showed a minimal distal M1–M2 subdivision flow signal at the depth of 50 mm (TIBI grade 1), positive diastolic flow in the proximal MCA/TICA, and a stenotic flow signal with harsh systolic bruits at the depths of the terminal ICA (70 mm, transtemporal approach) as well as at the depths of the posterior communicating and posterior cerebral arteries. The differential for the origin of this flow signal should include TICA stenosis and posterior communicating artery flow in the presence of an acute ICA obstruction. No flow signals were obtained from the right siphon and ophthalmic artery through transorbital window. On the contralateral side, TCD showed flow diversion to the ACA (MFV MCA < ACA, pulsatility MCA > ACA). Reproduced with permission from Alexandrov (2002).

artery, stenotic terminal ICA velocities (Figure 9.5), and/or reversed ophthalmic artery.

Bedside ultrasound examination in acute cerebral ischemia can help to

1. identify thrombus presence;
2. determine thrombus location(s);
3. assess collateral supply;
4. find the worst residual flow signal; and
5. monitor recanalization and reocclusion.

Chernyshev et al. evaluated the combined fast-track TCD and carotid/vertebral duplex to identify LAIT.

1. LAIT was defined as an occlusion or near-occlusion, or ≥50 percent stenosis or thrombi in an artery (arteries) supplying brain area(s) affected by ischemia.

2. The current definition of LAIT may include chronic lesions, and caution should be exercised if these lesions are directly responsible for current symptoms in the patient.
3. The ultrasound screening criteria for LAIT are shown in Table 9.2.

TCD monitoring

Prolonged TCD monitoring for emboli detection and vasomotor reactivity assessment has been performed for years without any evidence of harmful effects. No adverse biological effects have been documented for the frequencies and power ranges used in diagnostic ultrasound.

1. Previous work with TCD monitoring has shown that evolution of the MCA occlusion can be followed in real time and recanalization process measured.
2. The speed of clot lysis can be measured through the duration of flow improvement with real-time ultrasound monitoring with TIBI residual flow signals and other parameters such as intensity of flow signals, appearance of microembolic signals, velocity, and pulsatility changes.

To measure the *speed and completeness of intracranial clot lysis*, it is important to determine the beginning of arterial recanalization using the following five parameters:

1. waveform change by ≥ 1 TIBI residual flow grade (e.g., absent to minimal, minimal to blunted, and minimal to normal signal improvement);
2. appearance of embolic signals (transient high-intensity signals of variable duration);
3. flow velocity improvement by ≥ 30 percent at a constant angle of insonation;
4. signal intensity and velocity improvement of variable duration at constant skull/probe interface and gain/sample volume/scale settings;
5. appearance of flow signals with variable (≥ 30 percent) pulsatility indexes and amplitude of systolic peaks (Figure 9.6).

Once recanalization process started, TCD can detect the arrival of the highest TIBI flow grade that will indicate completion of recanalization. Using these sonographic parameters, TCD can measure the (Figure 9.7):

1. beginning,
2. duration (or speed),
3. timing to maximum completeness, and
4. amount of arterial recanalization (complete, partial, none).

Table 9.2: Ultrasound screening criteria for lesions amenable for intervention

Lesion location	TCD criteria (at least one present)	CD criteria
M1/ M2 MCA	Primary: Thrombolysis in brain infarction (TIBI) grades 0–4 (absent, minimmal, blunted, dampened, or stenotic) at depths <45 mm (M2) and 45–65 mm (M1) Secondary: Flow diversion to ACA, PCA, or M2 Increased resistance in unilateral TICA Embolic signals in MCA Turbulence, disturbed flow at stenosis Nonharmonic and harmonic covibrations (bruit or pure musical tones)	Extracranial findings may be normal or showing decreased ICA velocity unilateral to lesion
TICA	Primary: TIBI grades 0–4 at 60–70 mm Increased velocities suggest anterior cross-filling or collateral flow in posterior Communicating artery Secondary: Embolic signalsl in unilateral MCA Blunted unilateral MCA, MFV > 20 cm/s	Decreased ICA velocity unilateral to lesion or normal extracranial findings

(continued)

Table 9.2 (continued)

Lesion Location	TCD criteria (at least one present)	CD criteria
Proximal ICA	Primary: Increased flow velocities suggest anterior cross-filling through ACommA or collateral flow through PcommA Reversed OA Delayed systolic flow acceleration in or blunted ipsilateral MCA, MFV>20 cm/s Secondary: Embolic signals in unilateral MCA Normal OA direction due to retrograde filling of siphon	B-mode evidence of a lesion in ICA±CCA; Flow imaging evidence of no flow or residual lumen; ICA >50% stenosis: PSV >125 cm/s; EDV > 40 cm/s; ICA/CCA PSV ratio > 2 ICA near-occlusion or occlusion: Blunted, minimal, reverberating, or absent spectral Doppler waveforms in ICA
Tandem ICA/MCA stenosis/occlusion	Primary: TIBI grades 0–4 And: Increased velocities in contralateral ACA, MCA, or unilateral PCommA Or: Reversed unilateral OA	B-mode evidence of a lesion in ICA;± CCA; Or: Flow imaging evidence of residual lumen or no flow; ICA >50% stenosis: PSV >125cm/s; EDV > 40 cm/s; ICA/CCA PSV ratio > 2

	Secondary:	ICA near-occlusion or occlusion:
	Delayed systolic flow acceleration in proximal MCA or TICA	Blunted, minimal, reverberating, or absent spectral Doppler waveforms in ICA
	Embolic signals in proximal MCA or TICA	
Basilar artery	Primary:	Extracranial findings may be normal or showing decreased VA velocities or VA occlusion
	TIBI flow grades 0–4 at 75–100 mm	
	Secondary:	
	Flow velocity increase in terminal VA and branches, MCAs, or PCommAs	
	High resistance flow signals in VA(s)	
	Reversed flow direction in distal basilar artery (85 mm)	
Vertebral artery	Primary (intracranial VA occlusion):	Extracranial findings may be normal (intracranial VA lesion) or showing decreased VA velocities or VA occlusion
	TIBI flow grades 0–4 at 75–100 mm	
	Primary extracranial VA occlusion):	
	Absent, minimal, or reversed high resistance flow signals in unilateral terminal VA	
	Secondary:	
	Embolic signals	
	Increased velocities or low pulsatility in contralateral VA	

Notes: LAITs were defined as abstruction/near obstruction or ≥50% stenosis of (1) M1 or M2 segments of MCA, (2) ICA, (3) tandem ICA/MCA, or (4) vertebrobasilar (VB) arteries.

TICA indicates terminal carotid artery; TIBI, thrombolysis in brain infarction; ACommA, anterior communicating artery; and PCommA, posterior communicating artery.

Source: Reprinted with permission from Chernyshev et al. (2005).

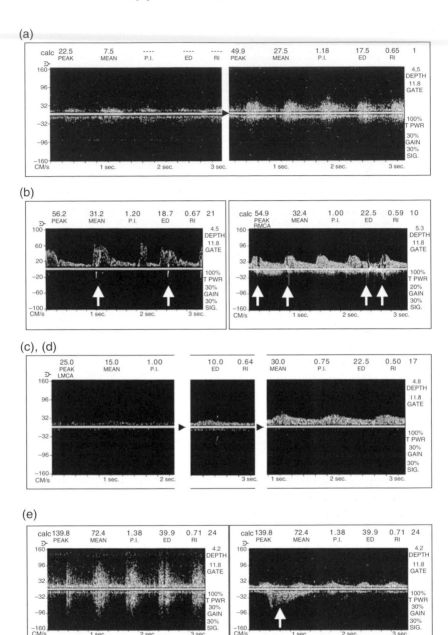

Figure 9.6 Signs of the beginning and continuation of arterial recanalization. (a) Waveform improvement by one or more TIBI residual flow grade: the first set illustrates flow changes from a minimal to blunted waveform (appearance of positive end-diastolic flow and rounded systolic complex). (b) Appearance of embolic signals: the second set of waveforms illustrate dampened and normal flow signals with multiple transient high intensity signals of variable duration with

In patients who experience partial or complete thrombus dissolution, arterial recanalization can be classified as

1. sudden (abrupt appearance of a normal or stenotic low-resistance signal),
2. stepwise (flow improvement over 1–29 min), and
3. slow ($\geq$ 30 min) (Figure 9.7).

In patients receiving intravenous thrombolysis, recanalization began at a median time of 17 min and reached maximum TIBI flow grades at 35 min after TPA bolus, with mean duration of recanalization of 23 $\pm$ 16 min. In this study, recanalization was sudden in 12 percent, stepwise in 53 percent, and slow in 35 percent patients. At 24 hr, 80, 30, and 13 percent of patients in these respective recanalization groups had NIHSS scores of 0–3 points.

Slow or partial recanalization with dampened TIBI flow signals was found in 53 percent of patients with total NIHSS scores $\geq$ 10 points at 24 hr. Complete recanalization occurred faster (median 10 min) than partial recanalization (median 30 min) most likely due to changing velocities and intensity of flow signals in the latter group.

1. Rapid arterial recanalization is associated with better short-term improvement.
2. Slow ($\geq$ 30 min) flow improvement and dampened TIBI flow signals are less favorable prognostic signs. This information on TCD may help with selection of patients for additional pharmacological or interventional treatment.
3. Recanalizations between 5 and 7 hr after cardioembolic stroke may lead to symptomatic hemorrhage.

Figure 9.8 shows a complete stepwise M1 MCA recanalization at 5.5 hr after stroke onset that preceded rapid clinical deterioration due to massive intracerebral hemorrhage leading to death within 24 hr after stroke onset. The last frame in Figure 9.8 shows a hyperemic signal with elevated mean flow velocities and low pulsatility of flow that may suggest failure of MCA autoregulatory response to late and relatively rapid reperfusion after cardioembolism.

Figure 9.6 *(continued)*
characteristic chirp or pop-like sounds (arrows). (c, d) Flow velocity improvement by 30 percent or more and the signal intensity or improvement: this set shows flow tracing obtained at a constant angle of insonation with mean flow velocity improvement from 15 to 30 cm/s preceded by the improvement in the strength (brightness) of the residual flow signal (middle set). (e) Appearance of flow signals with variable (> 30 percent) amplitude of systolic peaks and pulsatility: a turbulent high frequency, high resistance stenotic flow signal (bottom left); variable velocities with transient appearance of flow in a branching vessel below the baseline (arrow) (bottom right). Reproduced with permission from Kaps et al. (1990).

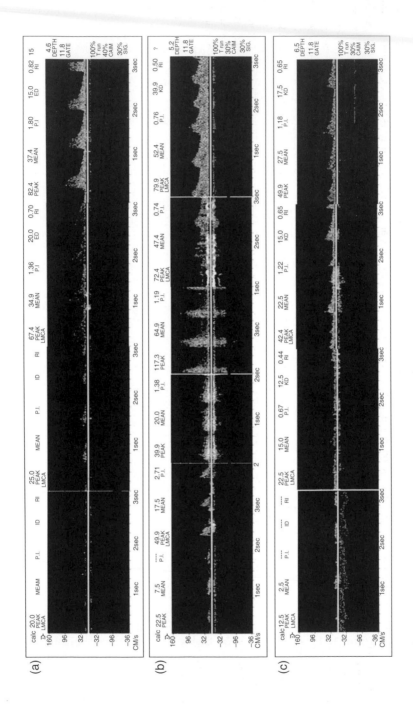

142

Figure 9.7 A "triple S" classification of the duration of arterial recanalization. (a) Sudden (abrupt appearance of a normal or stenotic low resistance signal): (1) TCD shows a minimal signal in the MCA at the time of TPA bolus. (2) At 31 min after bolus, the first improvement in signal intensity was noticed and marked as "beginning" of recanalization. (3) In less than 5 s, the first low resistance signal was detected with normal waveform, and 30 s later, (4) a strong normal flow velocity signal was detected. Recanalization started at 31 min after TPA bolus, its duration was 35 s, and timing of complete recanalization of the distal M1 MCA segment (TIMI grade III equivalent) was 32 min after TPA bolus. (b) Stepwise (flow improvement over 1–29 min): (1) TCD shows a minimal signal in the mid-to-distal M1 MCA at the time of TPA bolus. (2) Nine minutes later TCD shows the first improvement in the amplitude of systolic velocities (beginning of recanalization), however the absence of end-diastolic velocities still indicates minimal TIBI flow signal and persisting occlusion. (3) At 14 min, positive end-diastolic flow is detected with rounded systolic shape of the waveform (TIBI blunted signal) with flow improvement by 1 TIBI grade. Note high intensity bruits during each cardiac cycle with possible embolic signals. (4) At 16 min, TCD shows high resistance turbulent stenotic signals with elevated and variable systolic velocities that are replaced by normal waveforms at 18 min (5). At this point, TCD findings indicate that the M1 MCA patency at the site of insonation is restored. Further improvement in flow velocity, pulsatility, and strength of the signal was detected between the 18th and 20th min after bolus (6) indicating continuous flow recovery presumably due to distal clot migration beyond M2 MCA bifurcation. TCD shows the beginning of recanalization at 9 min, duration of 11 min, and timing of complete (TIMI grade III equivalent) recanalization at 20 min after TPA bolus. (c) Slow (30–60 min): (1) At the time of TPA bolus, TCD shows a minimal flow signal at the M1 MCA origin (above baseline) and a flow signal below baseline from the proximal A1 anterior cerebral artery (ACA) with mean flow velocity of 24 cm/s. (2) At 12 min after bolus, slow positive end-diastolic flow appears in the proximal M1 MCA indicating the beginning of recanalization. A decrease in the ACA flow signal may indicate clot movement or breakup at its proximal part. Variable M1 MCA and A1 ACA flow velocities with dampened TIBI flow grade are seen during the next 40 min (3) with arrival of the dampened flow signal with the highest mean flow velocity of 28 cm/s and improved A1 ACA velocities of 54 cm/s at 54 min after TPA bolus (4). TCD findings indicate the beginning of recanalization at 12 min, duration of 42 min and timing of partial (TIMI grade II equivalent) recanalization with continuing flow diversion to ACA at 54 min after TPA bolus. Reproduced with permission from Kaps et al. (1990).

143

Time 13.02 t-PA bolus

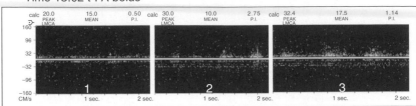

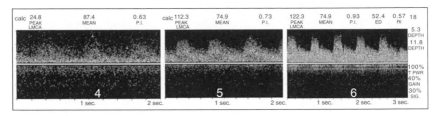

Time 13.38

Figure 9.8 TCD recordings were obtained via transtemporal approach at the depth of 53 mm with an 11.8 mm gate of insonation. Graphic below the spectra frames shows presumed clot location in the MCA main stem. Frame 1 – A minimal flow signal in the proximal MCA at the time of intravenous TPA bolus (13:02). After 30 min of continuous intravenous TPA infusion: Frames 2–3 – Early restoration of flow signals with increasing frequencies and microembolic signals (arrow). Frame 4 – A turbulent stenotic signal with audible chirping components suggesting continuing clot dissolution. Frame 5 – Hyperemic flow with velocities elevated above age-expected values and relatively low pulsatility (Gosling and King pulsatility index 0.73) indicating distal vasodilation. Frame 6 – Hyperemic flow with velocities elevated above age-expected values and normal pulsatility (Gosling and King pulsatility index 0.93) showing a proximal MCA reperfusion. Reproduced with permission from Demchuk et al. (1999).

It is important to remember that TIBI grades 2–3 indicate partial and TIBI grades 4–5 indicate complete recanalization.

1. Normal or increased diastolic flow velocities in patients with stenotic signals indicate low resistance in the distal circulatory bed and unobstructed distal contrast opacification at angiography (TIMI grade 3 flow equivalent).
2. A blunted signal with mean velocities usually exceeding 20 cm/s can be seen in patients with complete MCA recanalization but persisting proximal ICA occlusion (TIMI grade 3 flow equivalent).

Obtaining continuous information about the status of an arterial occlusion or reocclusion (Case report, Figure 9.9) in acute stroke has the potential to be very helpful in further decision making with thrombolytic therapy particularly if a combined intravenous/intraarterial drug delivery proves effective.

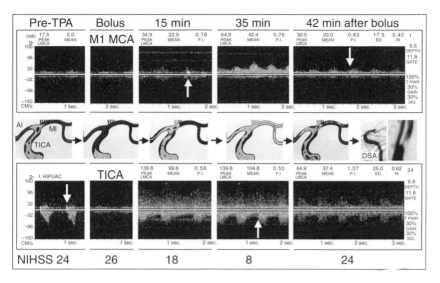

Figure 9.9 *Case report* – A 42-year-old right-handed woman was seen 80 min after the acute onset of right hemiplegia, global aphasia, eye deviation to the left, and a right homonymous hemianopsia (NIHSS score 24). Her past medical history included smoking, noninsulin-dependent diabetes mellitus, and peripheral vascular disease requiring bilateral femoral-popliteal bypasses with no history of cardiac or cerebral ischemia, and the patient was not on any antiplatelet regimen. Head CT showed a hyperdense left MCA and no hemorrhage.

At 90 min from symptom onset, TCD was performed with a single channel 2 MHz portable unit (Multigon 500M, Yonkers, NY), and monitoring started with a head-frame fixation (Marc 500, Spencer Technologies, Seattle, WA).

TCD showed a proximal M1 MCA and A1 anterior cerebral artery (ACA) occlusion (Figure 9.7, frame 1) followed by rapid progression to a terminal internal carotid artery (ICA) occlusion (frame 2). Within 5 min, she became drowsy (NIHSS score 26). Intravenous TPA was started at 120 min from symptom onset using a standard dose of 0.9 mg/kg (10 percent bolus, 90 percent infusion over 1 hr, maximum dose 90 mg).

At 10 min after TPA bolus, TCD showed terminal ICA recanalization with resumption of end-diastolic flow in the A1 ACA followed shortly by improvement in her level of consciousness. At 15 min of infusion, microembolic signals were heard in the M1 MCA accompanied with proximal M1 segment recanalization and resumption of low resistance end-diastolic flow toward the lenticulostriate perforating arteries (frame 3). Clinically, her right leg began to move followed by antigravity strength in the distal arm and improved facial weakness (NIHSS score 18).

TCD showed a continuing recanalization of the A1 ACA at 20 min, followed by resolution of her gaze preference and continued improvement in her right-sided weakness by 30 min (NIHSS score 15). At 35 min, she had complete M1 MCA recanalization with multiple microembolic signals **Figure 9.9** Continued from page 19 suggesting continuing proximal clot dissolution (frame 4). By 37 min, the patient could lift her arm with a mild drift, verbalize simple words, and follow axial and extraaxial commands (NIHSS score 8).

(continued)

Arterial reocclusion was not studied systematically in the NINDS rt-PA Stroke Study as no consistent vascular imaging protocol was implemented in this trial. However, deterioration following improvement (DFI) may represent a clinical surrogate of reocclusion; DFI was observed in 13 percent of patients in this trial:

1. We found that one-third of our patients with early recanalization experienced reocclusion within 2 hr of TPA bolus. Also, two-thirds of patients with DFI experienced early reocclusion and we believe that this is the main underlying mechanism of this phenomenon.

Figure 9.9 *(continued from page 145)*

At 42 min of infusion, TCD showed developing reocclusion of the M1 MCA and dampening of the terminal ICA flow (frame 5). At 44 min, the patient rapidly became drowsy and resumed her eye deviation, global aphasia, and right hemiplegia (NIHSS score 24). At the end of TPA infusion, a terminal ICA "T"-type occlusion was present on TCD (signal deterioration similar to frame 2). A post-TPA CT scan was unchanged.

Urgent angiography revealed a proximal ICA clot and a complete terminal ICA "T"-type occlusion with no flow in the M1 MCA and A1 ACA segments (frame 5 DSA). Under an approved experimental protocol, she received an additional 6 mg of intraarterial TPA with mechanical clot disruption leading to complete distal ICA, proximal M1 MCA, and A1 ACA recanalization with a remaining distal M1 MCA occlusion and a proximal ≥ 80 percent ICA stenosis. Diagnostic workup showed no other etiology for stroke. At two weeks, her major deficits included aphasia and arm plegia (NIHSS 18).

Sequential sonographic and clinical findings during intravenous TPA infusion are described below.

M1 MCA waveforms were obtained at 55 mm (upper row) and TICA at 68 mm (lower row) by switching between the depths at a constant angle of insonation. White arrows indicate high intensity, short duration microembolic signals (MES). The middle row is a graphic interpretation of TCD findings. The corresponding NIHSS scores are provided below each frame.

Frame 1 – Pre-TPA. High resistance flow signals in the M1 MCA, TICA, and A1 ACA segments. Frame 2 – Bolus. Progressive TICA occlusion with minimal flow signals in the M1, TICA , and A1 segments. Frame 3 – 15 min of infusion. Minimal flow signals with MES in the M1 MCA and the beginning of TICA/A1 ACA recanalization. Frame 4 – 35 min of infusion. Complete M1 MCA recanalization with low resistance flow, stenotic mean flow velocities (104 cm/s) in the TICA, and low resistance flow with MES in the A1 ACA. Frame 5 – 42 min of infusion. Developing M1 MCA and TICA reocclusion with dampened flow signals and decreased mean flow velocities compared to frame 4. Digital subtraction angiography (DSA) immediately after IV TPA infusion showed TICA "T"-type occlusion (lateral view) and a clot in the proximal ICA with a residual stenosis.

Abbreviations: TPA: tissue plasminogen activator; MCA: middle cerebral artery; TICA: terminal internal carotid artery; ACA: anterior cerebral artery; Peak: peak systolic velocity; Mean: mean flow velocity; PI: pulsatility index; ED: end diastolic flow; RI: resistance index; NIHSS: National Institutes of Health Stroke Scale. Reproduced with permission from Demchuk et al. (2000).

2. In the same study, we observed that patients with early reocclusion had better long-term outcomes than patients with no early renalization on TCD. One likely explanation may be that prior to reocclusion, these patients may have had some degree of early recanalization and reperfusion of the penumbral areas, resulting in additional time to tolerate further ischemia.

Therapeutic TCD

Recanalization is not achieved in a significant portion of coronary artery occlusions using systemic thrombolysis alone. Even lower recanalization rates have been demonstrated with intravenous thrombolysis in ischemic stroke.

1. del Zoppo et al. showed that only 26 percent of intracranial occlusions lyse partially or completely after 1 hr of intravenous duteplase infusion.
2. In the PROACT II trial, only 4 percent of MCA clots showed complete TIMI grade 3 recanalization when recombinant pro urokinase was infused at the clot surface for 1 hr.
3. Half of the patients remain moderately or severely disabled despite treatment with intravenous t-PA.
4. One of the major reasons for this poor rate of recovery is slow and incomplete thrombolysis.

Experimental evidence suggests that ultrasound substantially increases thrombolytic effect of TPA particularly if used in low megahertz to kilohertz frequency range.

1. The effect on lysis does not appear to be mediated by thermal or cavitational effects if the mechanical index is kept below one.
2. Even using 2 MHz frequency and power output less than 750 mW, TCD transmits some amount of ultrasound energy to the intracranial vessels raising the possibility that this diagnostic modality could also enhance TPA activity.

Diagnostic 2-MHz TCD is routinely used in patients with stroke to obtain spectral velocity measurements in intracranial arteries.

1. Continuous 2 MHz TCD energy transmission may promote thrombolysis by simply exposing more clot surface to residual flow.
2. When the worst residual flow signal is identified using TIBI grades, the ultrasound beam is usually focused at the intracranial clot location and its interface with surrounding, often minimal blood flow (Figure 9.2).
3. We observed high rate of complete recanalization and dramatic clinical recovery during TPA infusion when continuously monitored by 2 MHz TCD monitoring.

Our pilot clinical study assessed whether such a therapeutic effect is possible in stroke patients. Stroke patients receiving intravenous TPA were monitored with portable TCD starting at the time of TPA bolus.

1. Residual flow signals were obtained from the clot location identified by TCD.
2. Forty patients were studied with a mean baseline NIHSS score 19.
3. TCD monitoring occurred for the duration of TPA infusion.
4. Recanalization on TCD was found at 45 ± 20 min after TPA bolus. Recanalization was complete in 12 (30 percent) and partial in 16 (40 percent) patients.
5. Dramatic recovery during TPA infusion (NIHSS score ≤ 3 points) occurred in 8 (20 percent) patients, all with complete recanalization.
6. Lack of improvement or worsening was associated with no recanalization, late recanalization, or reocclusion on TCD.
7. Improvement by ≥ 10 NIHSS points or complete recovery was found in 30 percent of all patients at the end of TPA infusion and in 40 percent at 24 hr.
8. The unusually high frequency of "on the table" TPA responders and a high rate of early complete recanalization raised the possibility that ultrasonic energy transmission by TCD was facilitating more rapid thrombolysis.

This preliminary data provided enthusiasm to initiate a proper phase II randomized controlled trial, called CLOTBUST, to assess whether such therapeutic effect is clinically relevant.

1. In this trial we recruited 126 patients who were randomly assigned to receive continuous TCD monitoring or placebo (63 patients in each group) in addition to intravenous t-PA.
2. Complete recanalization or dramatic clinical recovery within 2 hr after the administration of a TPA bolus occurred in 49 percent in the target group as compared to 30 percent in the control group ($p = 0.03$).
3. Only 4.8 percent patients developed symptomatic intracerebral hemorrhage.
4. The rates of sustained complete recanalization within 2 hr are shown in Figure 9.10. Our results showed the positive effects of 2-MHz continuous TCD monitoring in acute stroke with no increase in the rate of intracerebral hemorrhage.

Eggers et al. evaluated the potential of transcranial color-coded sonography (TCCS)-guided, 2-MHz transcranial ultrasound in accelerating thrombolysis in acute stroke patients with occlusion of the MCA-M1 and with contraindications associated with thrombolytic therapy. They observed more frequent recanalization in the ultrasound group as compared to the control group ($p = 0.026$).

In the recently conducted TRUMBI trial, Daffertshofer et al. included 26 patients within 6-hr time window in a multicenter clinical trial.

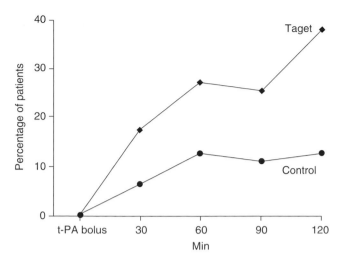

Figure 9.10 Rate of sustained complete recanalization within 2 hr after administration of a TPA bolus. From Alexandrov et al. (2004).

1. Twelve patients received TPA whereas fourteen patients were randomized to TPA plus 90 min of low-frequency (300 kHz) ultrasound exposure.
2. The study had to be stopped prematurely due to an increased incidence of intracranial hemorrhages (5 of 12 in TPA group versus 13 of 14 in TPA plus ultrasound group).
3. Parenchymal and even atypical hemorrhages occurred exclusively in the combined treatment group. They speculated that reverberations of the long wavelength ultrasound occurred inside the head, leading to "hot spots" in addition to the mechanical distortion of the brain microvessels.

Other bedside diagnostic applications

Emboli detection

Microembolic signals (MES) appear as signals of high intensity and short duration within the TCD spectrum, as a result of their different acoustic properties compared to the circulating blood.

1. MES have been proven to represent solid or gaseous particles within the blood flow.
2. They occur at random within the cardiac cycle and they can be acoustically identified by a characteristic "chirp," "click," or "whistle" sound.

Detection of MES is particularly important when stroke or TIA is believed to be due to embolism.

1. Doppler embolic signals detection is especially important in carotid stenosis. Clopidogrel and Aspirin for Reduction of Emboli in

Symptomatic Carotid Stenosis Study (CARESS) revealed that the combination of clopidogrel and aspirin was associated with a marked reduction in MES, compared with aspirin alone. Hence, TCD could be used to identify patients for early CEA.

2. In asymptomatic carotid stenosis, Spence et al. demonstrated that TCD negative cases for MES will not benefit from carotid endarterectomy or stenting unless the risk is < 1 percent. They suggested that asymptomatic carotid stenosis should be managed medically, with delay of surgical intervention until the occurrence of symptoms or emboli.

Intracranial stenosis

Intracranial arterial steno-occlusive lesions cause characteristic alterations in the Doppler signals, including

➠ focal increases in velocity
➠ local turbulence
➠ poststenotic drop in velocity
➠ collateral flow patterns

Sensitivity, specificity, positive predictive value, and negative predictive values of TCD are generally higher in anterior circulation than the vertebrobasilar circulation owing to the more reliable anatomy of the former and the technical problems in studying the latter.

1. One of the important limitations of TCD is an insufficient temporal acoustic window and this can be a limiting factor in a significant number of cases, depending upon the population being studied. The yield of TCD in cases with suboptimal acoustic windows can be enhanced with the help of various contrast agents.
2. Because no imaging is involved, the ability to assess the intracranial arteries by TCD remains as much an art as it is a science, and remains operator dependent.
3. Transcranial color-coded duplex study involves actual imaging of the intracranial vessels, making the identification of various arteries more reliable; the velocities can be assessed with proper angle correction.

Vasomotor reactivity

Although velocities in the MCA do not directly correlate with absolute values of cerebral blood flow, changes in velocity correlate with changes in the flow when MCA has a constant diameter. Vasomotor reactivity describes the ability of the cerebral circulation to respond to vasomotor stimuli, and the changes in cerebral blood flow in response to such stimuli can be studied by TCD.

1. The commonest agent to measure the cerebral vasomotor reactivity is CO_2.
2. Increased levels of CO_2 cause vasodilatation and increased cerebral blood flow, which is reflected by an increased velocity.
3. Measuring vasomotor reactivity requires a proper setup with controlled conditions regarding the concentration of CO_2.

Markus et al. described a simple measurement of the MCA velocity in response to 30 s of breath holding and termed it as breath-holding index (BHI).

$$BHI = \frac{MFV_{end} - MFV_{baseline}}{MFV_{baseline}} \times \frac{100}{\text{seconds of breath holding}}$$

where MFV is mean flow velocity.

1. Impaired vasomotor reactivity using BHI can help to identify patients at higher risk of stroke who have asymptomatic carotid stenosis or a previously symptomatic carotid occlusion.
2. A decreased vasomotor reactivity suggests failure of collateral flow to adapt to the stenosis progression.
3. Various studies, using different provocative measures for assessing the cerebral vasomotor reactivity, demonstrated a remarkable ipsilateral event rate of around 30 percent (30 percent risk of stroke/TIA during about 2 years).

Right-to-left shunt detection

Right-to-left shunts, particularly patent foramen ovale (PFO) are common in general population with a prevalence of 10–35 percent in various echocardiography and autopsy studies for PFO. The prevalence is even higher in certain selected populations, for example, in patients with cryptogenic stroke or TIA and especially in younger patients without an apparent etiology.

1. Different methods are used in clinical practice to diagnose a PFO. A contrast-enhanced transesophageal echocardiography (TEE) is still believed to be the gold standard for the diagnosis of PFO.
2. Since the early 1990s, contrast-enhanced TCD has been used as an optimal method for detecting the high-intensity transient signals (HITS) passing through the MCA, thus indicating the presence of a right-to-left shunt.
3. The sensitivity and specificity of contrast-enhanced TCD has been reported to be 68–100 and 67–100 percent, respectively.
4. In a recent study, Blersch et al. tested contrast-enhanced transcranial duplex sonography for the diagnosis of PFO and they found it to be as sensitive as contrast-enhanced TEE.

The above-mentioned tests such as emboli detection, vasomotor reactivity, and right-to-left shunt detection can be performed at bedside in the emergency room, observation, or stroke unit as part of fast diagnostic workup.

In conclusion, carotid ultrasound and TCD have established clinical value in diagnostic workup of stroke patients and are suggested as essential components of a comprehensive stroke center. TCD is also an evolving ultrasound method with increasing diagnostic value and a therapeutic potential. Validated occlusion criteria and TIBI classification of residual flow are aimed to ease its use in acute stroke, and technology advances will simplify bone window determination. Given the widespread availability of this equipment, increased use of this modality in acute stroke is expected and local validation of diagnostic criteria and test performance is required by vascular laboratory accreditation guidelines (www.icavl.org).

Bibliography

Albert MJ, Latchaw RE, Selman WR, Shephard T, et al. Recommendations for comprehensive stroke centers: A consensus statement from the brain attack coalition. *Stroke* 2005;36:1597–618.

Alexandrov AV. *Cerebrovascular ultrasound and stroke management*. Futura Publishing, New York. 2002.

Alexandrov AV, Burgin WS, Demchuk AM, El-Mitwalli A, Grotta JC. Speed of intracranial clot lysis with intravenous TPA therapy: Sonographic classification and short term improvement. *Circulation* 2001;103:2897–902.

Alexandrov AV, Demchuk A, Wein T, Grotta JC. The yield of transcranial Doppler in acute cerebral ischemia. *Stroke* 1999;30:1605–9.

Alexandrov AV, Demchuk AM, Felberg RA, et al. High rate of complete recanalization and dramatic clinical recovery during TPA infusion when continuously monitored by 2 MHz transcranial Doppler monitoring. *Stroke* 2000;31:610–14.

Alexandrov AV, Demchuk AM, Felberg RA, Grotta JC, Krieger D. Intracranial clot dissolution is associated with embolic signals on transcranial Doppler. *J Neuroimaging* 2000;10:27–32.

Alexandrov AV, Felberg RA, Demchuk AM, et al. Deterioration following spontaneous improvement: Sonographic findings in patients with acutely resolving symptoms of cerebral ischemia. *Stroke* 2000;31:915–19.

Alexandrov AV, Grotta JC. Arterial reocclusion in stroke patients treated with intravenous tissue plasminogen activator. *Neurology* 2002;59:862–7.

Alexandrov AV, Molina CA, Grotta JC, et al., for the CLOTBUST Investigators. Ultrasound-enhanced systemic thrombolysis for acute ischemic stroke. *N Engl J Med* 2004;351:2170–8.

Behrens S, Daffertshofer M, Spiegel D, Hennerici M. Low-frequency, low-intensity ultrasound accelerates thrombolysis through the skull. *Ultrasound Med Biol* 1999;25:269–73.

Blersch WK, Draganski BM, Holmer SR, et al. Transcranial duplex sonography in the detection of patent foramen ovale. *Radiology* 2002;225:693–9.

Braaten JV, Goss RA, Francis CW. Ultrasound reversibly disaggregates fibrin fibers. *Thromb Haemost* 1997;78:1063–8.

Burgin WS, Alexandrov AV. Deteriorations following improvement with TPA therapy: Carotid thrombosis and re-occlusion. *Neurology* 2001;56:568–70.

Burgin WS, Malkoff M, Felberg RA, et al. Transcranial Doppler ultrasound criteria for recanalization after thrombolysis for middle cerebral artery stroke. *Stroke* 2000;31:1128–32.

Chernyshev OY, Garami Z, Calleja S, et al. Yield and accuracy of urgent combined carotid/transcranial ultrasound testing in acute cerebral ischemia. *Stroke* 2005;36:32–7.

Daffertshofer M, Gass A, Ringleb P, et al. Transcranial low-frequency ultrasound-mediated thrombolysis in brain ischemia. *Stroke* 2005;36:1441–6.

Daffertshofer M, Hennerici M. Ultrasound in the treatment of ischemic stroke. *Lancet Neurol* 2003;2:283–90.

del Zoppo GJ, Poeck K, Pessin MS, et al. Recombinant tissue plasminogen activator in acute thrombotic and embolic stroke. *Ann Neurol* 1992;32:78–86.

Demchuk AM, Burgin WS, Christou I, et al. Thrombolysis in brain ischemia (TIBI) TCD flow grades predict clinical severity, early recovery and mortality in intravenous TPA treated patients. *Stroke* 2001;32:89–93.

Demchuk AM, Christou I, Wein TH, et al. Accuracy and criteria for localizing arterial occlusion with transcranial Doppler. *J Neuroimaging* 2000;10:1–12.

Demchuk AM, Wein TH, Felberg RA, Christou I, Alexandrov AV. Evolution of rapid middle cerebral artery recanalization during intravenous thrombolysis for acute ischemic stroke. *Circulation* 1999;100:2282–3.

Droste DW, Silling K, Stypmann J, et al. Contrast transcranial Doppler ultrasound in the detection of right-to-left shunt: Time window and threshold in microbubble numbers. *Stroke* 2000;31:1640–5.

Eggers J, Seidel G, Koch B, Konig IR. Sonothrombolysis in acute ischemic stroke for patients ineligible for rt-PA. *Neurology* 2005;64:1052–4.

Fieschi C, Argentino C, Lenzi GL, Sacchetti ML, Toni D, Bozzao L. Clinical and instrumental evaluation of patients with ischemic stroke within six hours. *J Neurol Sci* 1989;91:311–22.

Francis CW, Onundarson PT, Carstensen EL, et al. Enhancement of fibrinolysis in vitro by ultrasound. *J Clin Invest* 1992;90:2063–8.

Furlan AJ, Higashida RT, Wechsler LR, and PROACT II Investigators. PROACT II: Recombinant prourokinase (r-ProUK) in acute cerebral thromboembolism: Initial trial results. In *Highlights, 24th AHA International Conference on Stroke and Cerebral Circulation*. CD-ROM, AHA, 1999.

Grant EG, Benson CB, Moneta GL, et al. Carotid artery stenosis: Grey-scale and Doppler US diagnosis – Society of Radiologists in Ultrasound Consensus Conference. *Radiology* 2003;229:340–6.

Hankey GJ. Ongoing and planned trials of antiplatelet therapy in the acute and long term management of patients with ischemic brain syndromes: Setting a new standard of care. *Cerebrovasc Dis* 2004;17(Suppl 3):11–16.

Kaps M, Damian MS, Teschendorf U, Dorndorf W. Transcranial Doppler ultrasound findings in the middle cerebral artery occlusion. *Stroke* 1990;21:532–7.

Kaps M, Link A. Transcranial sonographic monitoring during thrombolytic therapy. *Am J Neuroradiol* 1998;19:758–60.

Lewandowski CA, Frankel M, Tomsick TA, et al. Combined intravenous and intra-arterial r-TPA versus intra-arterial therapy of acute ischemic stroke: Emergency Management of Stroke (EMS) Bridging Trial. *Stroke* 1999;30:2598–605.

Markus HS, Harrison MJ. Estimation of cerebrovascular reactivity using transcranial Doppler, including the use of breath-holding as the vasodilatory stimulus. *Stroke* 1992;23:668–73.

The National Institutes of Neurological Disorders and Stroke rt-PA Stroke Study Group. Tissue plasminogen activator for acute ischemic stroke. *N Engl J Med* 1995;333:1581–7.

Razumovsky AY, Gillard JH, Bryan RN, Hanley DF, Oppenheimer SM. TCD, MRA, and MRI in acute cerebral ischemia. *Acta Neurol Scand* 1999;99:65–76.

Sloan MA, Alexandrov AV, Tegeler CH, et al. Assessment: Transcranial Doppler ultrasonography: Report of the therapeutics and technology assessment subcommittee of the American Academy of Neurology. *Neurology* 2004;62:1468–81.

Spence JD, Tamayo A, Lownie SP, Ng WP, Ferguson GG. Absence of microemboli on transcranial Doppler identifies low-risk patients with asymptomatic carotid stenosis. *Stroke* 2005;36:2373–8.

Spencer MP, Thomas GI, Nicholls SC, Sauvage LR. Detection of middle cerebral artery emboli during carotid endarterectomy using transcranial Doppler ultrasonography. *Stroke* 1990;21:415–23.

Thomassen L, Waje-Andreassen U, Naess H, Aarseth J, Russel D. Doppler ultrasound and clinical findings in patients with acute ischemic stroke treated with intravenous thrombolysis. *Eur J Neurol* 2005;12:462–5.

The TIMI Study Group. The thrombolysis in myocardial infarction (TIMI) trial: Phase I findings. *N Engl J Med* 1985;312:932–6.

Zanette EM, Fieschi C, Bozzao L, et al. Comparison of cerebral angiography and transcranial Doppler sonography in acute stroke. *Stroke* 1989;20:899–903.

Management of Stroke Patients

10 Ischemic stroke in the first 24 hr

Magdy H. Selim

Time is brain. Every minute matters in patients with acute stroke. There is a limited time window for acute intervention since the ischemic tissue may no longer be salvageable after hours from stroke onset, in most patients. The first 24 hr of acute stroke are critical. An expansive and detailed evaluation may not be appropriate during the hyperacute phase. Rapid, efficient clinical examination, and diagnostic evaluation are necessary to deliver acute therapies in a timely fashion. Evaluations of increasing details can be performed at later stages to help formulate long-term treatment and prevention strategies. The management of acute stroke during the first 24 hr involves a chain of succeeding healthcare providers including ambulance personnel, emergency department (ED) physicians, neurologists, and nursing staff. Prehospital stroke evaluation and management in the field are covered in detail in the earlier chapters. This chapter focuses on in-hospital management.

The major goal of acute stroke management is resuscitation of the penumbral tissue to minimize the neurological deficits. If reperfusion of the penumbra occurs rapidly, neurons recover and the patient improves. With no reperfusion, a time-related cascade converts ailing neurons in salvageable penumbral tissue to permanent infarction. In order to achieve this goal, the management of acute stroke patients during the first 24 hr should aim to

1. stabilize the patient medical condition;
2. confirm the diagnosis of stroke rapidly and efficiently;
3. utilize laboratory and examination data to determine the best treatment option(s); and
4. prevent stroke worsening and complications.

Hospital door – ED phase

Once a patient with suspected stroke or Transient ischemic attack (TIA) has arrived at the ED, rapid triage and evaluation are of paramount importance.

The stroke team should be activated (if not already notified while the patient was en route), especially if the patient arrives within the time window for thrombolysis or other ongoing experimental therapies. It may even be worthwhile to activate the stroke team for all patients with suspected TIA to ensure adequate and timely evaluation of these patients who are at high risk for recurrent stroke. Management in the ED should proceed along the following steps, in parallel:

1. Place the patient in a telemetry monitored bed.
2. Check vital signs
   a) Administer supplemental oxygen (if needed).
   b) Do not treat high blood pressure, at this point in time, unless the suspicion for Intracerebral Hemorrhage (ICH) or aortic dissection is extremely high.
   c) Significant hypotension should always be treated.
   d) Always treat fever (if present).

1. Obtain a peripheral intravenous access.
2. Check glucose finger stick (if not done in the field).
3. Obtain a 12-lead electrocardiogram.
4. Send the following routine laboratory tests:
   a) Complete blood count.
   b) Electrolytes, renal functions (BUN and creatinine), and glucose.
   c) Coagulation studies (PT, PTT, and INR).
   d) Cardiac enzymes (CK, CK-MB, and troponin).

1. Obtain a focused history. Pay particular attention to the following key elements:
   a) Establishing the time of stroke onset (the last time the patient was known to be in his/her usual state of health) is important, as it determines available treatment options and the pace of subsequent evaluations and resources activation.
   b) Medications (anticoagulants, in particular).
   c) Exclusion criteria for intravenous thrombolysis (see Table 10.1).

1. Perform physical and neurological examinations. The initial examination should be focused, with particular attention to the following key elements:
   a) Level of consciousness.
   b) Severity and pattern of neurological deficits.
   c) Auscultation of the heart and carotid arteries.
   d) Fundus/visual fields.

1. Determine patient's weight.

Table 10.1: Summary of inclusion and exclusion criteria for IV t-PA in patients with acute ischemic stroke

Inclusion criteria
  Stroke onset-to-needle time <3 hr
  No evidence of ICH on CT/MRI
  A measurable deficit on examination, as assessed by NIHSS
Exclusion criteria
  Absolute
    History of stroke or serious head trauma within the prior 3 months
    Prior history of intracranial hemorrhage
    Major surgery within 14 days
    Pregnancy
    Persistent SBP > 185 or DBP > 110
    Platelets < 100,000
    INR > 1.7 if on warfarin – elevated PTT if on heparin
  Relative (depends on availability of advanced imaging techniques, stroke severity, and examiner's and patient's preferences)
    Genitourinary or gastrointestinal bleeding within the previous 21 days
    Arterial puncture or lumbar puncture within 7 days
    Improving stroke symptoms
    Seizure at stroke onset
    Serum glucose < 50 or > 400 mg/l
    NIHSS score < 4 or > 22

Neurological evaluation

Acute neurological evaluation and management of patients with stroke-like symptoms should be divided into four phases:

➡ Suspecting the diagnosis of stroke
➡ Confirming the diagnosis
➡ Determining stroke type and most likely etiology
➡ Determining the best treatment option(s)

The evaluation should proceed in a parallel, multistep manner, with minimal delay if any, to answer the following questions:

1. Are the patient's deficits attributed to a stroke or not (i.e., rule out stroke mimics)?
2. Is the patient a potential candidate for acute treatment (i.e., is the patient within the therapeutic time window)?
3. If it is a stroke, what is the stroke type (i.e., hemorrhagic versus non-hemorrhagic)?

4. Is the patient eligible for reperfusion therapy (i.e., does he/she meet all inclusion and none of the exclusion criteria for thrombolysis?), in case of a nonhemorrhagic stroke?
5. Does the patient require immediate surgical intervention, in case of a hemorrhagic stroke?
6. What is the suspected etiology for the stroke?

The diagnostic workup for stroke patients during the hyperacute phase should include

1. routine blood tests to determine eligibility for thrombolysis, and to exclude metabolic and infectious mimics of stroke;
2. brain imaging (computed tomography [CT] or magnetic resonance imaging [MRI]) to determine lesion location, its nature, and vascular distribution;
3. vascular imaging (CT angiography [CTA], MR angiography [MRA], ultrasound, or angiography) to determine the presence and location of arterial stenosis/occlusion;
4. cardiac evaluation (telemetry and ECG) to assess for heart disease or arrhythmias; and
5. additional tests may be required on a patient-by-patient basis.

Confirming the diagnosis of stroke

A few laboratory studies and brain imaging are always required during the initial evaluation of patients with suspected stroke. The results serve to rule out other conditions that can mimic stroke, provide clues to stroke etiology, guide the choice of subsequent tests, assist with therapeutic decision making, or reveal abnormalities that may require treatment or further work-up. These tests are especially valuable when the history is vague or inconclusive.

Laboratory tests

In addition to the list of routine laboratory studies mentioned above, a chest x-ray should be obtained in all stroke patients. Chest x-ray may show a widened mediastinum indicative of aortic dissection that can mimic stroke, a neoplastic process, pulmonary edema, or pneumonia requiring treatment.

The following laboratory studies are not routinely required during the hyperacute phase of stroke evaluation, but may be recommended on a case-by-case basis. These may serve an important role in determining stroke etiology and eligibility for thrombolytic therapy (if indicated):

1. Blood and urine toxicology screen.
2. Hypercoagulability assays. An assessment for a hypercoagulable state is recommended during the hyperacute phase only in young stroke patients, without apparent risk factors or with a personal/family history

of repeated miscarriages or vascular embolic events, in whom thrombolysis or anticoagulation is contemplated to avoid the confounding
effects of these therapies on test results.
a) Antithrombin III
b) Protein S and C
c) G20210A prothrombin gene mutation
d) Antiphospholipid antibodies (anticardiolipin antibody and lupus
    anticoagulant)
e) Factor V Leiden
3. Stool hemoccult.
4. Pregnancy test. Pregnancy test should be obtained in all women with
    child-bearing potential, since a positive result may influence the deci-
    sion making regarding the choice of imaging modality (CT versus MRI)
    and utility of intravenous thrombolysis. Generally speaking, CT and
    intravenous thrombolysis should be avoided in pregnant women.
5. Urine analysis.
6. Blood cultures (if endocarditis is suspected).
7. Lumbar puncture. Brain imaging, either CT or MRI, may miss small
    Subarachnoid hemorrhage (SAH) Therefore, lumbar puncture may be
    required during the hyperacute phase to confirm or exclude this
    diagnosis, in cases where the clinical suspicion is high.

Neuroimaging

Early triage of patients with acute stroke, as soon as possible, to brain CT or
MRI is a fundamental branch point in the evaluation. Imaging of the brain
parenchyma is crucial to exclude or confirm the presence of cerebral
hemorrhage. Early diagnosis of brain hemorrhage can be life saving. Brain
imaging also serves to exclude other conditions that mimic stroke or con-
traindicate thrombolysis, such as brain tumors, and to assess the extent of
brain injury. Advanced CT and MRI imaging, employing perfusion and/or
diffusion techniques, can provide additional information to identify brain
tissue that is potentially salvageable, allowing for better selection of patients
who are likely to benefit from reperfusion therapy particularly after the 3-hr
time window for thrombolysis. Imaging of the cerebral and cervical vasculature can identify the vascular lesion responsible for cerebral ischemia,
and may influence treatment strategy.

Both noncontrast CT and MRI with gradient-echo, susceptibility-
weighted images are highly sensitive for diagnosing brain hemorrhage in the
acute setting. The choice of the first imaging modality and additional use of
advanced and vascular imaging techniques varies from center to center
depending upon availability and specific clinical scenarios.

Careful inspection of location, size, and distribution of infarcts on CT or
MRI may help determine stroke cause and subtype. Visualization of

numerous infarcts in various arterial territories may suggest a proximal source for embolization. Similarly, identification of ipsilateral MCA and ACA ischemic lesions may indicate an underlying carotid artery occlusive disease. Small subcortical deep infarcts (lacunes) are usually located within the blood supply of a single penetrating artery. Cortical and cerebellar infarcts are usually embolic.

CT versus MRI in evaluation of hyperacute stroke

Although MRI has advantages over CT in stroke diagnosis, the utility of CT is probably of equal value to MRI in most patients presenting within 3 hr from stroke symptom onset.

1. A plain CT excluding hemorrhage and stroke mimics would suffice to assist thrombolysis decision making
2. However, MRI during the acute evaluation can play an important role in the following scenarios:
   a) cases where the diagnosis of stroke is in doubt.
   b) patients with history of prior stroke presenting with recurrent or worsening ipsilateral symptoms.
   c) cases where seizures occur at stroke onset.
   d) cases where focal deficits are associated with metabolic derangements such as blood sugar <50 or >300 mg/dl.
   e) TIA or rapidly resolving deficits.

Multimodal MRI with DWI, PWI, and T2*-weighted imaging, and MRA can help to confirm the diagnosis of new stroke in these various scenarios, thus extending the potential benefit of thrombolysis to patients who would have otherwise been excluded based on CT results alone. I recommend multimodal MRI in these situations, even in patients presenting within 3 hr of symptom onset.

Consideration for diffusion-perfusion MRI or perfusion CT, depending on availability, as first imaging modality should also be given to stroke patients who present between 3 and 9 hr of symptom onset. Thrombolysis, intravenous or intraarterial, may be an option in these patients, if the studies show a significant brain tissue at risk of infarction.

Vascular imaging

Wherever possible, dedicated noninvasive, vascular imaging studies (CTA, MRA, or ultrasound) of the intracranial and extracranial vessels should be performed during the initial evaluation of patients with suspected stroke- or TIA-like symptoms, especially in patients with recent TIA or rapidly resolving deficits. However, these tests should not delay initiation of treatment, if thrombolysis is contemplated.

The findings on exam and brain imaging should guide the choice of the vascular imaging modality. For example, duplex ultrasound of the neck may not be appropriate if the symptoms and infarcts are within the posterior circulation. Instead, MRA or CTA of the neck are preferable. Similarly, MRA of the head and neck with fat-suppressed images or CTA may be required in cases with high suspicion for arterial dissection.

These studies can provide valuable information regarding the site of arterial occlusion, if any, and may be important for therapeutic decision making. There is evidence that recanalization rates after intravenous versus intraarterial thrombolysis may differ depending upon the site of the arterial occlusion. For example, ICA occlusive lesions may recanalize less frequently after IV t-PA than intraarterial therapy.

Conventional angiography is rarely required during the acute phase of stroke evaluation. It is usually reserved for situations where intraarterial thrombolysis or mechanical clot disruption are contemplated in case of nonhemorrhagic strokes, diagnosis and coiling of cerebral aneurysm in case of SAH, or for follow-up when the above noninvasive studies are inconclusive.

Acute treatment(s) for Ischemic stroke in the first 24 hr

Once the working diagnosis of ischemic stroke is established, a decision will have to be made regarding suitable acute treatment options, and patient's eligibility for reperfusion therapy, which includes

⇒ IV thrombolysis (rt-PA)
⇒ IA thrombolysis
⇒ endovascular treatment – mechanical disruption of the clot
⇒ combination therapy
⇒ hypertensive therapy

The details of these various reperfusion strategies are covered elsewhere in this book. Table 10.1 lists all eligibility criteria for treatment of acute ischemic stroke with intravenous rt-PA, and is a fundamental branching point in decision making.

IV thrombolysis (rt-PA)

If an acute stroke patient fulfills all of the above inclusion and none of the absolute exclusion criteria, treatment with IV rt-PA at a dose of 0.9 mg/kg (maximum dose of 90 mg), with a 10 percent bolus over 1 min and the remainder of the dose over 60 min, should be considered in most cases.

IA thrombolysis

At present, no evidence is available to show that intra-arterial (IA) rt-PA is superior to IV treatment. Therapy should not be withheld from patients who are eligible for IV treatment so that medications can be administered IA.

IA is particularly helpful when IV is contraindicated, for example, in post-operative stroke. Patients are treated within a 6-hr window for anterior circulation strokes. This extends to 12–24 hr for basilar artery occlusion.

IV/IA combination therapy

An IV/IA rt-PA bridging approach is currently being evaluated in a multi-center trial. The IV rt-PA bolus is followed by 6.5 mg/kg and a cerebral angiogram. IA rt-PA may then be administered if there is evidence of persistent vascular occlusion. I currently reserve combined IV/IA rescue therapy for acute stroke patients with carotid occlusive lesions.

Mechanical disruption of the clot

This approach can be used in conjunction with IA thrombolysis and is helpful when IV is contraindicated, for example, in postoperative stroke, patients taking warfarin and pregnant women. Other promising new reper-fusion therapies are Desmoteplase, a plasminogen activator; Abciximab, a glycoprotein (GP) IIb/IIIa receptor inhibitor; use of external TCD; permissive hypertensive therapy; and high-dose albumin. These are ongoing active investigations.

In patients who are not eligible for any of the above acute reperfusion therapies:

1. Acute use of aspirin 160–300 mg daily, orally or rectally, is recommended unless there is a clear contraindication;
2. The use of intravenous heparin during the first 24 hr of acute ischemic stroke is rarely indicated. Its use may be reserved to
   a) patients with known source of embolism who present with ischemic stroke in the setting of subtherapeutic INR;
   b) patients with arterial dissection;
   c) patients with venous sinus thrombosis;
   d) patients with fluctuating deficits and documented large vessel stenosis as a bridge to definite surgical or endovascular intervention.
3. The decision of whether or not to continue anticoagulation therapy during the acute phase in patients who present with hemorrhagic transformation of ischemic stroke while on warfarin should be made on a patient-by-patient basis in view of the risk for recurrent embolism versus hemorrhage expansion. Most experts recommend withholding anticoagulation for 7–10 days.

The following general principles apply to the management of all stroke patients during the first 24 hr and subsequent days:

1. Admit to stroke unit (telemetry monitored bed).
2. Start an intravenous fluid drip.

3. Monitor vital signs and neurological examination.
4. Avoid arterial punctures, central venous lines, indwelling bladder catheters, nasogastric tube, antiplatelets, and anticoagulants for the first 24 hr in patients who receive thrombolytic therapy

Management of hydration and fluid status

1. Use isotonic crystalloids [0.9 percent NS]
2. Avoid hypovolemia in embolic and carotid strokes.
3. Hypotonic fluids (0.45 percent saline or D5W] aggravate cerebral edema and should be avoided.
4. Avoid hypervolemia in hemorrhagic or large strokes.

Management of fever

1. Fever worsens the neurologic outcome.
2. Fever should be treated aggressively with cooling blanket + Tylenol.

Management of blood sugar

1. Hyperglycemia promotes anaerobic metabolism and lactic acidosis within the ischemic tissue, thus worsening outcome; increasing the risk of hemorrhagic transformation after thrombolysis
2. Glucose should be <200 mg/dl (ideally, 150 mg/dl)
3. Management of hyperglycemia is best done by insulin sliding scale.

Management of blood pressure

The management of blood pressure is detailed in another chapter. Below is a summary of the key principles for blood pressure management during the first 24 hr of ischemic stroke onset:

1. Hypertension (HTN) in the setting of stroke is common. It often spontaneously resolves/improves over time.
2. High BP should not be treated within the first 24 hr after ischemic stroke, unless SBP > 220, DBP > 120, or mean BP >130 mmHg. However, there are two exceptions:
   a) Use of rt-PA: blood pressure should be lowered and maintained at <185/110 mmHg.
   b) Presence of myocardial infarction, aortic dissection, or heart failure.
3. Short-acting drugs, such as labetalol (IV drip), are preferred.
4. In non-rt-PA candidates, *do not* attempt to lower BP in the acute setting in patients with ischemic stroke without knowing the status of major cerebral vasculature.
   a) Areas of ischemia have pressure-dependent flow. Overly aggressive treatment to lower BP can decrease cerebral perfusion and lead to worsening of stroke.

b) The minimum cerebral perfusion pressure needed to maintain adequate cerebral perfusion is >55–60 mmHg, which corresponds a mean arterial pressure (MAP) of approximately 110–130 mmHg. Significantly low blood pressure should be treated in patients with ischemic stroke to maintain a MAP of 100–130 mmHg. In selected patients, pressor-induced hypertension (in 10 percent increments) may improve blood flow and lessen neurological consequences of stroke

In conclusion, the first 24 hr of stroke are critical in determining the patient's outcome. Acting quickly and efficiently, together with the use of advanced imaging and endovascular technology, can extend various treatment options to a larger number of patients to minimize the disability, complications, and mortality attributed to their strokes.

Bibliography

A systems approach to immediate evaluation and management of hyperacute stroke. Experience at eight centers and implications for community practice and patient care. The National Institute of Neurological Disorders and Stroke (NINDS) rt-PA Stroke Study Group. *Stroke* 1997;28(8):1530–40.

Adams H, Adams R, Del Zoppo G, Goldstein L B, Stroke Council of the American Heart Association, and American Stroke Association. Guidelines for the early management of patients with ischemic stroke: 2005 guidelines update a scientific statement from the Stroke Council of the American Heart Association/American Stroke Association. *Stroke* 2005;36(4):916–23.

Adams HP Jr, Adams RJ, Brott T, et al. Stroke Council of the American Stroke Association. Guidelines for the early management of patients with ischemic stroke: A scientific statement from the Stroke Council of the American Stroke Association. *Stroke* 2003;34(4):1056–83.

Alkawi A, Kirmani JF, Janjua N, et al. Advances in thrombolytics and mechanical devices for treatment of acute ischemic stroke. *Neurol Res* 2005;27(Suppl 1):S42–9.

Davalos A. Thrombolysis in acute ischemic stroke: Successes, failures, and new hopes. *Cerebrovasc Dis* 2005;20(Suppl 2):135–9.

Molina CA, Saver JL. Extending reperfusion therapy for acute ischemic stroke: Emerging pharmacological, mechanical, and imaging strategies. *Stroke* 2005;36 (10):2311–20.

Murugappan A, Coplin WM, Al-Sadat AN, et al. Thrombolytic therapy of acute ischemic stroke during pregnancy. *Neurology* 2006;66(5):768–70.

Selim M, Kumar S, Fink J, Schlaug G, Caplan LR, Linfante I. Seizure at stroke onset: Should it be an absolute contraindication to thrombolysis? *Cerebrovasc Dis* 2002;14(1):54–7.

Szabo K Lanczik O, Hennerici MG. Vascular diagnosis and acute stroke: What, when and why not? *Cerebrovasc Dis* 2005;20(Suppl 2):11–18.

11 Ischemic stroke beyond the first 24 hr

Eric Bershad and Jose I. Suarez

Introduction

Acute stroke treatment has changed tremendously in recent years as it continues to evolve from the nihilistic approach of yesterday to the active approach of today. After the hyperacute stage of stroke ends, the astute clinician needs to maintain continued vigilance to protect the patient from further ischemic injury. Specific neuroprotective measures must be instituted. The acute stroke patient faces a potential myriad of medical complications that must be managed efficiently. Thus, acute stroke management requires the clinician to take an interactive approach to enhance the patient's chances for a good long-term outcome.

In this chapter, we review the management of acute ischemic stroke from the time after the hyper acute phase (>24 hr) to hospital discharge. We address important factors that may significantly impact upon the patient's clinical outcome:

1. The role of a stroke unit or neuroscience critical care unit (neuro-ICU).
2. Neuroprotective measures including management of blood pressure (BP), temperature and hyperglycemia, airway management, and treatment of cerebral edema and elevated intracranial pressure (ICP).
3. The role of pharmacological management of stroke patients including the use of antithrombotics and statins in the acute hospital setting.
4. Institution of early nutrition and rehabilitation.
5. Prevention of pneumonia, deep venous thrombosis (DVT), urinary tract infection (UTI), and decubitus ulcers.
6. The utility of various surgical modalities in the treatment of the acute stroke patient.

Stroke centers and acute stroke units

Growing evidence supports the institution of comprehensive stroke centers to facilitate care for patients with acute stroke.

1. The Stroke Unit Trialists' Collaboration demonstrated that an organized stroke unit reduced the long-term mortality (OR 0.83), combined outcomes of death or dependency (OR 0.69), and death or institutionalization (OR 0.75). It also resulted in a shorter length of stay (LOS).

2. A Cochrane Database review found that organized stroke unit care provided by multidisciplinary teams improved long-term outcomes in stroke patients as compared to standard stroke care. At 1-year follow-up, significant reductions were found in odds of death (OR 0.86), odds of death or institutionalized care (OR 0.80), and death or dependency (OR 0.78).

3. The Stroke Care Outcomes: Providing Effective Services (SCOPES) group found that institution of organized stroke units in Australian hospitals allowed for significantly greater adherence to "standard processes of care" than hospitals providing conventional stroke care. Patients had significantly improved odds of surviving after hospital discharge when clinicians followed standard processes of care.

Neurointensive care unit

Many acute stroke patients develop complications that require management in a neuro-ICU. Some of the more common indications for ICU admission include BP management, control of cerebral edema and elevated ICP, and ventilatory support. The availability of a specialized neurocritical care team is associated with a significant reduction of in-hospital mortality and LOS in critically ill neurology and neurosurgical patients. Furthermore, the admission of critically ill acute ischemic stroke patients to a neurointensivist run neuro-ICU improves resource utilization while also improving outcome upon hospital discharge.

BP management

A large proportion of acute ischemic stroke patients, ranging from 69 to 84 percent, initially present to the hospital with elevated BP. In the first few days poststroke, BP usually declines in most patients spontaneously.

The reasons for elevated BP after acute ischemic stroke are multifactorial:

➤ A previous history of hypertension
➤ Abnormalities of the hypothalamic-pituitary-adrenal axis
➤ Endogenous catecholamine release
➤ "White-coat hypertension" effect
➤ Prior alcohol intake

Controversy exists over the management of BP in the acute setting of ischemic stroke. However, data suggests that the acute lowering of BP may

Table 11.1: Approach to elevated BP in acute ischemic stroke

BP level (mmHg)	Treatment if <u>not eligible</u> for thrombolytic therapy
Systolic ≤220 or diastolic ≤120	Observe unless other end-organ involvement (e.g., aortic dissection, acute myocardial infarction, pulmonary edema, hypertensive encephalopathy) Treat other symptoms of stroke (e.g., headache, pain, agitation, nausea, vomiting) Treat other acute complications of stroke, including hypoxia, increased ICP, seizures, or hypoglycemia
Systolic ≤220 or diastolic 121–140	Labetalol 10–20 mg IV over 1–2 min May repeat or double every 10 min (max dose 300 mg) or Nicardipine 5 mg/hr IV infusion as initial dose; titrate to desired effect by increasing 2.5 mg/hr every 5 min to max of 15 mg/hr Aim for a 10–15% reduction in BP
Diastolic >140	Nitroprusside 0.5 µg/kg/ min IV infusion as initial dose with continuous BP monitoring Aim for a 10–15% reduction in BP

Source: Adapted from Adams (2005).

worsen neurological outcome. Table 11.1 summarises the American Heart recommendations for BP management. After acute ischemic stroke, cerebral autoregulation mechanisms may fail and Central blood flow (CBF) then becomes directly related to the mean arterial pressure (MAP). Thus, a drop in the MAP will further reduce the already compromised CBF to the ischemic penumbra and may increase infarct size.

1. Early death increased by 17.9 percent for every 10 mmHg drop in systolic BP below 150 mmHg.
2. Ischemic stroke patients presenting to the emergency room with BP of less than 155/70 mmHg had double the mortality rate within 90 days (RR 2.2) as compared to patients with moderately elevated BP (155–220)/(70–105) mmHg.
3. In a trial of nimodipine for hypertension in acute stroke, the use of IV nimodipine was associated with higher risk of death or dependency (OR 10.16) compared to placebo-treated patients when BP fell by more than 20 percent.

An excessively elevated BP in acute stroke may also worsen patient outcome. In the analysis of the International Stroke Trial, early death increased by 3.8

percent for every 10 mmHg systolic BP increase above 150 mmHg. A recent phase II prospective randomized placebo-controlled trial found that, candesartan, an angiotensive I receptor blocking agent, given during the acute setting of ischemic stroke in excessively hypertensive patients may have a beneficial effect on mortality and reduction of vascular events in the long term.

Hypotension and hydration

Although not common, acute stroke patients may present with hypotension. The clinician must adequately hydrate these patients to protect the ischemic penumbra. Furthermore, one must identify the cause of hypotension. Potential causes may include

- aortic dissection
- sepsis
- acute blood loss
- myocardial infarction or cardiomyopathy

We routinely hydrate all ischemic stroke patients initially with normal saline at 75–100 cc/hr. This helps ensure adequate perfusion to the ischemic penumbra and may prevent extension of an infarct.

1. One should avoid hypotonic solutions as these may lead to increased cerebral edema.
2. Once patients have demonstrated stable BP and maintain adequate oral hydration, intravenous fluids can be discontinued.

In some cases, it may be necessary to induce hypertension with vasopressor agents if hydration alone is not adequate.

1. We prefer phenylephrine, an alpha-adrenergic agonist, to raise the BP to a level that is at least at the patient's baseline. In some cases it may be necessary to raise the BP even further, if it is determined that the patient is having "pressure-dependent" symptoms.
2. For example, a patient with an ischemic stroke in a border-zone territory related to a critically stenosed ipsilateral carotid artery may become symptomatic only if the MAP drops below a critical level. If pressure dependence is found, we titrate the BP to an MAP of about 10–20 percent above the threshold level that produces the ischemic symptoms. Note that there is no solid randomized literature to support the safety of induced hypertension in stroke patients.

Prevention of DVT and pulmonary embolism

DVT occurs very frequently in stroke patients and may lead to a fatal pulmonary embolism.

1. DVT is found in 50 percent of acute stroke patients within the first 2 weeks in the absence of heparin prophylaxis.
2. Peak incidence of DVT occurs within the first week after stroke.
3. About 3 percent of stroke patients will die from a pulmonary embolus (PE) within 3 months of the initial stroke. This makes up about 13–25 percent of all cases of early mortality after stroke.
4. Peak incidence of PE occurs 2–4 weeks poststroke.

Both pharmacological and mechanical methods can help prevent DVT.

➠ Unfractionated heparin (UFH)
➠ Low-molecular weight heparin (LMWH)
➠ Elastic compression stockings
➠ Intermittent pneumatic compression devices

DVT prophylaxis using combination therapy with anticoagulation, elastic stockings, and pneumatic sequential compression devices may reduce risk of DVT by 40-fold. In our institution, we institute DVT prophylaxis for all immobile stroke patients with low-dose heparin SQ anticoagulation (5,000 units q8–q12 hr), elastic compression stockings, and pneumatic compression devices.

1. Duration of anticoagulant or mechanical prophylaxis required to prevent DVT and PE is unclear.
2. Continuing prophylaxis for 2–4 weeks after a stroke or until the patient is fully mobilized seems prudent.

The clinician must actively search for DVT in stroke patients with an unexplained fever or local symptoms of leg swelling, pain, or redness. Ultrasound scanning noninvasively detects symptomatic DVT with high sensitivity and specificity; however it has low sensitivity for the detection of asymptomatic DVT. The D-dimer has high sensitivity (97 percent) for DVT, but very low specificity (35–45 percent), and provides no localizing information. MR venography, can directly visualize DVT and also detect pelvic vein thrombosis, an area not imaged by ultrasound; however, this technique is relatively expensive.

The diagnosis of PE in stroke patients requires a high index of suspicion, coupled with key clinical findings.

1. Some of the red flags for PE include dyspnea, cough, chest pain or discomfort, hemoptysis, or hypotension.
2. Some of the more common clinical exam findings include tachypnea, rales, tachycardia, and fever; however, the patient may be asymptomatic.
3. The arterial blood may show hypoxemia, hypocapnia, and respiratory alkalosis. The EKG may show sinus tachycardia or evidence of right heart strain.

4. The diagnostic imaging test of choice in stable patients with suspected PE is a CT angiogram of the pulmonary vessels.
5. A ventilation/perfusion scan may be obtained if a CT angiogram is not obtainable.
6. We do not recommend the use of anticoagulation in patients with hemorrhagic stroke, or in patients with an acute stroke larger than one-third of the middle cerebral artery territory. In this setting, the placement of an inferior vena cava filter should be considered.

Maintenance of normoglycemia

Hyperglycemia occurs in about 20–40 percent of acute stroke patients. Many of these patients are not previously diabetic. Investigators do not yet understand the factors resulting in hyperglycemia in the acute phase of stroke; however, stress is not thought to play a major role. Initial hyperglycemia portends a worse outcome in acute ischemic stroke patients. Glucose levels >140 mg/dl were found to be associated with worse neurological outcome.

The management of hyperglycemia in acute ischemic stroke patients is controversial, however strong prospective randomized data supports tight glucose management in some critically ill patients.

1. Based on the available data, we choose an aggressive approach to control hyperglycemia in our institution.
2. We adapted the continuous intravenous insulin protocol used by Krinsley (2004) (Table 11.2).
3. We found the protocol to be easily instituted and highly effective in maintaining strict glucose control in the neuro-ICU setting. Once we transfer ischemic stroke patients out of the neuro-ICU, we use a traditional insulin sliding scale to control glucose.

Temperature control: Normothermia or hypothermia

The clinician must strictly manage hyperthermia in acute ischemic stroke as it may worsen outcome.

1. In a retrospective analysis of 110 patients with acute ischemic stroke, temperature above 37.5°C predicted more severe symptoms.
2. In a recent prospective study of 390 consecutive acute stroke patients, admission hyperthermia strongly correlated with initial stroke severity, infarct size, mortality, and poor outcome.
3. For each 1°C increase in temperature, mortality increased by 2.2-fold.

Table 11.2: University Hospitals of Cleveland Neurosciences Critical Care Unit Protocol for hyperglycemia, management

Goal: The goal of the protocol is to maintain serum glucose <120 mg/dl. Monitoring: Serum glucose levels will be monitored through fingerstick testing, or if available, blood testing in the lab, every 4 hr.
Treatment of hyperglycemia (on first evaluation of the serum glucose in the neurointensive care unit)

Glucose value (mg/dl)	Action (subcutaneous insulin dose)
<120	None
120–140	2 units subcutaneous regular insulin; recheck serum glucose in 4 hr
140–169	3 units; recheck in 4 hr
170–199	4 units; recheck in 4 hr
200–249	6 units; recheck in 4 hr
250–299	8 units; recheck in 4 hr
≥ 300	10 units; recheck in 4 hr

If glucose value is greater than 140 mg/dl on three successive measurements, then the continuous insulin drip should be started. Monitoring of serum glucose will be hourly while the patient is maintained on an insulin drip.
Management of the insulin infusion (drip)
Initial infusion rate

Glucose value (mg/dl)	Insulin drip rate (units/hr)
140–169	2
170–199	3
200–249	4
250–299	6
300–399	8
≥400	10

Progressive management, as determined by the serum glucose level every hour

<140	Stop infusion and recheck in 1 hr a low dose (<2 units/hr) may be continued to avoid rebound hyperglycemia, as determined by the judgment of the treating physician
140–169	2
170–199	3
200–249	4
250–299	6
300–399	8

(continued)

Table 11.2: *(continued)*

Glucose value (mg/dl)	Insulin drip rate (units/hr)
≥400	10

Instruction to nursing will be that should this protocol either
not l ead to a decrease in the patient's serum glucose level or if
the protocol causes dramatic and rapid shifts in the glucose level (such
as serum glucose fluctuating every 1–2 hr between hypoglycemia,
<80 mg/dl, and extreme hyperglycemia, >400 mg/dl), the treating
physician should be contacted.

Hyperthermic-related ischemic damage probably occurs by multiple mechanisms:

1. Facilitation of toxic neurotransmitters such as glutamate.
2. Oxygen free-radical production.
3. Worsening of blood-brain barrier opening, ischemic membrane depolarizations, and cytoskeletal degradation.

Normothermia or hypothermia in acute ischemic stroke patients can be achieved through different means:

⟹ administration of antipyretics
⟹ passive or active external cooling
⟹ internal endovascular cooling

Reported use of hypothermia:

⟹ malignant ischemic middle cerebral artery (MCA) stroke
⟹ severe ischemic stroke NIHSS >19

In several small pilot studies, hypothermia induction to 32–33°C may have been successful in lowering ICP but improving long-term clinical outcome remains controversial. Potential complications with hypothermia:

⟹ pneumonia
⟹ bradycardia
⟹ ventricular ectopy
⟹ hypotension
⟹ melena
⟹ infection
⟹ myocardial infarction

Despite a clear association between hyperthermia and poor outcome in acute ischemic stroke patients, it is unknown whether aggressive treatment to lower body temperature will improve clinical outcome. Although, there is solid data to support the use of hypothermia in global cerebral ischemia following cardiac arrest, we consider the use of hypothermia in acute ischemic stroke patients experimental and do not routinely employ it in our institution. Our protocol consists of the following:

1. Aggressively lowering temperature to maintain normothermia in all acute ischemic stroke patients.
2. Use a threshold of 37.5°C to initiate treatment.
3. Start with acetaminophen 650 mg every 4–6 hr. If temperature persists, we initiate external cooling

The underlying cause of a fever must always be thoroughly investigated. An exhaustive search should be made before attributing a fever to a medication effect or a central cause. Potential causes of fever include

➠ chemical aspiration pneumonia and other respiratory infection
➠ UTIs or line infections
➠ viral infections
➠ cndocarditis
➠ DVT or pulmonary embolism
➠ drug fever, blood product reaction
➠ cocaine intoxication
➠ retroperitoneal hemorrhage
➠ central fever

Initial diagnostic modalities for a fever workup include chest roentgenogram (CXR), sputum cultures, urinalysis and culture, and blood cultures. One should send stool for clostridium difficile toxin in patients who have received antibiotics, have diarrhea, or have had a prolonged hospitalization. All lines should be carefully examined for signs of infection. Screening for DVT and PE should also be considered, especially in febrile patients with leg pain or swelling, or hypoxemia. It is also necessary to carefully review all new medications. A skin rash or eosinophilia may suggest a drug fever. Phenytoin and beta-lactamase antibiotics may cause drug fever. In patients with an unexplained decreased level of consciousness and fever, a lumbar puncture is mandatory.

Airway management

Following acute ischemic stroke, approximately 8–10 percent of patients will require mechanical ventilation. Some of the indications may include

➠ decreased level of consciousness
➠ compromised airway integrity
➠ hypoxemic or hypercarbic respiratory failure
➠ management of elevated ICP
➠ elective intubation before angiography or a surgical procedure.

The clinician should intubate the patient promptly after making the decision, as the stroke patient may quickly deteriorate. Before intubation, the clinician should bag-mask the patient to keep $SaO_2 > 97$ percent, administer intravenous 0.9 percent saline to avoid hypotension, and continuously monitor BP. We recommend using a rapid sequence intubation with etomidate, lidocaine, and vecuronium.

1. Etomidate (0.2–0.3 mg/kg) provides short sedation without significantly lowering BP.
2. Intravenous lidocaine (1–2 mg/kg) will help blunt the cough response and thus prevent a dangerous rise in ICP.
3. Vecuronium (0.1 mg/kg), a nondepolarizing neuromuscular blocking agent, provides muscle paralysis for about 30–40 min and has no significant risk of producing elevated ICP.
4. Oral intubation is preferred to nasal intubation due to less risk of nosocomial sinusitis, a risk factor for nosocomial pneumonia.
5. After intubation, one can maintain sedation with short-acting sedatives such as propofol or midazolam.

Initial ventilator settings usually include

1. Assist control (AC) or synchronous intermittent mechanical ventilation (SIMV) of 12, tidal volume (VT) of 6 ml/kg of ideal body weight, positive end-expiratory pressure (PEEP) of 5–10 cm H_2O, and 100 percent oxygenation.
2. PEEP may benefit the patient by improving residual function capacity, lung compliance, and decreasing the risk of developing acute respiratory distress syndrome (ARDS) by preventing alveolar derecruitment.
3. In clinical practice, levels of PEEP from 5 to 15 cm H_2O are not shown to affect ICP or cerebral perfusion pressure (CPP) in critically ill neurological patients.
4. The oxygen should be titrated down from 100 percent as soon as possible. Hyperoxia may increase the production of free radicals and induce cerebral vasoconstriction, which may reduce CBF.

During mechanical ventilation, precautions must be instituted to protect the patient from potentially fatal iatrogenic complications, most notably ventilator-associated pneumonia (VAP). Institution of nonpharmacologic precautions can minimize the risk of VAP. (Table 11.3)

Weaning parameters

1. Ability to maintain good oxygenation ($PaO_2 > 60$ mmHg with $FiO_2 < 50$ percent and PEEP < 5 cm H_2O).
2. Increased level of alertness.
3. Minimal upper airway secretions and possess an adequate cough reflex.
4. Vital capacity > 15 mg/kg.

Table 11.3: Recommended protocol for prevention of VAP in patients requiring mechanical ventilation

---

Handwashing before and after entering patient's room
Maintain adequate staffing levels of nurses and respiratory therapists
Head elevation 30–45° at all times
Chlorhexadine 0.12% oral rinse, 15 ml for 30 s twice daily
Inline continuous suctioning of tracheal secretions
Minimize unnecessary manipulations of the ventilator circuit
Avoid gastric distention by closely monitoring gastric residuals
Wean and extubate patients as soon as feasible

---

5. Patient hemodynamically stable and possesses normal electrolytes.
6. Rapid shallow breathing index (RSBI) should be measured.
   a) RSBI equals the respiratory rate over TV in liters (RR/V_t).
   b) RSBI less than 105 helps predict successful extubation.

The most effective method to help successfully extubate patients may be via spontaneous breathing trials (SBTs). We perform a daily SBT on ventilated patients by switching the mode to continuous positive airway pressure (CPAP). Once patients tolerate CPAP for at least 120 consecutive min, we extubate them.

Cerebral edema and elevated ICP

Following acute ischemic stroke, cerebral edema and elevated ICP may pose a direct threat to the patient's survival. About 10 percent of ischemic stroke patients will have a complete MCA infarction that almost always leads to severe potentially fatal cerebral edema. The clinician must identify and effectively manage these complications to avoid a potentially fatal outcome.

1. The risk of cerebral edema is highest following an occlusion of a large artery such as the internal carotid or middle cerebral artery.
2. The usual peak brain edema occurs between 48 and 72 hr poststroke; however, a subset of patients may deteriorate early.
3. The acute treatment of cerebral edema and elevated ICP following stroke involves a combination of medical and surgical management.
4. Medical management includes controlled hyperventilation, osmotherapy, and neuroprotective measures.

Controlled hyperventilation rapidly reduces the ICP by lowering the arterial carbon dioxide pressure ($PaCO_2$) and causing cerebral vasoconstriction.

1. Effects only last for several hours; thus, hyperventilation serves as only a temporizing measure to prevent neurological deterioration.
2. Target $PaCO_2$ level is controversial, but a level of 28–32 mmHg seems reasonable.

3. Excessive hyperventilation to a $PaCO_2$ below 25 mmHg may result in increasing cerebral ischemia in some patients. The clinician should measure blood gases regularly or use continuous end-tidal-CO_2 monitoring during hyperventilation to avoid this complication.

Osmotherapy for management of cerebral edema and elevated ICP usually begins with mannitol. In the setting of acutely elevated ICP or brain herniation, we use an initial bolus dose of mannitol of 0.5–1 g/kg.

1. Serum osmolality should be checked after 1 hr and then every 4–6 hr with a goal of about 300–320 mOsm/l.
2. Repeat boluses of mannitol 0.25–0.50 g/kg can be given if the serum osmolality is below the target range.
3. The clinician should pay close attention to the urine output and electrolytes during mannitol administration as a profound diuresis may lead to hypotension and cardiovascular collapse if fluid and electrolyte losses are not carefully repleted.
4. Renal failure is a potential risk of mannitol use.
5. In patient with elevated ICP or impending herniation refractory to mannitol, continuous or bolus hypertonic saline to keep serum sodium 145–155 mmol/l may be useful.
6. In patients, with elevated ICP and markedly elevated MAP (>150 mmHg), thiopental may be useful; however, the CPP may also decrease.
7. Corticosteroids, which reduce vasogenic edema, have no role in reducing the predominantly cytotoxic cerebral edema in ischemic stroke patients, and likely worsen outcome due to systemic complications.

Some neuroprotective measures may help limit cerebral edema and ICP elevation.

1. Hyperthermia may worsen cerebral edema, thus close monitoring and treatment is essential.
2. Hyperglycemia must be controlled as it is associated with increased cerebral edema.
3. The head of the bed should generally be elevated to a 30° angle to help lower ICP.
4. The neck should be positioned midline to avoid jugular venous compression, which can worsen ICP.

After instituting urgent medical therapy and neuroprotective measures to reduce cerebral edema and ICP, a definitive surgical decompression must be considered.

1. Hemicraniectomy markedly reduces ICP and can even reverse brain herniation in some cases. The long-term outcome of patients undergoing hemicraniectomy requires further study.
2. In patients with cerebellar infarction, edematous brain may compress the fourth ventricle and lead to fatal hydrocephalus. A ventriculostomy must

be rapidly placed to prevent fatal increases in ICP if hydrocephalus occurs. Furthermore, the edema from a cerebellar stroke can result in downward displacement of the cerebellar tonsils leading to a fatal brainstem compression. A posterior fossa decompression may prevent death in these patients and may lead to a good functional outcome in some.

Nutrition management

Nutrition management is an important issue that is often neglected in the acute stroke patient; however, it has critical importance in helping facilitate a good outcome. Critically ill patients undergo a hypercatabolic state due to the acute stress of their illness. Furthermore, many patients have baseline malnutrition, placing them at an increased risk for infection and complications. Nutritional support in the ICU has been shown to improve wound healing, decrease catabolic response to injury, enhance immune system function, improve gastrointestinal structure and function, and improve clinical outcome.

1. Enteral feeding should be the primary method of feeding for patients with an intact gastrointestinal tract.
2. The timing of when to start enteral feeding is debatable; however, the Canadian Clinical Practice Guidelines for Nutrition Support suggest initiating enteral nutrition in ICU patients within 24–48 hr after admission.
3. Before initiating feeding, the clinician must evaluate the patient's swallowing function to assess the risk of aspiration.
4. In patients with a dysfunctional swallowing mechanism, a Dobhoff or NG tube should be carefully placed and verified with a portable abdominal roentgenogram.
5. All stroke patients receiving enteral feeding should have the head of the bed angled up 30° or higher to help minimize the risk of aspiration.
6. Nursing staff should regularly check gastric residuals in patients receiving tube feedings, as a distended stomach can result in aspiration of contents into the airway.
7. A nutritionist can be helpful in tailoring the nutritional plan for an individual patient, as caloric requirements may vary widely, including amount and type of enteral feeding and whether to give additional nutritional supplementation.

Prevention of pressure ulcers

Stroke patients have an especially strong propensity for developing pressure ulcers in the hospital due to multiple intrinsic factors. These factors may include

➡ immobility
➡ urinary and fecal incontinence

⮚ malnutrition
⮚ impaired sensation
⮚ diminished level of consciousness
⮚ increased age

In addition to the intrinsic factors of the patient, several important extrinsic mechanisms lead to pressure ulcers including pressure, friction, shearing, and moisture. Complications of pressure ulcers include pain, cellulitis, osteomyelitis, and sepsis. Sepsis may lead to endocarditis, septic arthritis, abscesses, and death.

Prevention of pressure ulcers requires a multifaceted approach:

1. Frequent turning and careful repositioning of patients every 2 hr to avoid prolonged pressure on bony prominences.
2. Pillows under the calves should be placed to avoid heel pressure.
3. A low degree of head elevation can minimize shearing forces.
4. The use of specialized pressure-reducing bed mattresses lowers the incidence and severity of pressure ulcers.
5. Moisture from urine, stool, and perspiration can lead to breakdown of skin integrity. Meticulous attention should be directed toward maintaining dry skin. A moisture barrier using transparent adhesive dressings or a moisture barrier with petroleum jelly or a liquid spray may be helpful after skin cleansing.
6. A careful skin inspection should be made daily. The skin should be cleansed at regular intervals and every time it is soiled. Hot water and drying soaps should be avoided.
7. Early mobilization and physical therapy will help reduce the incidence of pressure ulcers.

Prevention of UTIs

UTI occurs frequently in acute stroke patients with an incidence of about 15–20 percent. An indwelling Foley catheter carries about a 5-percent daily risk of developing bacteruria in hospitalized patients. We recommend limiting the use of an indwelling urinary catheter to patients requiring strict fluid management. The indwelling catheter should be removed as soon as possible.

Early poststroke seizures

Early seizures, within 1 week of acute ischemic stroke occur in about 2–6 percent of patients. Independent risk factors for early poststroke seizures include a cortical location and worse initial stroke severity. The stroke subtype does not appear to be an independent risk factor for early poststroke seizure.

1. Most early poststroke seizures (50–90 percent) are reported to be simple partial seizures; however, complex partial seizures may be underreported due to lack of detection of the seizure. One study reported a high frequency (50 percent) of generalized tonic-clonic seizures.

2. There are no randomized controlled data to help clinicians decide whether anticonvulsants should be started after one isolated seizure. Furthermore, there are no strong data to guide the choice of what anticonvulsant to use. Some retrospective data suggest that dilantin, phenobarbital, and benzodiazepines may interfere with poststroke recover (Gubitz et al., 2000). We generally prefer to use the newer generation anticonvulsants such as oxcarbazepine, levetiracetam, topiramate, or lamotrigine due to a more favorable side-effect profile and less drug interactions.

Early rehabilitation

The clinician should plan for rehabilitation as soon as possible in the stroke patient. Multiple randomized controlled studies support early rehabilitation and hospital discharge in medically stable stroke patients. We advocate early discharge planning of stroke patients for rehabilitation services.

1. It is important to stress to the patient and family the importance of early rehabilitation in enhancing the patient's long-term functional outcome.

2. A social worker and rehabilitation team can help facilitate the creation of an appropriate outpatient rehabilitation plan.

3. The possible options for rehabilitation include home, outpatient, and acute or subacute rehabilitation.

Early antithrombotics

Anticoagulation versus antiplatelet agents

After elucidation of the mechanism of stroke, the clinician must institute measures to reduce the incidence of a recurrent stroke. Antithrombotic therapy usually includes either anticoagulation or antiplatelet agents. The role of antithrombotic therapy in the acute stroke period is controversial. The clinician often ponders whether to start the patient on antithrombotic with anticoagulation or an antiplatelet agent.

1. Abundant data from randomized clinical trials demonstrates that warfarin anticoagulation markedly reduces the long-term risk of recurrent stroke in patients with atrial fibrillation; however, evidence

from well-conducted clinical trials does not support the use of heparin
therapy to prevent early recurrent ischemic stroke.

2. In contrast, early aspirin use modestly improves early outcome in
   stroke patients as shown by several large trials.

In order to clarify the confusion on the use of early anticoagulants or
antiplatelets in acute ischemic stroke, the American Academy of Neurology
(AAN) and American Stroke Association reviewed the available literature
and concluded that "there is no reliable evidence that dose-adjusted, IV,
UFH reduces the risk of early recurrent stroke." Furthermore, the AAN
committee concluded that "although patients with atrial fibrillation do
benefit from long-term anticoagulation for secondary stroke prevention,
there are limited data addressing the optimal time for beginning anticoagulation after an acute ischemic stroke". Furthermore, a Cochrane review
of 23,427 patients enrolled in 21 trials concluded that immediate anticoagulation of patients with acute ischemic stroke did not significantly
reduce the odds of death or dependency at final follow-up (OR 0.99).

1. In the acute setting of ischemic stroke, we recommend starting aspirin
   162–325 mg daily based on the results of the CAST and IST trials.
2. In terms of starting other antiplatelets agents in the acute setting, no
   randomized data supports a benefit for early clopidogrel or the combination of aspirin and extended-release dipyridamole. The American
   Stroke Association in 2003 with regard to early antiplatelet use besides
   aspirin stated, "data reflecting the efficiency of other platelet anti-
   aggregants are too limited to support any conclusions." Nevertheless,
   in patients with an allergy to aspirin or who previously failed aspirin
   therapy, we will initiate clopidogrel 75 mg daily or aggrenox in the
   acute setting, 24 hr after tPA use.

Surgical and endovascular management

Neurosurgical procedures may be required in some acute ischemic stroke
patients. These include decompressive hemicraniectomy, cerebellectomy
and posterior fossa decompression, external ventricular drainage, removal
of intracerebral hemorrhage, and surgical revascularization.

Decompressive hemicraniectomy

In patients with massive hemispheric cerebral infarction refractory to
medical management, hemicraniectomy may be a life-saving measure.

1. In hemicraniectomy, the neurosurgeon creates a large bone flap,
   usually involving parts of the frontal, parietal, and temporal bones and
   then opens the dura overlying the infarcted hemisphere.

2. The large opening in the skull and dura allows the edematous brain to swell outward instead of the usual downward path that leads to brainstem compression and death.

3. The timing of hemicraniectomy needs to be established; however, some evidence supports early hemicraniectomy.

4. The long-term functional outcome of patients receiving a hemicraniectomy varies; however, younger patients seem to have a better long-term outcome than older patients. Currently there is no clinical evidence to support the routine use of hemicraniectomy.

Posterior fossa decompression and cerebellectomy

Cerebellar infarction may lead to severe edema with resulting hydrocephalus or brainstem compression with brain death.

1. Any deterioration of level of consciousness should prompt immediate decompressive craniotomy in patients with cerebellar infarct or hemorrhage.

2. Neuroimaging may help guide the clinician to determine appropriate surgical candidates in patients with cerebellar infarction and mass effect.

3. Radiological features more likely to be found in deteriorating patients compared to stable patients include
   a) fourth ventricular shift
   b) hydrocephalus
   c) brainstem deformity
   d) basal cistern compression.

Ventricular drainage

Ventricular drainage in the setting of acute ischemic stroke usually occurs after cerebellar infarction; however, some case reports indicate a possible use in patients with large cerebral hemispheric infarcts.

1. In cerebellar infarction, edema with mass effect may compress the fourth ventricle and lead to rapidly progressive hydrocephalus. In this case, an emergent ventriculostomy with external drainage can be life saving; however, the patient may require further definitive treatment with posterior fossa decompression.

2. Although not a usual indication, external ventricular drainage has been reported in the literature in the case of a large cerebral hemispheric infarction.

Evacuation of intracerebral hemorrhage

1. Early hemorrhagic transformation (HT) of ischemic stroke occurs frequently. Based on computerized axial tomography (CT scan) criteria from recent randomized stroke trials, about 3–37 percent of non-tPA-treated patients and about 10–44 percent of tPA-treated patients will have HT within the first 5 days after ischemic stroke.
2. Symptomatic HT results in substantial morbidity due to mass effect and increased ICP. In the National Institute of Neurological Disorders and Stroke (NINDS) trial, the 6.4 percent of patients experiencing symptomatic HT after receiving IV tPA had a 75 percent mortality rate by 3 months.
3. The surgical indications for patients with symptomatic HT of ischemic stroke remain unclear; however, we recommend correcting coagulopathy with fresh-frozen plasma, vitamin K, protamine sulfate, cryoprecipitate, or platelet transfusion as necessary to avoid potential worsening of hemorrhage.

Large vessel revascularization

Symptomatic extra or intracranial vessel stenosis carries a high recurrent stroke risk. Much of the risk of recurrent stroke from large vessel disease comes early after the initial event. In one study, 18 percent of patients had a recurrent stroke within 30 days of a large vessel atherothrombotic stroke.

The timing of carotid revascularization after acute stroke has been a subject of debate. Early revascularization may lead to a "hyperperfusion syndrome," which involves excessive reperfusion of an area previously adapted to low cerebral blood flow. Although this syndrome is rare, some patients may develop seizures, cerebral edema, and intracerebral hemorrhage. On the other hand, delaying carotid revascularization means subjecting patients to the risk of early recurrent ipsilateral stroke.

Most of the benefit from Carotid endarterectomy (CEA) in symptomatic patients comes from early intervention, within 2 weeks after symptoms.

1. The number needed to treat (NNT) to prevent one ipsilateral stroke was only five in patients randomized within 2 weeks of their symptoms; however, in patients randomized after 2 weeks, the benefit of CEA rapidly dropped off.
2. The NNT to prevent one ipsilateral stroke increased to 125 when randomization of patients occurred more than 12 weeks after last ischemic symptoms.

   Based on this data, we suggest early carotid revascularization within 2 weeks in patients with a stable nondisabling ischemic deficit who meet similar criteria as patients who participated in the North American Symptomatic Carotid Endarterectomy Trial.

Table 11.4: Summary of acute stroke management

Manage acute ischemic stroke patients in a dedicated stroke unit or neuro-ICU

Closely monitor BP to avoid hypotension

Keep patients well hydrated

Prevent DVT with subcutaneous heparin, elastic hose, and pneumatic sequential compression boots

Prevent pressure ulcers

Avoid urinary catheters if possible or remove promptly to avoid UTI

Maintain strict normoglycemia

Avoid hyperthermia

Identify and treat early poststroke seizures

Institute precautions to prevent VAP

Promptly treat cerebral edema and elevated ICP to prevent neurological deterioration

Institute early nutrition

Institute early rehabilitation to prevent complications of immobilization

Institute early antiplatelet agents or anticoagulation to help reduce recurrent stroke risk

Consider early use of statins

Consider early hemicraniectomy for patients with large hemispheric stroke

Consider posterior fossa decompression for patients with large cerebellar stroke

Ventricular drainage should be performed promptly in patients with hydrocephalus

Consider removal of intracerebral hemorrhage in deteriorating patients

Consider early carotid revascularization in stable patients to reduce recurrent stroke risk

---

3. (NASCET) and The European Carotid Surgery Trial (ECST) trials.
4. In addition to early carotid endarterectomy, there is some data suggesting that early carotid angioplasty and stenting may be safely performed within 1 week after a mild ischemic stroke.

In order to minimize risk of developing the hyperperfusion syndrome after carotid revascularization, we recommend strictly controlling the BP. At this point, we do not recommend urgent CEA in patients with ongoing ischemia, mass effect or midline shift on imaging study, or medically unstable patients.

Conclusions

The management of patients with acute ischemic stroke has advanced tremendously. As we have reviewed, the treatment of acute ischemic stroke involves more than thrombolytic administration. The focus of in-hospital care of ischemic stroke patients must involve the timely institution of neuroprotective measures, anticipation and prevention of complications, and initiation of secondary stroke prevention (Table 11.4).

Bibliography

Adams HP, Jr, Brott T, del Zoppo GJ, et al. Guidelines for the early management of patients with ischemic stroke: A scientific statement from the Stroke Council of the American Stroke Association. *Stroke* 2003;34(4):1056–83.

Aslanyan S, Weir CJ, Diener HC, Kaste M, Lees KR, et al. Pneumonia and urinary tract infection after acute ischaemic stroke: A tertiary analysis of the GAIN International trial. *Eur J Neurol* 2004;11(1):49–53.

Camilo O, Goldstein LB. Seizures and epilepsy after ischemic stroke. *Stroke* 2004;35(7):1769–75.

Carlberg B, Asplund K, Hagg E. Factors influencing admission blood pressure levels in patients with acute stroke. *Stroke* 1991;22(4):527–30.

Delashaw JB, Broaddus WC, Kassell NF, Haley EC, et al. Treatment of right hemispheric cerebral infarction by hemicraniectomy. *Stroke* 1990;21(6):874–81.

Esteban A, Frutos F, Tobin MJ, Alia I, et al. A comparison of four methods of weaning patients from mechanical ventilation. Spanish Lung Failure Collaborative Group. *N Engl J Med* 1995;332(6):345–50.

Ginsberg MD, Busto R. Combating hyperthermia in acute stroke: A significant clinical concern. *Stroke* 1998;29(2):529–34.

Gubitz G, Counsell C, Sandercock P, Signorini D. Anticoagulants for acute ischaemic stroke. *Cochrane Database Syst Rev* 2000;(2):CD000024.

Heyland DK. Nutritional support in the critically ill patients. A critical review of the evidence. *Crit Care Clin* 1998;14(3):423–40.

Jaillard A, Cornu C, Durieux A, Moulin T. Hemorrhagic transformation in acute ischemic stroke. The MAST-E study. MAST-E Group. *Stroke* 1999;30(7):1326–32.

Kase CS, Norrving B, Levine SR, Babikian VL, et al. Cerebellar infarction. Clinical and anatomic observations in 66 cases. *Stroke* 1993;24(1):76–83.

Krieger DW, De Georgia MA, Abou-Chebl A, et al. Cooling for acute ischemic brain damage (cool aid): An open pilot study of induced hypothermia in acute ischemic stroke. *Stroke* 2001;32(8):1847–54.

Krinsley JS. Effect of an intensive glucose management protocol on the mortality of critically ill adult patients. *Mayo Clin Proc* 2004;79(8):992–1000.

Leigh R, Zaidat OO, Suri MF, Lynch G, et al. Predictors of hyperacute clinical worsening in ischemic stroke patients receiving thrombolytic therapy. *Stroke* 2004;35(8):1903–7.

Leonardi-Bee J, Bath PM, Phillips SF, Sandercock, PA, et al. Blood pressure and clinical outcomes in the International Stroke Trial. *Stroke* 2002;33(5):1315–20.

Mild therapeutic hypothermia to improve the neurologic outcome after cardiac arrest. *N Engl J Med* 2002;346(8):549–56.

Oliveira-Filho J, Silva SC, Trabuco CC, et al. Detrimental effect of blood pressure reduction in the first 24 hours of acute stroke onset. *Neurology* 2003;61(8):1047–51.

Organised inpatient (stroke unit) care for stroke. *Cochrane Database Syst Rev* 2002;(1): CD000197.

Poor nutritional status on admission predicts poor outcomes after stroke: Observational data from the FOOD trial. *Stroke* 2003;34(6):1450–6.

Qureshi AI, Suarez JI. Use of hypertonic saline solutions in treatment of cerebral edema and intracranial hypertension. *Crit Care Med* 2000;28(9):3301–13.

Reith J, Jorgensen HS, Pedersen PM, et al. Body temperature in acute stroke: Relation to stroke severity, infarct size, mortality, and outcome. *Lancet* 1996;347 (8999):422–5.

Rothwell PM, Eliasziw M, Gutnikov SA, et al. Analysis of pooled data from the randomised controlled trials of endarterectomy for symptomatic carotid stenosis. *Lancet* 2003;361(9352):107–16.

Schwab S, Steiner T, Aschoff A, Schwarz S, et al. Early hemicraniectomy in patients with complete middle cerebral artery infarction. *Stroke* 1998;29(9):1888–93.

Suarez JI, Zaidat OO, Suri MF, Feen ES, et al. Impact of a specialized neurocritical care team on outcome and length of stay of critically ill acute ischemic stroke patients. *J Neurol Sci* 2005;238:205.

Suarez JI, Qureshi AI, Bhardwaj A, Williams MA, et al. Treatment of refractory intracranial hypertension with 23.4% saline. *Crit Care Med* 1998;26(6):1118–22.

Tapson VF, Carroll BA, Davidson BL, Elliott CG, et al. The diagnostic approach to acute venous thromboembolism. Clinical practice guideline. American Thoracic Society. *Am J Respir Crit Care Med* 1999;160(3):1043–66.

Thorsen AM, Holmqvist LW, de Pedro-Cuesta, J, von Koch L, et al. A randomized controlled trial of early supported discharge and continued rehabilitation at home after stroke: Five-year follow-up of patient outcome. *Stroke* 2005;36(2):297–303.

van den Berghe G, Wouters P, Weekers F, Verwaest C. Intensive insulin therapy in the critically ill patients. *N Engl J Med* 2001;345(19):1359–67.

Viitanen M, Winblad B, Asplund K. Autopsy-verified causes of death after stroke. *Acta Med Scand* 1987;222(5):401–8.

Zaidat OO, Alexander MJ, Suarez JI. Early carotid artery stenting and angioplasty in patients with acute ischemic stroke. *Perspect Vasc Surg Endovasc Ther* 2005;17 (3):273–4.

12 Intracerebral hemorrhage

Katja Elfriede Wartenberg and Stephan A. Mayer

Epidemiology

Intracerebral hemorrhage (ICH) is defined as acute, extravasation of blood into the brain parenchyma that may extend to the ventricular system and the subarachnoid space.

1. ICH is responsible for 10–15 percent of stroke cases in the United States and up to 20–30 percent in Asian populations.
2. In the United States, approximately 37,000–52,400 people experience an ICH per year.
3. Worldwide incidence is 10–20 cases per 100,000 people. The incidence doubles with each decade of life above 45 years.

Despite all advances in management and neurocritical care, ICH remains the least treatable form of stroke and, therefore, carries the highest risk of severe morbidity and mortality compared to ischemic stroke or sub-arachnoid hemorrhage.

Risk factors

Several risk factors for ICH have been identified in epidemiological studies. They include the following:

1. Hypertension (HTN) is the single most common risk factor and accounts for 60–70 percent of all cases.
   a) Chronic HTN causes degeneration, fragmentation, fibrinoid necrosis, lipohyalinosis, and small Charcot Bouchard aneurysms of small penetrating arteries in the brain, predisposing them to rupture.
   b) The most common locations of hypertensive ICH occur in the basal ganglia, thalamus, pons, cerebellum, or deep hemispheric white.
2. Amyloid angiopathy accounts for 15 percent of ICH. Deposition of beta amyloid protein in small- to medium-sized blood vessels of the brain and leptomeninges leads to vascular friability.

a) The location of the bleed is mainly lobar, and most patients are older than 70 years.
b) The annual risk of recurrence is 10.5 percent.
c) The presence of the e2 and e4 alleles of the apolipoprotein E gene is associated with a tripling of the risk of hemorrhage recurrence.
d) The likelihood of ICH recurrence in amyloid angiopathy is augmented in the presence of a larger number of baseline chronic hemorrhages on the gradient-echo sequence of magnetic resonance imaging (MRI).

3. Advancing age.
4. Serum cholesterol <4.1 mmol/l.
5. Excessive alcohol intake.
6. Anticoagulation and antiplatelet agents.
7. Genetic mutations such as in genes encoding for factor XIII.

Clinical presentation

The diagnosis of ICH should be considered when a patient presents with a rapid onset of a focal neurological deficit and clinical signs of elevated intracranial pressure (ICP), such as progressively declining mental status, headache, nausea, and vomiting. Symptoms are usually maximal within minutes of onset, which may suggest ICH rather than acute ischemic stroke. However, the presentation is variable and may be indistinguishable from ischemic stroke on clinical grounds alone.

Diagnosis

Computed tomography (CT) remains the diagnostic imaging test of choice (Figure 12.1). The location and size of the hematoma, presence of ventricular blood, and hydrocephalus should be noted. The pattern and topography of the hemorrhage may reveal a secondary cause of ICH (Figure 12.2), such as

1. subarachnoid blood suggesting the presence of a ruptured aneurysm;
2. multiple inferior frontal and temporal hemorrhages pointing to brain trauma; and
3. fluid-fluid levels within the hematoma indicative of coagulopathy.

The ICH volume can be estimated at the bedside utilizing the ABC/2 formula after multiplying the greatest diameter of the hematoma in all three dimensions and dividing the multiplication product by two.

⟹ A corresponds to the largest diameter of the bleed on CT.
⟹ B perpendicular to A on the CT plane.
⟹ C is the number of slices showing hematoma multiplied by the slice thickness.

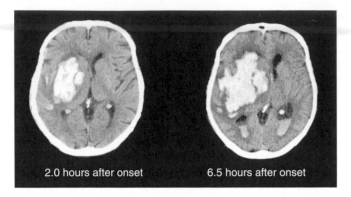

2.0 hours after onset   6.5 hours after onset

Figure 12.1 Early hematoma growth in a 48-year-old chronically hypertensive woman. (a) The baseline CT scan performed shows a moderate-sized right putamen ICH. At this point she is stuporous with a left hemiparesis. (b) A followup CT performed after she deteriorated to coma with bilateral deceretrate posturing shows massive expansion of the hematoma as well as new intraventricular hemorrhage and obstructive hydrocephalus. Within 24 hr she was declared brain dead. From Mayer and Rincon (2005), with permission.

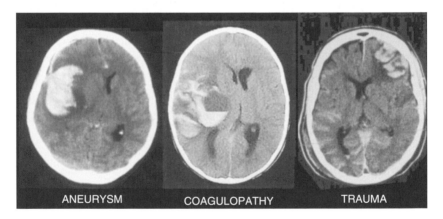

ANEURYSM   COAGULOPATHY   TRAUMA

Figure 12.2 CT clues to common causes of secondary ICH. (a) A thin rim of subdural blood of the right frontal region, and sulci adjacent to the medial aspect of the clot, are suggestive of bleeding into the sylvian subarachnoid space, characteristic of a middle cerebral artery aneurysm. (b) The presence of fluid-fluid levels, indicative of nonclotting blood, is highly suggestive of coagulopathic hemorrhage. This patient bled during cardiac surgery while anticoagulated for cardiopulmonary bypass. (c) Traumatic contusion of the left frontal lobe, which represents contre coup bleeding in relation to extracranial soft tissue swelling over the right parietal region. A small amount of subarachnoid hemorrhage is also present within the sulci of the right parietal and bilateral occipital regions. From Mayer and Rincon (2005), with permission.

Pathophysiology and hematoma enlargement

Two decades ago bleeding was thought to stop within minutes of onset. Now ICH is considered to be a more dynamic and complex process that involves several phases, such as expansion of the hematoma for several hours after initial symptom onset, and an inflammatory process following formation of the hematoma leading to secondary injury.

Retrospective observational studies then began to reveal that intracerebral hemorrhages undergo substantial growth within the first 24 hr (Figure 12.1). In a prospective study, at least 38 percent of 103 patients experienced a >33 percent growth in the ICH volume during the first 24 hr after symptom onset. Follow-up CT scans found that 26 percent of patients had progressed within 1 hr, and 12 percent within 1–20 hr. This was accompanied by neurological deterioration in one-third of patients within 1 hr of the baseline CT, and in an additional 25 percent of patients within the next 20 hr. These findings have been substantiated by CT angiography (CTA), gadolinium-enhanced MRI, and cerebral angiography studies demonstrating contrast extravasation that indicates active bleeding, and by ultraearly ICH surgery trials showing an association between fatal postsurgical bleeding and poor outcome.

Several multivariate analyses have identified the following factors to increase the likelihood of hematoma enlargement and early neurological deterioration:

⇒ shorter time from symptom onset to first CT (<6 hr) (4.9 hr)
⇒ hematoma volume on first CT <25 mm^3
⇒ irregular hematoma shape
⇒ acute blood pressure elevation
⇒ depressed level of consciousness
⇒ history of cerebral infarction
⇒ liver disease
⇒ fasting plasma glucose $\geq$141 mg/dl and hemoglobin A_{1c} $\geq$5.1 percent
⇒ alcohol consumption (>46 g/d)
⇒ low (<87 mg/dl) or high (>523 mg/dl) serum fibrinogen levels
⇒ body temperature >37.5°C
⇒ neutrophil count elevation
⇒ intraventricular hemorrhage

Evidence from pathological and neuroimaging studies demonstrated that secondary multifocal bleeding into tissue surrounding the initial clot leads to hematoma enlargement. These observations suggest that early hematoma growth may result from bleeding into congested tissue surrounding the hematoma. Postulated mechanisms for secondary bleeding include

1. increased intravascular hydrostatic pressure;
2. increased local tissue pressure resulting in mechanical injury;
3. reduced cerebral blood flow;

4. plasma protein induction resulting in secondary inflammation and fluid extravasation.

For several years, the development of an ischemic penumbra around the hematoma leading to secondary injury and cytotoxic edema was a major concern. However, multiple trials utilizing positron emission tomography (PET), diffusion-weighted imaging (DWI) failed to demonstrate true ischemia in hypoperfused brain tissue surrounding the initial hematoma. Animal and human studies have found an inflammatory response induced by plasma rich in thrombin and other coagulation end products released during the coagulation process of the hematoma instead. The inflammatory process incorporates activation and expression of cytotoxic and inflammatory mediators, induction of matrix metalloproteases, leukocyte recruitment, and disruption of blood-brain barrier. By contrast, ICH in the setting of anticoagulants, antifibrinolytic agents, or thrombin inhibitors does not clot, which reduces the amount of surrounding brain swelling and tissue injury.

Several days after onset, perihematomal edema may result in an increase in mass effect, ICP, and herniation.

1. Perihematomal brain edema is the primary cause of neurological deterioration beyond 12 hr of symptom onset.
2. According to conventional beliefs the brain edema reaches its point of maximal swelling at 72 hr.
3. Neuroimaging studies have shown progression of the extent of edema and midline shift early and late up to 2 weeks after symptom onset, although later edema formation might not be clinically significant.
4. Proposed mechanisms of perihematomal brain edema include compression of intraparenchymal microcirculation, inflammation, and vasoconstriction secondary to metabolites released in the process of hematoma formation, and extravasation of plasma from damaged blood vessels, eliciting a neuroinflammatory response.

Outcome and prognostic indicators

The average mortality of ICH ranges from 30 to 50 percent. Of all the patients who suffered an ICH in 1997, 35–52 percent had died at 1 month, 10 percent were independent at 1 month, and 20 percent reached a state of independent living by 6 months. Early mortality in ICH is higher compared to ischemic infarctions, but surviving patients are just as likely to recover to functional independence.

Independent predictors of 30-day and 1-year mortality include

⇒ large ICH volume
⇒ depressed level of consciousness

Table 12.1: The ICH Score

Component	Points	Total points	30-day mortality%
Glasgow Coma Scale score			
3–4	2	5±	100
5–12	1		
13–15	0	4	97
ICH volume (ml)			
≥30	1	3	72
<30	0		
Intraventricular hemorrhage		2	26
Yes	1		
No	0	1	13
Age (years)			
≥80	1	0	0
<80	0		
Infratentorial origin			
Yes	1		
No	0		

Adapted with permission from Hemphill JC 3rd, Bonovich DC, Besmertis L, Manley GT, Johnston SC. The ICH score: a simple, reliable grading scale for intracerebral hemorrhage. Stroke. 2001; 32:891–897

- older age
- Intraventricular hemorrhage (IVH)
- infratentorial location
- relative edema volume

Broderick identified hematoma volume as the single most powerful predictor of 30-day mortality after ICH. The ICH score is a clinical grading scale that includes most independent predictors of long-term outcome after ICH that allows estimation of 30-day mortality on admission (Table 12.1). However, a very poor prognosis should be communicated with caution as studies have shown that physicians frequently underestimate the likelihood of a better outcome. Poor outcome may represent self-fulfilling prophecies, as shown in a California study in which do-not-resuscitate orders written within 24 hr were the most important determinant of mortality. Mortality of ICH may be decreased by referring the patient to a dedicated neurological intensive care unit where the patient receives standardized treatment, early rehabilitation, and is cared for by an interested team of specialists.

Emergency management

Treatment of ICH starts with management of airway, respiration, and circulation, followed by evaluation of the level of consciousness. Initial laboratory tests should include

➠ complete blood count (CBC)
➠ comprehensive metabolic panel
➠ coagulation studies
➠ troponin I
➠ urine toxicology screen
➠ electrocardiogram
➠ chest x-ray

Airway

Patients who experience neurological decline with depressed level of consciousness have difficulties maintaining their airway due to loss of reflexes that keep the airway open. This can lead to aspiration, hypoxemia, or hypercapnia that may increase ICP by induction of cerebral vasodilatation. Intubation and mechanical ventilation are required under these circumstances.

1. For rapid sequence intubation, midazolam, IV or topical lidocaine, propofol, or etomidate and nondepolarizing neuromuscular blocking agents such as rocuronium, vecuronium, or atracurium that do not raise ICP should be utilized.
2. The initial respiratory rate and tidal volume should be set to achieve a pCO_2 of 35 mmHg.
3. Early aggressive hyperventilation to target pCO_2 levels below 25 mmHg is not recommended because it can potentially result in excessive vasoconstriction and exacerbation of ischemia.

Blood pressure

Optimal target blood pressure levels during the acute phase of ICH remain controversial. The guidelines for management of ICH recommend decreasing the MAP to less than 130 mmHg and greater than 90 mmHg based on anecdotal and nonrandomized trials. Given current evidence indicating the lack of a true ischemic penumbra surrounding the clot and evidence that elevated blood pressure is a powerful predictor of early hematoma growth and poor outcome, it seems increasingly plausible that early aggressive blood pressure reduction might be justified.

1. In a recent nonrandomized study, lowering blood pressure to less than 160/100 mmHg with intravenous labetalol or hydralazine within 6 hr

of onset of ICH was safe, feasible, and more likely to result in decreased hematoma expansion and functional independence at 1 month.

2. A trial of blood pressure control (MAP 100–120 mmHg) within 3 hr of symptom onset was given the highest priority by a recent National Institute of Health (NIH) consensus panel.

3. In patients undergoing ICP monitoring, cerebral perfusion pressure (CPP), which is calculated as mean arterial pressure (MAP) minus ICP, should be maintained above 60 mmHg at all times.

4. In the presence of chronic hypertension, cerebral autoregulation adapts to higher blood pressures. Additionally, cerebral autoregulation can become compromised in regions adjacent to the hematoma. The result is that cerebral perfusion brain tissue oxygenation can become compromised at blood pressures that might under ordinary circumstances be acceptable.

5. For patients that undergo craniotomy, MAP should be maintained at 100 mmHg.

6. Most patients require placement of an arterial catheter for adequate treatment of hypertension.

7. Intravenous boluses of labetalol every 10 min dosed from 20 to 80 mg can be used for treatment of hypertension in the emergency department. Continuous infusions of labetalol, esmolol, or nicardipine are used in the ICU setting (Table 12.2).

Management of increased ICP

ICP control is essential for patients who acutely present in stupor or coma, or with clinical signs of brain stem herniation. The following should be applied to lower ICP quickly and effectively before a neurosurgical intervention can be performed.

1. Head elevation at 30°.

2. Administration of 1.0–1.5 g/kg of 20 percent mannitol as a bolus.

3. Hyperventilation to a pCO_2 of 28–35 mmHg.

4. Infusion of hypertonic saline solution (23.4 percent) at a dose of 0.5–2.0 ml/kg is a valuable alternative to mannitol, particularly in the setting of hypotension, but requires central venous access.

   a) In a canine model of ICH administration of 23.4 percent saline was more effective than infusion of 10 percent saline or mannitol during impending transtentorial herniation.

5. Definite neurosurgical ICP management requires craniotomy and hematoma evacuation, ventriculostomy for hydrocephalus, or decompressive hemicraniectomy.

6. Placement of an ICP monitor may be useful to guide therapy.

Table 12.2: Intravenous Antihypertensive Agents for Acute ICH

Drug	Mechanism	Dose	Adverse effects
Labetalol	Alpha-1, beta-1, beta-2 receptor antagonist	20–80 mg bolus every 10 min, up to 300 mg; 0.5–2.0 mg/min infusion	Bradycardia, congestive heart failure, bronchospasm
Esmolol	Beta-1 receptor antagonist	0.5 mg/kg bolus; 50–300 µg/kg/min	Bradycardia, congestive heart failure, bronchospasm
Nicardipine	L-type calcium channel blocker (dihydropyridine)	5–15 mg/hr infusion	Severe aortic stenosis, myocardial ischemia
Enalaprilat	ACE inhibitor	0.625 mg bolus; 1.25–5 mg every 6 hrs	Variable response, precipitous fall in BP with high-renin states
Fenoldopam	Dopamine-1 receptor agonist	0.1–0.3 µg/kg/min	Tachycardia, headache, nausea, flushing, glaucoma, portal hypertension
Nitroprusside*	Nitrovasodilator (arterial and venous)	0.25–10 µg/kg/min	Increased ICP, variable response, myocardial ischemia, thiocyanate and cyanide toxicity

*Nitroprusside is not recommended for use in acute ICH because of its tendency to increase ICP.

Hemostatic therapy

Recombinant activated factor VII (rFVIIa, NovoSeven®; Novo Nordisk, Bagsvaerd, Denmark) facilitates hemostasis during spontaneous and surgical bleeding in patients with hemophilia A and B and inhibitors to factors VIII or IX and is currently approved for patients with hemophilia whose bleeding is resistant to factor VIII therapy. Considerable evidence also suggests that rFVIIa can enhance local hemostasis even in the absence of a coagulopathy.

1. In a randomized, double-blind, placebo-controlled study of 399 patients, treatment with rFVIIa at doses of 40, 80, or 160 µg/kg within 4 hr after ICH onset limited growth of the hematoma by approximately 50 percent.
2. The mean percent increase was 29 in placebo versus 16, 14, and 11 in the 40, 80, and 160 µg/kg rFVIIa groups, respectively ($P=0.011$, rFVIIa versus placebo). This was associated with a 38 percent reduction in mortality ($P=0.025$, rFVIIa versus placebo) and significantly improved functional outcomes at 90 days, despite a 5 percent increase in the frequency of arterial thromboembolic adverse events. However, a larger phase III trial comparing doses of placebo, 20 and 80 µg/kg did not show a reduction in mortality or severe disability at 90 days.
3. Another pilot trial of an antifibrinolytic agent, epsilon aminocaproic acid, could not demonstrate a benefit for hemostasis.
4. The results from a larger confirmatory phase III study are yet to be published. However, a recent press release reported that initial results from the phase III trial were negative. Although, ultra-early treatment with factor VIIa decreased hematoma expansion, the treatment had no effect on long-term clinical outcomes and mortality after 90 days.

Reversal of anticoagulation

1. Anticoagulation with warfarin carries a 5–10-fold higher risk of spontaneous ICH compared to the general population.
2. Warfarin use doubles the risk of death in ICH victims due to increased risk of bleeding.
3. Insufficient normalization of the international normalized ratio (INR) to <1.4 in anticoagulated ICH patients results in an increased risk of neurological deterioration and mortality.

Patients on warfarin who present with an ICH should receive fresh frozen plasma (FFP) or prothrombin-complex concentrate (PCC) and vitamin K (Table 12.3) immediately, even before the results of coagulation tests are available.

1. Normalization of the INR with FFP or vitamin K takes several hours.
2. Infusions of FFP are associated with volume load and may exacerbate congestive heart failure with underlying cardiac or renal disease.

Table 12.3: Emergency Management of ICH in a coagulopathic patients

Scenario	Agent	Dose	Comments	Level of Evidence*
Warfarin	Fresh frozen plasma (FFP)	15 ml/kg	Usually 4 to 6 units (200 ml) each are given	II
	or		Works faster than FFP, but carries risk of DIC	II
	Prothrombin complex concentrate *and* IV Vitamin K	15–30 U/kg 10 mg	Can take up to 24 hr to normalize INR	II
Warfarin and emergency neurosurgical intervention	*Above plus* Recombinant factor VIIa	20–80 µg/kg	Contraindicated in acute thromboembolic disease	III
Unfractionated or low molecular weight heparin†	Protamine sulfate	1 mg per 100 units of heparin, or 1 mg of enoxaparin	Can cause flushing, bradycardia, or hypotension.	III
Platelet dysfunction or thrombocytopenia	Platelet transfusion *and/or*	6 units	Range 4–8 units based on size; transfuse to >100,000	III
	Desmopressin (DDAVP)	0.3 µg/kg	Single dose required	III

In general anticoagulants should be discontinued immediately, and can be safely restarted approximately two weeks after presentation (see text for further discussion).

* Class I = based on one or more high quality randomized controlled trials; Class II = based on 2 or more high quality prospective or retrospective cohort studies; Class III = Case reports and series, expert opinion.

† Protamine has minimal efficacy against danaparoid or fondaparinux

DIC, disseminated intravascular coagulation; INR, international normalized ratio.

3. PCC, a concentrate of the vitamin K–dependent coagulation factors II, VII, IX, and X, can be given in smaller volumes and normalizes the INR more rapidly, but carries the risk of triggering disseminated intravascular coagulation.

4. Use of rFVIIa can speed the reversal of anticoagulation in ICH.
   a) A single dose of rVIIa normalizes the INR within minutes, and larger doses result in longer duration of INR suppression.
   b) Doses of rVIIa ranging from 10 to 90 µg/kg have been used to promote hemostasis in anticoagulation-related ICH with good clinical results, primarily in the setting of a planned neurosurgical intervention.
   c) Due to its short half-life (2.3 hr), rFVIIa should always be used in conjunction with FFP and vitamin K to attain a sustained reversal of anticoagulation.

5. Protamine sulfate is used to reverse the effects of unfractionated or low-molecular weight heparin in ICH.

6. A single dose of desmopressin (DDAVP) and platelet transfusions is used for hemostasis in patients with thrombocytopenia or platelet dysfunction.

In patients with a strong indication for anticoagulation, such as atrial fibrillation and a prior history of cardioembolic stroke or a prosthetic heart valve, anticoagulation can be restarted 10–14 days after ICH in most cases. Deep ICH might have a lower rate of recurrence on anticoagulation (0.04/ year) than lobar ICH (0.3/year).

Critical care management

Patient positioning

The head of the bed should be elevated at 30° for ICP control to reduce the risk of aspiration in nonintubated patients, and to reduce the risk of ventilator-associated pneumonia in mechanically ventilated patients.

ICP management

Large volume ICH is often accompanied by increased ICP, brain tissue shifts related to mass effect, and obstructive hydrocephalus from IVH. To effectively manage these problems, an ICP monitor or external ventricular drain (EVD) should be placed in all patients in coma (Glasgow Coma Scale ≤8). Placement of an EVD can be life saving in patients with hydrocephalus or IVH and impending brainstem herniation. However, the relationship between changes of ventricular size and level of consciousness in ICH patients treated with EVD is less clear.

1. An ICP of less than 20 mmHg along with CPP greater than 60 mmHg should be maintained.

Table 12.4: Stepwise Treatment Protocol for Elevated ICP in a
Monitored Patient

1. **Surgical decompression**. Consider repeat CT scanning, and definitive
   surgical intervention or ventricular drainage
2. **Sedation**. Intravenous sedation to attain a motionless, quiet state
3. **CPP optimization**. Pressor infusion if CPP is <70 mm Hg, or reduction of
   blood pressure if CPP is >110 mm Hg,
4. **Osmotherapy**. Mannitol 0.25–1.5 g/kg IV or 0.5–2.0 ml/kg 23.4 percent
   hypertonic saline (repeat every 1–6 hr as needed)
5. **Hyperventilation**. Target pCO_2 levels of 26–30 mm Hg.
6. **High dose pentobarbital therapy**. Load with 5–20 mg/kg, infuse
   1–4 mg/kg/hr.
7. **Hypothermia**. Cool core body temperature to 32–33°C.

Reproduced with permission from Mayer SA, Chong J. Critical care management of
increased intracranial pressure. J Int Care Med 2002;17:55–67

2. When ICP is monitored, a standard management algorithm should be
   used (Table 12.4).
3. There is no role for corticosteroids, such as dexamethasone, in the
   treatment of ICH due to a lack of efficacy, especially since corticosteroid therapy is complicated by hyperglycemia, immunosuppression,
   impaired wound healing, and protein catabolism.

Fluid resuscitation

1. A central venous catheter should be placed for large volume access and
   monitoring of central venous pressure (CVP) in patients who require
   mechanical ventilation or ICP management.
2. Standard intravenous fluid management for patients with ICH consists
   of isotonic fluids such as 0.9 percent saline or hypertonic saline solution (2 or 3 percent sodium chloride/acetate, 1 ml/kg/hr) in the presence of increased ICP or significant perihematomal mass effect.
   a) Hypertonic saline is administered to maintain a target serum
      osmolarity of 300–320 mosms/l and hypernatremia (150–155 meq/l),
      which may decrease cellular swelling and ICP peaks.
   b) When treatment with hypertonic saline is discontinued, caution
      has to be given to avoid large drops in osmolarity that may trigger
      rebound edema and ICP elevations.
   c) The serum sodium concentrations should not be allowed to drop
      more than 6–8 mmol/l in 24 hr. The use of hypertonic saline is
      limited by renal failure and severe congestive heart failure.
3. Free water in the form of 0.45 percent saline or 5 percent dextrose
   in water may exacerbate cerebral edema and increase ICP because

of the osmotic gradient between the intravascular space and brain parenchyma.

4. In general, the patient should be maintained in a euvolemic state as assessed by fluid balance, CVP, and body weight.

Anticonvulsants

Clinically evident seizures occur in about 8–12 percent of patients with ICH by 30 days, and approximately half of these seizures occur in the first 24 hr. One to two percent of patients develop convulsive status epilepticus, and five to twenty percent of ICH survivors develop chronic epilepsy. Lobar location of ICH independently predicts the occurrence of early seizures. Nonconvulsive posthemorrhagic seizures are associated with neurological deterioration and increased midline shift, and might worsen outcome.

1. Treatment of acute seizures begins with intravenous lorazepam (0.05–0.1 mg/kg) followed by an intravenous load with fosphenytoin or phenytoin (15–20 mg/kg), valproic acid (15–45 mg/kg), or phenobarbital (15–20 mg/kg).
2. Prophylactic anticonvulsant therapy may be beneficial, especially in large, supratentorial ICH and in patients with depressed level of consciousness, but has not been studied in a controlled, randomized trial. However, there is evidence that prophylaxis with phenytoin reduces the frequency of seizures from 14 to 4 percent during the first week after severe traumatic brain injury.
3. Anticonvulsant therapy is recommended for selected patients for up to 1 month after ICH according to the AHA guidelines, a policy that is supported by an observational study demonstrating a lower seizure frequency in patients with lobar ICH on anticonvulsant therapy.
4. Continuous electroencephalographic (cEEG) monitoring may be helpful in patients with ICH in persistent stupor or coma.
   a) In one observational study, nonconvulsive seizures or status epilepticus were detected by cEEG in 28 percent of stuporous or comatose patients with ICH.
   b) It is our policy to perform surveillance cEEG for at least 48 hr in all comatose ICH patients. When detected, nonconvulsive seizures can be treated with intravenous midazolam infusion (starting at 0.2 mg/kg/hr).

Fever

Fever occurs commonly after intracranial bleeds and is particularly common with IVH. Persistent fever after ICH impacts negatively on mortality and outcome, and even small temperature elevations have been shown to worsen neuronal injury and death in experimental models.

1. Fever should be treated aggressively, starting with acetaminophen and cooling blankets for all patients with sustained temperatures exceeding 38.3°C (101.0°F).
2. Newer adhesive surface cooling systems (Arctic sun, Medivance Inc.) and endovascular heat exchange catheters (Cool Line System, Alsius, Inc.; Innercool, Innercool Therapies) may be more effective for maintaining normothermia, but their association with outcome after ICH requires further studies.

Nutrition

1. Enteral feeding should be started within 48 hr of admission to decrease the risk of malnutrition. Small-bore nasoduodenal feeding tubes are preferred to lower the risk of aspiration.
2. As hyperglycemia may worsen outcome after brain injury, glucose- or dextrose-containing solutions should be avoided. Persistent hyperglycemia should be treated vigorously by means of an insulin protocol utilizing continuous insulin infusions.

Deep venous thrombosis prophylaxis

Patients with ICH tend to be immobilized for a prolonged period of time, which puts them at high risk for deep venous thrombosis and pulmonary embolism.

1. Pneumatic compression devices and elastic stockings have been shown to decrease the incidence of thromboembolic events in neurosurgical patients and can be placed on admission.
2. Low dose subcutaneous heparin starting 48 hr after ICH is protective as well and was not associated with increase in intracranial bleeding. Alternatively, low molecular weight heparins such as enoxaparin can be used.

Surgical management of ICH

The benefit of emergent hematoma evacuation has long been controversial. Many small controlled and uncontrolled trials of early craniotomy for supratentorial hemorrhages showed either a small potential benefit on outcome or an increased rate of rebleeding. Premorbid condition, level of consciousness, laterality of the hemorrhage, and medical comorbidities have traditionally influenced the decision to perform surgery in ICH. A recently published large randomized landmark trial, the STICH trial, compared immediate surgical clot evacuation with initial conservative management in 1,033 patients with ICH and found no difference in impact on outcome and mortality at 6 months.

1. The time window for randomization was 72 hr, and there was a high degree of crossover, with over 20 percent of those randomized to initial medical management eventually undergoing a salvage neurosurgical procedure.
2. Enrollment in STICH was based on the condition of clinical equipoise: patients were only enrolled if the investigator was uncertain whether surgery or conservative management would be of more benefit. Therefore, the results of STICH might not be applicable for patients with a well-accepted indication for surgical intervention, such as patients who are younger and present with large lobar hemorrhages and early deterioration related to symptomatic mass effect.
3. Craniotomy was the preferred method of clot evacuation in 75 percent of patients in the surgical group in the STICH trial.

Minimally invasive stereotactic surgery with and without clot thrombolysis with recombinant tissue plasminogen activator (rtPA), streptokinase, or urokinase showed promising results in uncontrolled single-center and small multicenter reports and one promising clinical trial. However, in the STICH trial, patients treated with these so-called minimally invasive surgical techniques tended to fare worse than those treated with open craniotomy.

Intraventricular thrombolysis

Injection of rtPA (3 mg every 12 hr) or urokinase (25,000 units every 12 hr) via a ventricular catheter into one or both lateral ventricles can accelerate the clearance of intraventricular blood on CT. A pilot prospective randomized, double-blinded, controlled trial of intraventricular injection of urokinase in 12 patients with IVH demonstrated a 44 percent reduction of clot half-life in 12 patients. Unfortunately the procedure carries with it a fairly significant risk of intracranial bleeding. Further studies investigating smaller doses given at more frequent intervals are underway.

Surgical treatment for cerebellar hemorrhage

Cerebellar hemorrhage can be followed by sudden and dramatic neurological deterioration due to swelling, causing obstructive hydrocephalus and brainstem compression up to 2 weeks after the initial bleed. Effacement or asymmetry of the fourth ventricle, effacement or obliteration of the ambient cistern, and early hydrocephalus on CT warrant close neuromonitoring and consideration of a surgical intervention. Occasionally placement of EVD is sufficient for treatment of hydrocephalus. Since patients can abruptly deteriorate to coma and death, surgical evacuation based on a wait-and-see approach in patients with a large hemorrhage is not advisable.

1. Most cerebellar hemorrhages larger than 3 cm in diameter benefit from surgical evaluation with decompressive suboccipital craniectomy.
2. Reversal of coma with advanced signs of brain stem herniation (i.e., fixed pupils) after this procedure is well documented.

Future directions

New treatment options to prevent neurological deterioration and, therefore, improve long-term neurological function, such as aggressive blood pressure reduction, intraventricular thrombolysis, and minimally invasive surgical techniques, are currently under investigation and may soon be available. The combination of administration of rFVIIa with early surgical blood clot removal might minimize the risk of postoperative bleeding and improve outcome. For now, aggressive and meticulous ICU care seems to be the most effective approach for improving outcomes from this devastating disease.

Bibliography

Broderick JP, Adams HP, Jr, Barsan W, et al. Guidelines for the management of spontaneous intracerebral hemorrhage: A statement for healthcare professionals from a special writing group of the Stroke Council, American Heart Association. *Stroke* 1999;30(4):905–15.

Broderick JP, Brott T, Tomsick T, Miller R, Huster G. Intracerebral hemorrhage more than twice as common as subarachnoid hemorrhage. *J Neurosurg* 1993;78 (2):188–91.

Broderick JP, Brott TG, Duldner JE, Tomsick T. Huster G. Volume of intracerebral hemorrhage. A powerful and easy to use predictor of 30 day mortality. *Stroke* 1993;24(7):987–93.

Brott T, Broderick J, Kothari R, et al. Early hemorrhage growth in patients with intracerebral hemorrhage. *Stroke* 1997;28(1):1–5.

Brott T, Thalinger K, Hertzberg V. Hypertension as a risk factor for spontaneous intracerebral hemorrhage. *Stroke* 1986;17(6):1078–83.

Chong J, Mayer SA. Critical care management of increased intracranial pressure. *J. Intensive Care Med* 2002;17:55–67.

Claassen J, Mayer SA, Kowalski RG, Emerson RG, Hirsch LJ. Detection of electrographic seizures with continuous EEG monitoring in critically ill patients. *Neurology* 2004;62(10):1743–8.

Diringer MN, Edwards DF. Admission to a neurologic/neurosurgical intensive care unit is associated with reduced mortality rate after intracerebral hemorrhage. *Crit Care Med* 2001;29(3):635–40.

Eckman MH, Rosand J, Knudsen KA, Singer DE, Greenberg SM. Can patients be anticoagulated after intracerebral hemorrhage? A decision analysis. *Stroke* 2003;34 (7):1710–16.

Fujii Y, Takeuchi S, Sasaki O, Minakawa T, Tanaka R. Multivariate analysis of predictors of hematoma enlargement in spontaneous intracerebral hemorrhage. *Stroke* 1998;29(6):1160–6.

Gebel JM, Jr, Jauch EC, Brott TG, et al. Relative edema volume is a predictor of outcome in patients with hyperacute spontaneous intracerebral hemorrhage. *Stroke* 2002;33(11):2636–41.

Gujjar AR, Deibert E, Manno EM, Duff S, Diringer MN. Mechanical ventilation for ischemic stroke and intracerebral hemorrhage: Indications, timing, and outcome. *Neurology* 1998;51(2):447–51.

Hedner U. Recombinant activated factor VII as a universal haemostatic agent. *Blood Coagul Fibrinol* 1998;9(Suppl 1):S147–52.

Hemphill JC, 3rd, Bonovich DC, Besmertis L, Manley GT, Johnston SC. The ICH score: A simple, reliable grading scale for intracerebral hemorrhage. *Stroke* 2001;32:891–7.

Hemphill JC, 3rd, Newman J, Zhao S, Johnston SC. Hospital usage of early do not resuscitate orders and outcome after intracerebral hemorrhage. *Stroke* 2004;35 (5):1130–4.

Juvela S. Risk factors for impaired outcome after spontaneous intracerebral hemorrhage. *Arch Neurol* 1995;52(12):1193–200.

Kidwell CS, Chalela JA, Saver JL, et al. Comparison of MRI and CT for detection of acute intracerebral hemorrhage. *JAMA* 2004;292(15):1823–30.

Kothari RU, Brott T, Broderick JP, et al. The ABCs of measuring intracerebral hemorrhage volumes. *Stroke* 1996;27(8):1304–5.

Mayer SA, Brun NC, Begtrup K, et al. Recombinant activated factor VII for acute intracerebral hemorrhage. *N Engl J Med* 2005;352(8):777–85.

Mayer SA, Lignelli A, Fink ME, et al. Perilesional blood flow and edema formation in acute intracerebral hemorrhage: A SPECT study. *Stroke* 1998;29(9):1791–8.

Mayer SA, Rincon F. Treatment of intracerebral hemorrhage. *Lancet Neurol* 2005;4:662–72.

Mendelow AD, Gregson BA, Fernandes HM, et al. Early surgery versus initial conservative treatment in patients with spontaneous supratentorial intracerebral haematomas in the International Surgical Trial in Intracerebral Haemorrhage (STICH): A randomised trial. *Lancet* 2005;365(9457):387–97.

Morgenstern LB, Demchuk AM, Kim DH, Frankowski RF, Grotta JC. Rebleeding leads to poor outcome in ultra early craniotomy for intracerebral hemorrhage. *Neurology* 2001;56(10):1294–9.

Ott KH, Kase CS, Ojemann RG, Mohr JP. Cerebellar hemorrhage: Diagnosis and treatment. A review of 56 cases. *Arch Neurol* 1974;31(3):160–7.

Powers WJ, Zazulia AR, Videen TO, et al. Autoregulation of cerebral blood flow surrounding acute (6 to 22 hours) intracerebral hemorrhage. *Neurology* 2001;57 (1):18–24.

Qureshi AI, Mohammad YM, Yahia AM, et al. A prospective multicenter study to evaluate the feasibility and safety of aggressive antihypertensive treatment in patients with acute intracerebral hemorrhage. *J Intensive Care Med* 2005;20(1):34–42.

Qureshi AI, Safdar K, Weil J, et al. Predictors of early deterioration and mortality in black Americans with spontaneous intracerebral hemorrhage. *Stroke* 1995;26 (10):1764–7.

Qureshi AI, Tuhrim S, Broderick JP, Batjer HH, Hondo H, Hanley DF. Spontaneous intracerebral hemorrhage. *N Engl J Med* 2001;344(19):1450–60.

Qureshi AI, Wilson DA, Hanley DF, Traystman RJ. No evidence for an ischemic
    penumbra in massive experimental intracerebral hemorrhage. *Neurology* 1999;52
    (2):266–72.
van den Berghe G, Wouters P, Weekers F, et al. Intensive insulin therapy in the
    critically ill patients. *N Engl J Med* 2001;345(19):1359–67 First trial to demonstrate
    the impact of strict glucose control on mortality and long–term outcome in
    critically ill patients.
Zazulia AR, Diringer MN, Derdeyn CP, Powers WJ. Progression of mass effect after
    intracerebral hemorrhage. *Stroke* 1999;30(6):1167–73.
Zhu XL, Chan MS, Poon WS. Spontaneous intracranial hemorrhage: Which patients
    need diagnostic cerebral angiography? A prospective study of 206 cases and review
    of the literature. *Stroke* 1997;28(7):1406–9.

13 Subarachnoid hemorrhage

Katja Elfriede Wartenberg and Stephan A. Mayer

Epidemiology and risk factors

Subarachnoid hemorrhage (SAH) occurs most commonly from rupture of an intracranial aneurysm and accounts for 2–5 percent of all strokes with an annual incidence of 1 per 10,000. In 10–20 percent of SAH cases, an aneurysm cannot be found and the prognosis is good. This disease affects nearly 21,000–33,000 individuals per year in the United States, with an annual incidence of 1 per 10,000. Saccular (or berry) aneurysms at the base of the brain cause the majority of cases of SAH.

1. Most common between the ages of 40 and 60 years.
2. Risk is 1.6 times higher for women compared to men and 10 times higher for African Americans than for Caucasians.
3. Approximately 12 percent of patients die before receiving medical attention, and 25 percent of patients die during hospitalization.

Risk factors for the initial rupture of an aneurysm include

➡ large aneurysm size
➡ age
➡ prior SAH from a separate aneurysm
➡ basilar apex and posterior communicating artery location
➡ cigarette smoking
➡ aneurysm-related headache or cranial nerve compression
➡ heavy alcohol use
➡ family history of SAH
➡ female sex (especially postmenopausal)
➡ multiple aneurysms
➡ hypertension
➡ exposure to cocaine or any other sympathomimetic agents
➡ connective tissue disease associated with intracranial aneurysms such as polycystic kidney disease, Ehlers-Danlos syndrome (type IV), pseudoxanthoma elasticum, fibromuscular dysplasia

Clinical presentation

Patients with SAH present with an explosive "thunderclap" generalized headache followed by neck stiffness and back pain, photophobia, nausea and vomiting, loss of consciousness, and seizures.

1. More than one-third of patients experience "sentinel headaches," symptoms from minor leaking of blood from an aneurysm, days or weeks before SAH, that last for minutes or hours.
2. Sudden onset of neck stiffness and the Kernig sign are hallmarks of SAH. However, these signs are not invariably present, and confusion and low back pain are sometimes more prominent than headache.
3. Preretinal or subhyaloid hemorrhages – large, smooth bordered, and on the retinal surface – occur in up to 25 percent of patients.

Although aneurysmal rupture often occurs during periods of exercise or physical stress, SAH can occur at any time, including sleep. Initial misdiagnosis of SAH occurs in approximately 15 percent of patients, and those with the mildest symptoms are at greatest risk. Reasons for initial misdiagnosis include not obtaining an imaging study in 73 percent and/or not performing or wrongly interpreting a spinal tap in 23 percent. This often leads to delayed treatment after rebleeding or neurological deterioration has occurred, with increased morbidity and mortality.

Diagnosis

Computed tomography (CT) remains the diagnostic imaging test of choice for the diagnosis of SAH.

1. Most commonly, CT shows diffuse blood in the basal cisterns (Figure 13.1); with more severe hemorrhages, blood extends into the sylvian and interhemispheric fissures and ventricular system.
2. CT may also demonstrate a focal intraparenchymal or subdural hemorrhage, hydrocephalus, a large thrombosed aneurysm, focal or global cerebral edema, or infarction due to vasospasm.
3. Sensitivity of CT for SAH is 90–95 percent within 24 hr, 80 percent at 3 days, and 50 percent at 1 week.
4. The location of the intraparenchymal blood on CT can occasionally predict the site of the aneurysm.

Magnetic resonance tomography (MRT) can also be used to make the initial diagnosis of SAH or to detect a completely thrombosed aneurysm when the initial angiogram is negative.

A lumbar puncture should always be performed with suspected SAH if the CT is negative.

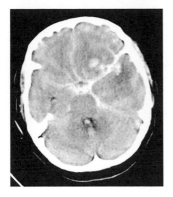

Figure 13.1 Noncontrast CT demonstrating hyperdensity within the lateral sylvian, anterior interhemispheric, supracellar, and ambient cisterns, characteristic of acute aneurysmal SAH. The predominance of blood in the left sylvian fissure is characteristic of a middle cerebral artery aneurysm in that region.

1. Cerebrospinal fluid (CSF) should be collected in four consecutive tubes.
2. SAH can be diagnosed by spinal tap demonstrating xanthochromia (yellow-tinged appearance) after centrifugation, which differentiates SAH from a traumatic tap.
   a) Xanthochromia may take up to 12 hr to appear after aneurysm rupture. The erythrocyte count is elevated and does not diminish from tube 1 through 4.
3. CSF pressure is nearly always high and the protein elevated.
4. Initially, the proportion of CSF leukocytes to erythrocytes is that of the peripheral blood, with a usual ratio of 1:700; after several days a reactive pleocytosis and low glucose levels may develop due to sterile chemical meningitis caused by the blood.
5. Red blood cells and xanthochromia disappear in about 2 weeks, unless hemorrhage recurs.
6. Spectrophotometry is another method to evaluate CSF for subarachnoid blood and was shown to have a sensitivity of 100 percent and a specificity of only 75.2 percent.

Cerebral angiography is the definitive diagnostic procedure for detecting intracranial aneurysms and delineating their anatomy (Figure 13.2). The increasing availability and image quality of CT and MR angiography – and having a sensitivity and specificity comparable to angiography – have decreased the utilization of invasive testing for initial diagnosis. However, a four vessel (bilateral internal carotid and vertebral artery injections) is mandatory when these tests are negative. Moreover, cerebral angiography during coiling or after surgical clipping can evaluate the adequacy of

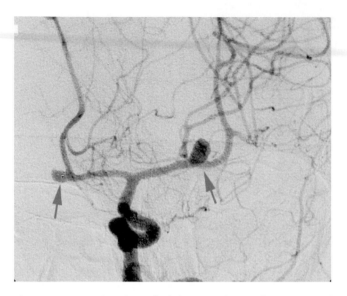

Figure 13.2 Anterior view of a left internal carotid angiogram demonstrates a giant aneurysm of the left middle cerebral artery at the level of trifurcation and an aneurysm of the left anterior communicating artery (see arrows).

aneurysm repair screen for smaller secondary aneurysms that may be missed by CT or MRT. Vasospasm, local thrombosis, or poor technique can lead to a false-negative angiogram. For this reason, patients with a negative angiogram at first should have a follow-up study 1–2 weeks later; an aneurysm will be demonstrated in about 5 percent of these cases. The exception to this rule is "perimesencephalic" SAH, which implies no risk of rebleeding; these patients do not require follow-up angiography.

Aneurysm features

Saccular aneurysms commonly arise from the circle of Willis, especially at the bifurcations, whenever the arterial elastic lamina and tunica media sustain a defect. The aneurysm wall consists of the intima and adventitia of the blood vessel and is, therefore, prone to rupture, which results in SAH. The point of rupture is usually the dome of the aneurysm.

1. Most aneurysms (85–90 percent) are located in the anterior circulation, at the junction of the internal carotid and posterior communication artery (40 percent), the anterior communicating artery complex (30 percent), and the middle cerebral artery at the bifurcation or tri-furcation (20 percent).
2. The apex of the basilar artery or the junction of the vertebral and posterior inferior cerebellar arteries are the preferred locations in the posterior circulation.

3. About 20 percent of patients have two or more aneurysms, occasionally on the same artery contralaterally, so-called mirror aneurysms, and 20 percent have a family history of aneurysms.

Intracranial aneurysms are also associated with arteriovenous malformations, polycystic kidney disease, coarctation of the aorta, fibromuscular dysplasia, Marfan syndrome, Moya Moya disease, Ehlers-Danlos syndrome, pseudoxanthoma elasticum, and pituitary gland tumors.

Outcome and prognostic indicators

SAH carries a mortality rate of 12 percent before medical attention. The in-hospital mortality rate is 20–25 percent. Of the two-thirds of patients who survive, approximately 50 percent are permanently disabled, mainly due to neurocognitive deficits, anxiety, and depression that occur in up to 80 percent. Many patients do not return to work or retire early, and their relationships are affected. The most important factor impacting outcome is the patient's neurological condition on arrival at the hospital as graded by the Hunt and Hess grading scale (Table 13.1). Other major independent determinants of outcome after SAH include

⟩ age
⟩ large aneurysm size >10 mm
⟩ aneurysm rebleeding
⟩ delayed cerebral ischemia from vasospasm
⟩ fever, anemia, and hyperglycemia

Table 13.1: Hunt and Hess grading scale for aneurysmal SAH

Grade	Clinical findings	Hospital Mortality (%)[a]	
		1968	1997
I	Asymptomatic or mild headache	11	1
II	Moderate to severe headache or oculomotor palsy	26	5
III	Confused, drowsy, or mild focal signs	37	19
IV	Stupor (localizes to pain)	71	42
V	Coma (posturing or no motor response to pain)	100	77
TOTAL		35	18

Note: [a] Data from 275 patients reported by Hunt and Hess in 1968, and 214 patients reported by Oshiro et al. in 1997; mortality figures do not include out-of-hospital deaths.

General emergency and critical care management

Immediate treatment of SAH starts with management of airway, respiration, and circulation, followed by evaluation of the level of consciousness. A complete blood count (CBC), metabolic panel, coagulation studies, troponin I, urine toxicology screen, electrocardiogram, and a chest x-ray should be obtained. Our management protocol for SAH is summarized in Table 13.2.

1. The efficacy of early blood pressure reduction for prevention of rebleeding is not established.
2. A relationship between rebleeding and persistent hypertension has been described.
   a) Treatment for systolic blood pressure (SBP) > 140–160 mmHg is generally practiced until the aneurysm is secured.
   b) Useful continuous infusion intravenous agents for blood pressure control include labetolol and nicardipine.
3. Administration of corticosteroids in SAH is controversial.

Dexamethasone 4–6 mg IV every 6 hr with a taper over 7–10 days is often used perioperatively to counteract the effects of intraoperative brain retraction injury and to treat headaches. However, this practice is not supported by controlled trials in the literature.

Treatment of hydrocephalus

The development of acute hydrocephalus is primarily related to the volume of intraventricular and subarachnoid blood in the basal cisterns.

1. SAH is complicated by significant hydrocephalus in 15–25 percent of cases.
2. Clinical findings of hydrocephalus include lethargy, psychomotor slowing, impaired short-term memory, limitation of upgaze, sixth cranial nerve palsies, and lower extremity hyperreflexia.
3. When obstructive hydrocephalus leads to increased intracranial pressure (ICP), the patient may be found stuporous or comatose with signs of brainstem compression.

Insertion of an extraventricular drain (EVD) is life saving with a prompt clinical response such as improvement of consciousness, but is complicated by a high risk of infection (up to 15 percent). If there is no improvement in 36–48 hr and the ICP is low, a poor neurological state is likely due to primary brain injury related to the acute effects of hemorrhage. Weaning of the EVD should begin after ICP is controlled for 48 hr either by trials of intermittent clamping with ICP monitoring. Serial lumbar puncture or placement of a spinal drain is an alternative to prolonged or repeated EVD placement if the basal cisterns are open.

Table 13.2: Columbia University Medical Center Management
Protocol for Acute SAH

Blood pressure	⬛➤ Control elevated blood pressure during the preoperative phase (systolic BP <140 mmHg) with IV labetolol or nicardipine to prevent rebleeding
Pre operative	⬛➤ Administer Amicar 4 g IV as a bolus, followed by a continuous infusion at 1 g/hr to prevent rebleeding in the absence of history of systemic thromboembolism and coronary artery disease
IV hydration	⬛➤ Preoperative: Normal (0.9%) saline at 80–100 ml/hr ⬛➤ Postoperative: Normal (0.9%) saline at 80–100 ml/hr, and 250 ml 5% albumin every 2 hr if the CVP is ≤5 mmHg
Laboratory testing	⬛➤ Periodically check complete blood count; transfuse for hematocrit <21% in stable patients, or <30% in patients with symptomatic vasospasm ⬛➤ Periodically check electrolytes to detect hyponatremia ⬛➤ Obtain serial ECGs and check admission cardiac troponin I (cTI) level to evaluate for cardiac injury; perform echocardiography in patients with abnormal ECG findings or cTI elevation
Seizure prophylaxis	⬛➤ Fosphenytoin or phenytoin IV load (15–20 mg/kg); discontinue on post-op day 2 unless patient has seized or is unstable
Vasospasm prophylaxis	⬛➤ Nimodipine 60 mg PO every 4 hr for 21 days
Physiologic homeostasis	⬛➤ Cooling blankets, systemic adhesive surface cooling, or intravenous heat exchange catheter to maintain T≤37.5°C ⬛➤ Insulin drip to maintain blood glucose ≤120 mg/dl
Ventricular ICP drainage	⬛➤ Begin trials of clamping external ventricular drain and monitoring on day 3 after placement
Vasospasm diagnosis	⬛➤ Transcranial Doppler sonography every 1–2 days until the eighth day after SAH

(continued)

Table 13.2: (continued)

	➠ CT or MR perfusion on day 4–8 after SAH if high risk
Therapy for symptomatic vasospasm	➠ Place patient in Trendelenberg (head down) position
	➠ Infuse 500 ml 5% albumin over 15 min
	➠ If the deficit persists, raise the systolic BP with phenylephrine or dopamine until the deficit resolves, up to a maximum of 200–220 mmHg
	➠ 250 ml 5% albumin solution every 2 hr if the CVP is ≤8 mmHg or the PADP is ≤14 mmHg
	➠ If refractory, place pulmonary artery catheter and add milrinone or dobutamine to maintain cardiac index ≥4.0 l/min/m²
	➠ Emergency angiogram for possible cerebral angioplasty and/or intraarterial verapamil injection unless the patient responds well to the above measures

Late hydrocephalus after SAH creates a clinical syndrome indistinguishable from normal pressure hydrocephalus and is closely correlated with a prolonged duration of EVD treatment. The symptoms encompass dementia, gait disturbance, and urinary incontinence that respond to shunting. About 20 percent of all SAH patients require a ventriculoperitoneal shunt for persistent hydrocephalus.

Fluid management

A central venous catheter should be placed for large volume access and monitoring of central venous pressure (CVP) in all patients with poor grade aneurysmal SAH.

Standard intravenous fluid management for patients with SAH consists of

1. isotonic fluids such as 0.9 percent saline at 1–1.5 ml/kg/hr;
2. supplemental 250 ml boluses of crystalloid (0.9 percent saline) or colloid (5 percent albumin) solution can be given every 2 hr if the CVP is ≤5 mmHg;
3. hypertonic saline solution (2 or 3 percent sodium chloride/acetate, 1 ml/kg/hr) is an alternative to normal saline for patients suffering from refractory ICP or symptomatic intracranial mass effect. The infusion is adjusted to maintain a sodium level of 155 meq/l and serum osmolality of 320 mosms/l.

Seizures

The incidence of seizures in SAH has been reported to be 6–25 percent at onset, although many of these events may represent tonic posturing. Approximately 5 percent experience seizures during hospitalization, and 7 percent will experience repeated seizures during the first year after discharge. The most important risk factors for seizure is focal pathology, such as large subarachnoid clots, subdural hemotoma, or cerebral infarction. A seizure at the onset of SAH does not predict an increased risk for epilepsy.

1. Intravenous anticonvulsant therapy with phenytoin or fosphenytoin is recommended in patients with SAH initially to prevent rebleeding related to seizures.
2. if the patient is stable and has not experienced a seizure, the anticonvulsant therapy may be stopped on the second postoperative day.
3. Some practitioners continue prophylactic anticonvulsant therapy during the period of critical illness in high risk patients.
4. Patients should be not continued on anticonvulsant therapy after discharge unless they have experienced seizures in the hospital, since anticonvulsants such as phenytoin may have a negative impact on long-term cognitive outcome.
5. Continuous electroencephalographic (cEEG) monitoring is recommended in poor-grade SAH patients in stupor or coma.
   a) Nonconvulsive seizures or status epilepticus can be detected with cEEG in 8–13 percent of poor grade patients with SAH.
   b) Midazolam infusion 0.2 mg/kg/hr titrated to background suppression is the first line of therapy for nonconvulsive status epilepticus.

ICU management

Fever and hyperglycemia after SAH impact negatively on mortality and outcome and should be treated. Prophylaxis for deep vein thrombosis is crucial, but subcutaneous heparin should not be started until the aneurysm is protected.

Special considerations in the management of SAH

Cerebral edema

Brain edema is common after SAH, especially in poor grade patients. Global cerebral edema occurs in up to 12 percent of SAH patients and may be explained by autoregulatory breakthrough in the setting of hypertension.

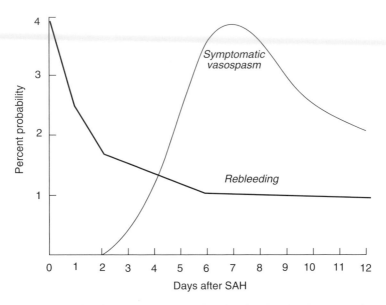

Figure 13.3 The daily percentage probability for the development of symptomatic vasospasm (solid line) or rebleeding (dashed line) after SAH. Day 0 denotes day of onset of SAH. From Mayer SA, et al. 2005, with permission.

There is an association with loss of consciousness at ictus and with poor outcome. Focal brain edema is found around large hematomas and can elicit mass effect with subsequent herniation.

Rebleeding

The risk of rebleeding is highest in the first 24 hr after initial aneurysm rupture (4 percent), but remains 1–2 percent per day for the next 4 weeks (Figure 13.3). The cumulative risk of rebleeding in untreated patients is high (20 percent at 2 weeks, 30 percent at 1 month, 40 percent at 6 months), but decreased after 6 months to 2–4 percent per year. An increased risk of rebleeding is associated with

- poor clinical grade
- loss of consciousness at ictus
- larger aneurysm size
- ventricular drainage

Rebleeding leads to poor outcome: about 50 percent of those who rebleed die immediately, and up to another 30 percent die from complications of rebleeding. Therefore, the initial treatment of SAH is targeted at securing the aneurysm in order to prevent rebleeding.

Craniotomy and aneurysm clipping

Craniotomy and aneurysm clipping with microsurgical technique and preservation of the parent artery and its branches has long been considered the gold standard of aneurysm therapy.

1. Early clipping within 48–72 hr of presentation as well as safer microsurgical techniques result in permanent aneurysm obliteration in over 90 percent confirmed by intra- or postoperative angiogram and low morbidity and mortality of 5–15 percent excluding giant aneurysms.
2. The risk of surgery is highest when the aneurysm is large or located on the basilar artery.

Endovascular coiling

With the introduction of Guglielmi Detachable Coils (soft thrombogenic detachable platinum coils, GDC, Target Therapeutics, Fremont, CA) for endovascular therapy of aneurysm, coil embolization became an essential alternative to craniotomy and aneurysm clipping. Obliteration of small-necked aneurysms can be achieved in 80–90 percent of the cases with a complication rate of 9 percent. The decision between surgical clipping and endovascular coiling should be based on clinical and radiological factors such as

1. clinical status of the patient;
2. anticipated surgical difficulty based on anatomical location;
3. anatomy of the access vessels (tortuosity, extent of arteriosclerotic change);
4. breadth of aneurysm neck in comparison to the dome and the parent artery (wide neck aneurysms are difficult to completely obliterate with coils – coils may migrate and be a source for emboli).

Recent advances in technique including the balloon remodeling technique that holds the coils in the aneurysm cavity, liquid embolic agents, and endovascular stents through which coils can be employed into the aneurysm make treatment of broad neck aneurysm feasible.

For a short-term period endovascular coiling seems to be safer than clipping as demonstrated by the International Subarachnoid Hemorrhage Aneurysm Trial (ISAT).

1. The ISAT study enrolled 2,134 good-grade patients with mostly small aneurysms <10 mm in the anterior circulation in a randomized fashion to undergo aneurysm clipping or intraoperative rebleeding coiling.
2. At 1 year, death and dependency was 23.7 percent after coiling and 30.6 percent after clipping, which may be attributed to a lower

frequency of brain retraction injury or rebleeding with coiling compared to clipping. This finding is further substantiated by previous
and followup studies.

3. The main concern about endovascular therapy is potential rebleeding
   after several years due to coil compaction and aneurysm regrowth at
   the residual neck. Serial followup angiographic studies every 6–24
   months are recommended until long-term results are available.

Electrolyte disturbances

Hyponatremia has been reported in 5–30 percent of SAH patients. Hyponatremia is usually the result of inappropriate secretion of antidiuretic
hormone (SIADH) and free water retention and/or excessive renal sodium
excretion due to increased atrial natriuretic factor, so-called cerebral salt
wasting syndrome.

1. Intravascular volume depletion and sodium loss may increase the risk
   of ischemia during the vasospasm period.
2. Administration of large volume isotonic crystalloids and restriction of
   free water intake should be applied to counteract potential hypovolemia and to prevent inappropriate free water retention.
3. Central venous catheters or pulmonary artery catheters can be used
   to maintain normal cardiac filling pressures and to prevent hypovolemia.

Neurogenic cardiac and pulmonary complications

Poor grade SAH may be further complicated by cardiac dysfunction and
pulmonary edema due to a catecholamine surge, resulting in neurogenic
"stunned myocardium" and neurogenic pulmonary edema. Cardiac dysfunction is accompanied by transient electrocardiographic abnormalities,
troponin leaks, reversible wall motion abnormalities on echocardiogram,
hypotension, and reduction of cardiac output. Neurogenic pulmonary
edema results from increased permeability of the pulmonary vasculature
and may occur isolated or in conjunction with neurogenic cardiac injury.
Hypotension, reduced cardiac output, and impaired oxygenation may
impair cerebral perfusion in the setting of increased ICP or vasospasm.

Vasospasm

Delayed cerebral ischemia from vasospasm is an independent predictor of
poor outcome after SAH.

1. Arterial narrowing can be demonstrated angiographically in 50–70
   percent and leads to delayed ischemia in 19–46 percent after SAH (see
   Figure 13.4).

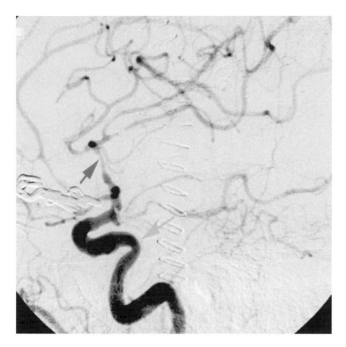

Figure 13.4 Cerebral angiogram demonstrates vasospasm of the basilar artery (black arrow), the right vertebral artery (white arrow), and branches of the left posterior cerebral artery (grey arrow).

2. Development of vasospasm begins on day 3 after SAH, is maximal at 5–14 days, and is diminishing by day 21.
3. Presence of thick blood seen on admission CT and severe IVH are strongly associated with higher risk for vasospasm (Table 13.3).

The underlying pathophysiology involves subintimal edema and infiltration of the arterial wall with leukocytes due to substances released from the subarachnoid blood such as oxyhemoglobin (possesses intrinsic vasoconstrictive properties), hydroperoxides, leukotrienes, free radicals, prostaglandins, thromboxane A_2, serotonin, endothelin, platelet-derived growth factor, and other inflammatory mediators.

Decreased level of consciousness and focal signs such as aphasia or hemiparesis should prompt the clinician to take immediate action. Transcranial Doppler (TCD) ultrasonography is a noninvasive method used to diagnose vasospasm in the larger cerebral arteries.

1. A mean flow velocity (Vm) of greater than 120 cm/s in the middle cerebral artery (MCA) is concerning for vasospasm, Vm above 200 cm/s is considered to be predictive, but dynamic changes of the mean flow velocities such as a two-fold increase might be more sensitive for the diagnosis of vasospasm.

Table 13.3: Modified Fisher CT rating scale for the prediction of symptomatic vasospasm

Grade	Criteria	Percentage of patients (%)	Frequency of DCI (%)	Frequency of Infarction (%)
0	No SAH or IVH	5	0	0
1	Minimal/thin SAH, no biventricular IVH	30	12	6
2	Minimal/thin SAH, *with* biventricular IVH	5	21	14
3	Thick SAH, no biventricular IVH	43	19	12
4	Thick SAH, *with* biventricular IVH	17	40	28
	All patients	100	20	12

*Notes:*Thick SAH refers to subarachnoid clot >5 mm in width that completely fills at least one cistern or fissure.

DCI, delayed cerebral ischemia (defined as symptomatic deterioration, cerebral infarction, or both resulting from vasospasm).

Data are based on a prospectively studied cohort of 276 patients at Columbia University Medical Center. From claassen et al. (2001) with permission.

2. Overall, prediction of vasospasm by serial TCD is not reliable, dependent on operator, and other systemic conditions.

Nimodipine, a calcium channel blocker, is administered orally for prevention of vasospasm on day 1 and was found to improve neurological outcome after SAH. However, nimodipine does not change the arterial diameter. A neuroprotective effect is postulated as the underlying mechanism. The treatment for acute vasospasm encompasses aggressive volume expansion and augmentation of blood pressure and cardiac output in order to improve cerebral blood flow through arteries in spasm and without autoregulatory capacity.

1. Crystalloid or colloid solutions provide volume to maintain CVP greater than 8 mmHg or pulmonary artery diastolic pressure greater than 14 mmHg.
2. Vasopressors, usually starting with phenylephrine, are used to elevate SBP up to 180–220 mmHg.
3. In the presence of cardiac dysfunction, dobutamine or milrinone infusions can be applied to maintain sufficient cardiac output as measured by cardiac index. Hypertensive, hypervolemic hemodilution,

so-called triple H therapy, leads to clinical improvement in about 70 percent of patients.

4. If the neurological symptoms are refractory to maximized triple H therapy, cerebral angioplasty and/or administration of intraarterial papaverine, nicardipine, or verapamil may lead to reversal of the neurological deterioration.

Future therapies

New endovascular techniques to secure aneurysms including biologically active coils and stents and to treat vasospasm with intraarterial vasodilators and intraaortic balloon placement, neurosurgical techniques such as intracisternal application of thrombolytic therapy to decrease the clot burden are currently under investigation. Administration of statins on day 1 after SAH or human albumin might decrease the incidence of vasospasm and improve neurological outcome. Improvement of ICU care including continuous control of hyperglycemia and hyperthermia may impact long-term neurological outcome.

Bibliography

Broderick JP, Brott TG, Duldner JE, Tomsick T, Leach A. Initial and recurrent bleeding are the major causes of death following subarachnoid hemorrhage. *Stroke* 1994;25(7):1342–7.

Broderick JP, Viscoli CM, Brott T, et al. Major risk factors for aneurysmal subarachnoid hemorrhage in the young are modifiable. *Stroke* 2003;34(6):1375–81.

Claassen J, Bernardini GL, Kreiter K, et al. Effect of cisternal and ventricular blood on risk of delayed cerebral ischemia after subarachnoid hemorrhage: The Fisher scale revisited. *Stroke* 2001;32(9):2012–20.

Claassen J, Carhuapoma JR, Kreiter KT, Du EY, Connolly ES, Mayer SA. Global cerebral edema after subarachnoid hemorrhage: Frequency, predictors, and impact on outcome. *Stroke* 2002;33(5):1225–32.

Claassen J, Peery S, Kreiter KT, et al. Predictors and clinical impact of epilepsy after subarachnoid hemorrhage. *Neurology* 2003;60(2):208–14.

Edlow JA, Caplan LR. Avoiding pitfalls in the diagnosis of subarachnoid hemorrhage. *N Engl J Med* 2000;342(1):29–36.

Fisher CM, Kistler JP, Davis JM. Relation of cerebral vasospasm to subarachnoid hemorrhage visualized by computerized tomographic scanning. *Neurosurgery* 1980;6(1):1–9.

Hunt WE, Hess RM. Surgical risk as related to time of intervention in the repair of intracranial aneurysms. *J Neurosurgery* 1968;28:14–20.

Janjua N, Mayer SA. Cerebral vasospasm after subarachnoid hemorrhage. *Curr Opin Crit Care* 2003;9(2):113–19.

Kassell NF, Torner JC, Haley EC, Jr, Jane JA, Adams HP, Kongable GL. The International Cooperative Study on the Timing of Aneurysm Surgery. Part 1: Overall management results. *J Neurosurg* 1990;73(1):18–36.

Kassell NF, Torner JC, Jane JA, Haley EC, Jr, Adams HP. The International Cooperative Study on the Timing of Aneurysm Surgery. Part 2: Surgical results. *J Neurosurg* 1990;73(1):37–47.

Klopfenstein JD, Kim LJ, Feiz– Erfan I, et al. Comparison of rapid and gradual weaning from external ventricular drainage in patients with aneurysmal subarachnoid hemorrhage: A prospective randomized trial. *J Neurosurg* 2004;100 (2):225–9.

Kowalski RG, Claassen J, Kreiter KT, et al. Initial misdiagnosis and outcome after subarachnoid hemorrhage. *JAMA* 2004;291(7):866–9.

Kreiter KT, Copeland D, Bernardini GL, et al. Predictors of cognitive dysfunction after subarachnoid hemorrhage. *Stroke* 2002;33(1):200–8.

Latchaw RE, Silva P, Falcone SF. The role of CT following aneurysmal rupture. *Neuroimaging Clin N Am* 1997;7(4):693–708.

Mack WJ, King RG, Ducruet AF, et al. Intracranial pressure following aneurysmal subarachnoid hemorrhage: Monitoring practices and outcome data. *Neurosurg Focus* 2003; 14(4):e3. This review evaluates management of hydrocephalus and increased intracranial pressure after subarachnoid hemorrhage.

Mayberg MR, Batjer HH, Dacey R, et al. Guidelines for the management of aneurysmal subarachnoid hemorrhage. A statement for healthcare professionals from a special writing group of the Stroke Council, American Heart Association. *Circulation* 1994;90(5):2592–605.

Mayer SA, Bernadini GL, Solomon RA, Brust JCM. Subarachnoid hemorrhage. In LP Rowland (ed.), *Merritt's textbook of neurology*, 11th edition, chapter 46. Lippincott Williams & Wilkins 2005 (1271 pages)

Molyneux A, Kerr R, Stratton I, et al. International Subarachnoid Aneurysm Trial (ISAT) of neurosurgical clipping versus endovascular coiling in 2143 patients with ruptured intracranial aneurysms: A randomised trial. *Lancet* 2002;360 (9342):1267–74.

Naidech AM, Kreiter KT, Janjua N, et al. Phenytoin exposure is associated with functional and cognitive disability after subarachnoid hemorrhage. *Stroke* 2005;36 (3):583–7.

Oshiro EM, Walter KA, Piantadosi S, Witham TF, Tamargo RJ. A new subarachnoid hemorrhage grading system base on the Glasgow Come Scale: A comparison with the Hunt–Hess Scale and World Federation of Neurological Surgeons Scales in a clinical series. *Neurosurgery* 1997; 41(1): 140–7.

Petruk KC, West M, Mohr G, et al. Nimodipine treatment in poor–grade aneurysm patients. Results of a multicenter double–blind placebo–controlled trial. *J Neurosurg* 1988;68(4):505–17.

Qureshi AI, Suarez JI, Bhardwaj A, Yahia AM, Tamargo RJ, Ulatowski JA. Early predictors of outcome in patients receiving hypervolemic and hypertensive therapy for symptomatic vasospasm after subarachnoid hemorrhage. *Crit Care Med* 2000;28 (3):824–9.

Qureshi AI, Suri MF, Yahia AM, et al. Risk factors for subarachnoid hemorrhage. *Neurosurgery* 2001;49(3):607–12; discussion 12–3.

Rinkel GJ, Djibuti M, Algra A, van Gijn J. Prevalence and risk of rupture of intracranial aneurysms: A systematic review. *Stroke* 1998;29(1):251–6.

Schievink WI. Intracranial aneurysms. *N Engl J Med* 1997;336(1):28–40.

Schievink WI, Michels VV, Piepgras DG. Neurovascular manifestations of heritable connective tissue disorders. A review. *Stroke* 1994;25(4):889–903.

Treggiari MM, Walder B, Suter PM, Romand JA. Systematic review of the prevention of delayed ischemic neurological deficits with hypertension, hypervolemia, and hemodilution therapy following subarachnoid hemorrhage. *J Neurosurg* 2003;98 (5):978–84.

Tseng MY, Czosnyka M, Richards H, Pickard JD, Kirkpatrick PJ. Effects of acute treatment with pravastatin on cerebral vasospasm, autoregulation, and delayed ischemic deficits after aneurysmal subarachnoid hemorrhage: A phase II randomized placebo–controlled trial. *Stroke* 2005;36(8):1627–32.

Wartenberg KE, Schmidt JM, Claassen J, et al. Impact of medical complications on outcome after subarachnoid hemorrhage. *Crit Care Med* 2006;34(3):617–23.

Wermer MJ, Greebe P, Algra A, Rinkel GJ. Incidence of recurrent subarachnoid hemorrhage after clipping for ruptured intracranial aneurysms. *Stroke* 2005; 36(1): 2394–9.

Wiebers DO, Whisnant JP, Huston J, 3rd, et al. Unruptured intracranial aneurysms: Natural history, clinical outcome, and risks of surgical and endovascular treatment. *Lancet* 2003;362(9378):103–10.

14 Dural and cerebral sinus thrombosis

James S. Castle and Romergryko G. Geocadin

Although quite rare, cerebral venous thrombosis (CVT) is responsible for 1–9 percent of all cerebrovascular deaths in the United States. CVT results from blockage of blood flow in the intracranial venous system. The spectrum of causes, locations, signs, and symptoms can be quite varied, making the diagnosis of CVT quite difficult. Not infrequently, the venous system is overlooked while working up neurologic symptoms, being overshadowed by the more common diseases of the arteries and parenchyma. Contrary to popular belief, CVT does not necessarily carry a poor prognosis, and treatment can be effective. Therefore, despite the difficulties involved in making a diagnosis, it is important for the clinician to quickly identify the disease, and initiate treatment in a timely manner.

This chapter provides a review of CVT, giving an explanation of the anatomy, pathophysiology, clinical presentation, diagnostic tools, and treatment necessary to effectively tackle this challenging disease.

A basic overview of venous anatomy

The venous drainage of the brain (as diagrammed in Figure 14.1) consists of two groups of venous systems that drain into larger sinuses, which then eventually drain into the internal jugular veins. The veins can be divided into superficial and deep groups. The superficial veins drain the surface of the brain into the deep veins, which then drain into the larger sinuses and finally into the internal jugular veins. Of particular clinical relevance are the larger sinuses that include

1. superior sagittal sinus:
   a) runs posteriorly along the midline roof of the skull in the midsagittal line;
   b) empties into the confluence of sinuses located on the very posterior aspect of the skull.

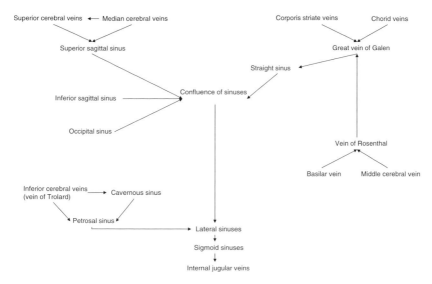

Figure 14.1 Diagram of the basic outflow pathway of venous blood from the brain out of the cranium.

2. inferior sagittal sinus:
   a) runs posteriorly along the midline on the bottom portion of the falx cerebri;
   b) receives drainage from the falx cerebri and mesial portions of the cerebral hemispheres and eventually drains into the straight sinus.
3. straight sinus:
   a) runs posteriorly along the intersection of the falx cerebri and the tentorium in a posterior direction into the confluence of sinuses;
   b) receives drainage from the vein of Galen, inferior sagittal sinus, and superior cerebellar veins.
4. lateral sinuses:
   a) start at the confluence of sinuses (one running along the tentorium to the right, one to the left);
   b) one sinus is typically larger than the other (one being fed predominantly from the larger superior sagittal sinus, the other being fed predominantly from the smaller straight sinus);
   c) collect additional drainage from the superior petrosal sinuses and then travel to the base of the brain where they become the internal jugular veins after passing through the jugular foramen.
5. occipital sinus:
   a) runs from the foramen magnum to the confluence of sinuses;
   b) has collateral flow with the spinal veins.
6. cavernous sinus:
   a) bilateral sinuses supplied by the ophthalmic veins, some cerebral veins, and the sphenoparietal sinus;

    b) drain into the lateral sinuses through the petrosal sinuses and collateralize with the other cavernous sinus through the circular sinus;

    c) are clinically very important because through them runs the internal carotid artery, CN III, CN IV, CN VI, and the ophthalmic and maxillary divisions of CN V. Pathology in these sinuses can often present with palsies of those nerves.

7. inferior petrosal veins:

    a) are located one on each side of the skull and receive flow from the internal ear, brainstem, and cerebellum.

    b) drain into the lateral sinuses to form the internal jugular veins.

8. also clinically relevant are numerous emissary veins that pass through the skull at various points and collateralize the intracranial and extracranial circulation.

Signs and symptoms

CVT can affect a wide variety of age groups with mean age of onset in the third decade of life. Incidence in women outnumbers men 1.5–5:1. The most common symptom on presentation is headache. But the headache presentation may have wide variability (see Table 14.1).

1. The headache is believed to be caused either by increased intracranial pressure (ICP) and/or local irritation of pain-sensitive fibers in the dura by an expanding sinus.

2. Of particular concern is the overlap between symptoms of CVT and pseudotumor cerebri. Both diseases are seen more frequently in women, and both can be seen in the obese. It is very important to rule out CVT when evaluating any patient prior to diagnosing pseudotumor cerebri.

3. The headache of CVT may also be misdiagnosed as originating from a more benign source such as migraine, tension, or sinus. Often, a falsely normal head CT will reassure the physician that there are no structural lesions.

4. The consideration of CVT needs to be entertained in headache patients, particularly in association of focal neurologic deficits or a significant change in headache quality.

5. In addition to headache, CVT may be heralded by focal neurologic deficits, seizures, or changes in mental status.

Etiology

Classically, the etiology of CVT is broken into two types: septic and nonseptic. The vast majority of cases are nonseptic. In the case of septic thrombi, infection is often spread from nearby tissue – generally from the

Table 14.1: Headache and other symptoms on presentation with CVT (from Agostoni 2004 *Neurol Sci* and Iurlaro et al. 2004 *Neurol Sci.*)

Symptom	Presentation I
Headache	77–86
Focal neurologic deficit	53–54
Seizure	35–40
Altered consciousness	24–30
In those with headache, nature of headache	
Acute (< 48 hours)	39–45
Subacute (48 hours to 1 month)	40–50
Chronic (> 1 month)	11–15
Localized	67–75
Generalized	25–33
Mild	11–15
Moderate	37–45
Severe	40–52
Continuous	69–78
Nausea and vomiting	57
Responded to analgesic	17

sinuses of the cranium, the periorbital region, or the ear. Therefore, in cases of septic CVT, there is often a history of sinus, periorbital, or ear infection in the days prior to the onset of neurologic signs and symptoms.

Several of the underlying conditions associated with nonseptic thrombi are summarized in Table 14.2. Many are similar to risk factors associated with general venous thromboses.

Establishing the diagnosis

Radiological diagnostic tests

COMPUTERIZED TOMOGRAPHY (CT)

Generally, a noncontrast CT of head is the first diagnostic image used in CVT patients. CVT findings on head CT include

1. parenchymal hypodensities that do not respect arterial distributions.
2. parenchymal hyperdensities indicative of hemorrhage, particularly in patients without other risk factors such as severe hypertension, amyloid angiopathy, tumor, recent illicit drug use, or bleeding diathesis (see Figure 14.2). These hemorrhages, unlike their primary arterial counterparts, are believed to be caused by venous occlusion leading to increased capillary pressure and diapedesis of red blood cells.
3. subarachnoid hemorrhage.

Table 14.2: Possible etiology of CVT

⇒ **Pregnancy and/or recent pregnancy**
⇒ **Oral contraceptive pills**
⇒ **Clotting disorders**:

- abnormalities of Protein C or S, nephrotic syndrome, hyperhomocysteinemia, antiphospholipid antibody syndrome, antithrombin III deficiency
- activated protein C resistance
- Factor V Leidin mutation
- Prothrombin G 20210 mutation
- elevated Factor VIII levels
- MTHFR (methylene tetrahydrofolate reductase) gene mutation
- elevated lipoprotein(a)

⇒ **Autoimmune diseases**:

- Inflammatory bowel disease
- Bechets syndrome
- anti-Phospholipid antibody syndrome
- Wegener's Granulomatosis

⇒ **Cancer**
⇒ **Chemotherapy**:

- Tamoxifen
- l-Asparaginase

⇒ **Hematologic disorders**:

- Polycythemia Vera, blood doping in athletes
- Dehydration
- Paroxysmal nocturnal hemoglobinuria
- Sickle cell disease
- Malarial infection

⇒ **Recent trauma**
⇒ **Recent lumbar puncture**
⇒ **History of intracranial hypotension**: no clear etiology for this association
⇒ **Anabolic steroid use**
⇒ **High dose corticosteroids**: particularly at doses >500mg of methylprednisolone

However, head CT is typically not a very sensitive test to diagnose CVT. Sensitivity is only 70 percent. CT with intravenous contrast may show an "empty delta sign" in one of the large venous sinuses. This results from contrast-filled blood flowing around a central clot, giving the contrast a triangular shape similar to the Greek letter delta. CT venography is generally accepted as also being excellent for identifying CVT.

CEREBRAL ANGIOGRAPHY

This is the gold standard for diagnosing CVT (see Figures 14.3 and 14.4). When other tests are unavailable or nondiagnostic, conventional angiogram can be extremely useful for identifying a thrombus. However, given the risks of stroke, arterial dissection, contrast induced nephropathy, and the like, associated with angiography, it has been largely replaced by magnetic resonance (MR) imaging.

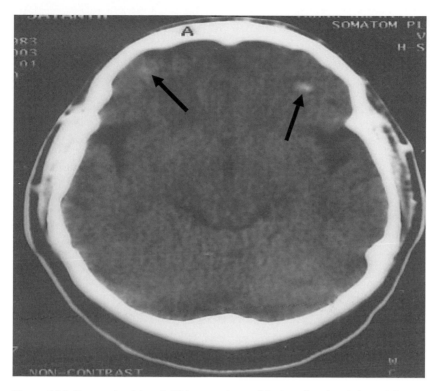

Figure 14.2 Noncontrast head CT in a patient with CVT showing bilateral frontal lobe hyperdensities (arrows) indicating acute intraparenchymal hemorrhage (Courtesy of Murphy K, *Interventional neuroradiology*, Johns Hopkins Hospital.)

MR

MR venography is considered a reliable tool for the diagnosis of CVT (see Figure 14.5). MR imaging can help determine the temporal onset of CVT.

1. An isodense T1 signal coupled with a dark T2 signal in the occluded sinus is suggestive of an acute disease.
2. Brightness on both T1 and T2 could be seen in subacute presentation.
3. T2 STAR imaging is particularly good at visualizing shifts from hemoglobin to deoxyhemoglobin within clots, and, therefore, may be helpful in showing signal loss in the affected sinus or vein and in areas of venous infarct.

Other diagnostic tests

1. *D-dimer blood level* When <500 ng/ml is used as a reference for a negative test, the negative predictive value is 95 percent and sensitivity is 83 percent.

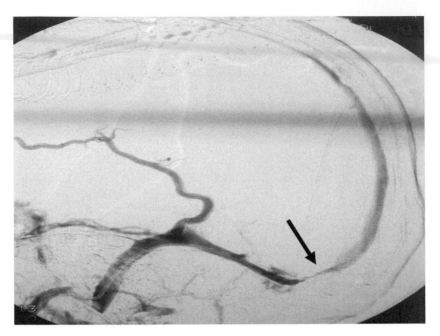

Figure 14.3 Venous phase of conventional angiogram showing no filling in the inferior sagittal sinus and poor flow in the confluence of sinuses (see arrow) (Courtesy of Murphy K, *Interventional neuroradiology*, Johns Hopkins Hospital and Dr. Richard Berger.)

2. *Lumbar puncture* may indicate elevated opening pressure, evidence of subarachnoid blood as seen in the cell count and differential (performed on two tubes of CSF to check for clearing of RBCs), xanthochromia, and elevated CSF bilirubin

Workup of hypercoagulable state

Given the risk factors discussed, depending on the level of clinical suspicion, a screen for the cause of CVT may include

1. complete blood count, ESR, ANA, ANCA;
2. antiphospholipid antibody screen (prothrombin time, partial thromboplastin time, lupus anticoagulant, anticardiolipin antibody, β2 glycoprotein-I);
3. protein C and S, antithrombin III, activated protein C resistance, Factor V Leidin mutation, G20210A transition of prothrombin gene mutation, homocysteine, Factor VIII level, lipoprotein(a) level, methylene tetrahydrofolate reductase (MTHFR) gene mutation;
4. hemoglobin electropheresis to rule out sickle cell disease;

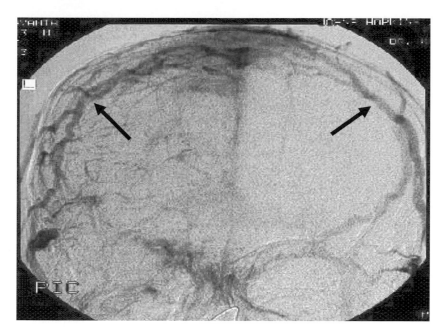

Figure 14.4 Venous phase of conventional angiogram showing no filling in the bilateral sigmoid sinuses with good collateralization of flow (see arrows) indicating chronic thrombosis (Courtesy of Murphy K, *Interventional neuroradiology*, Johns Hopkins Hospital.)

5. heparin-induced thrombocytopenia panel in patients exposed to heparin prior to formation of the thrombus;
6. malignancy screen;
7. urine for βHCG;
8. the yield of similar panels has been in the range of 41–75 percent;
9. blood should be drawn prior to initiation of any anticoagulation.

Treatment

Anticoagulation

Anticoagulation should be used as first-line therapy for treating CVT as recommended by Cochrane Reviews and the American College of Chest Physicians (ACCP). The ACCP grades the strength of evidence for this recommendation as 1B (very certain that benefits outweigh risks based on inconsistent results from randomized controlled trials) for heparin and 1C (very certain that benefits outweigh risks based on observational studies) for warfarin. Few randomized controlled trials support these recommendations.

1. Recommended therapy for patients with CVT is IV heparin or LMWH.
2. Intracranial hemorrhage is *not* a contraindication.
3. Target activated partial thromplastin time (APTT) should be around 80–100 s.
4. For long-term treatment, oral anticoagulation should be continued for 3–6 months with INR goal of 2.0–3.0.
5. Optimum duration of therapy is still not firmly established. Some evidence indicates that if recanalization is to occur, it will only occur within the first 4 months of therapy. However, if a patient has an ongoing clotting disorder, they may benefit from longer term therapy.

Thrombolysis

Currently, there are no randomized controlled trials showing a benefit from thrombolysis in CVT. Although many of the published case series dealing with thrombolysis in CVT have reported a benefit, others have reported mixed results. The use of local fibrinolysis should only be considered in cases where the patient's condition is deteriorating despite standard anticoagulation. Of some interest recently is the potential for mechanical disruption of the clot together with intravenous thrombolysis. A handful of patients have benefited from these techniques, and the

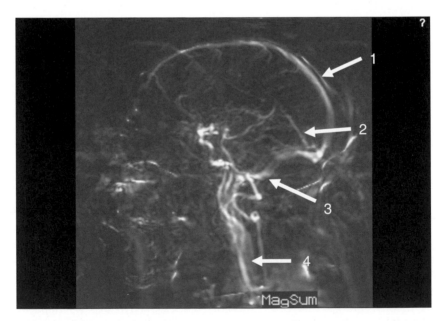

Figure 14.5 Magnetic resonance venogram of the cerebral venous system. Evident is the superior sagittal sinus (arrow #1), straight sinus (arrow #2), lateral and sigmoid sinuses (arrow #3), and internal jugular veins (arrow#4).

outcomes show a low complication rate with generally good neurological outcome.

Treatment of CVT complications

In cases where neurologic deterioration is likely, patients should be cared for in an ICU setting. As the presentation is varied, supportive neurologic therapies can be individualized for patients.

1. Signs and symptoms due to increased ICP should be treated accordingly.
2. In cases with focal mass effect and impending neurologic deterioration, aggressive therapy may include securing of the airway by endotracheal intubation, especially in those with impaired mentation, providing adequate oxygenation and acute hyperventilation (generally effective for only a few hours) with a goal pCO_2 of 25–35 mmHg. It is worthwhile mentioning that prophylactic hyperventilation provides no benefit and has been found to cause harm.
3. With continued ICP elevation or significant mass effect, mannitol as intravenous boluses or hypertonic saline infusion should be considered. Neurosurgical consultation for ICP monitoring and/or shunting may be required.
4. Acetazolamide may be used, especially after the acute period to reduce CSF production; however, in more acute cases, aggressive therapy should be used.
5. In cases with no focal mass effect in the brain, lumbar puncture, lumbar shunting, and optic fenestration should be considered if visual loss is imminent.
6. Finally, in case of infectious thrombosis from a local source, immediate neurosurgical and/or ENT consult should be obtained, and appropriate antibiotics initiated.
7. In patients with seizures or cortical disease secondary to CVT, antiepileptics should be used for seizure control and prophylaxis. Phenytoin (loading dose 20 mg/kg) has classically been first-line therapy in hospitalized patients for its ease of loading and monitoring. In emergent situations, IV loading should be done with fosphenytoin. Rapid phenytoin IV loads can lead to hypotension, heart block, and venous irritation.

Prognosis

Several studies have been done examining the outcomes of patients with CVT. When treated precipitously, patients with CVT could achieve full recovery. Sixty-four to eighty-two percent can have full recovery, while less than ten percent may die from the disease. Factors that portend a poor prognosis include focal deficits, cancer, encephalopathy, and/or coma. Isolated ICP is associated with a good prognosis.

Conclusion

The clinical manifestations of CVT are quite varied and can mimic several other diseases. One must have a high index of suspicion to make the diagnosis. The development of neuroimaging provides the clinician a wide range of ability to confirm this disorder. In patients with confirmed CVT, anticoagulation is still the therapy of choice. Aggressive supportive care must be provided. Overall, if identified early, treated appropriately and supported aggressively, there is a high likelihood for a good outcome in patients with CVT.

Bibliography

Agostoni E. Headache in cerebral venous thrombosis. *Neurol Sci* 2004;25(Suppl 3): S206–10.

Albers GW. Antithrombotic and thrombolytic therapy for ischemic stroke: The Seventh ACCP Conference on Antithrombotic and Thrombolytic Therapy. *Chest* 2004;126(Suppl 3):483–512.

Baumgartner RW, Studer A, Arnold M, Georgiadis D. Recanalisation of cerebral venous thrombosis. *J Neurol Neurosurg Psychiatry* 2003;74(4):459–61.

Berroir S, Grabli D, Heran F, Bakouche P, Bousser MG. Cerebral sinus thrombosis in two patients with spontaneous intracranial hypotension. *Cerebrovasc Dis* 2004;17 (1):9–12.

Bousser MG. Cerebral venous thrombosis: Nothing, heparin, or local thrombolysis? *Stroke* 1999;30:481–3.

Bradley W, Daroff R, Fenichel G, Jankovic J. *Neurology in clinical practice*, 4th edition. Massachusetts: Butterworth Heinemann, 2000.

Breteau G, Mounier-Vehier F, Godefroy O, et al. Cerebral venous thrombosis 3 year clinical outcome in 55 consecutive patients. *J Neurol* 2003;250(1):29–35.

Cakmak S, Derex L, Berruyer M, et al. Cerebral venous thrombosis: Clinical outcome and systematic screening of prothrombotic factors. *Neurology* 2003;60 (7):1175–8.

Cantu C, Alonso E, Jara A, et al. Hyperhomocysteinemia, low folate and vitamin B12 concentrations, and methylene tetrahydrofolate reductase mutation in cerebral venous thrombosis. *Stroke* 2004;35(8):1790–4.

Crassard I, Bousser MG. Cerebral venous thrombosis. *J Neuroophthalmol* 2004;24 (2):156–63.

Einhaupl K, Villringer A, Meister W, et al. Heparin treatment in sinus venous thrombosis. *Lancet* 1991;338(8767):597–600.

Fernandes A, Ribeiro C, Marques C, Reis J. Venous cerebral thrombosis. Mechanical and chemical thrombolysis. *Acta Med Port* 2003;16(3):213–15.

Ferro JM, Lopes MG, Rosas MJ, Ferro MA, Fontes J. Long term prognosis of cerebral vein and dural sinus thrombosis. Results of the VENOPORT study. *Cerebrovasc Dis* 2002;13(4):272–8.

Gray H. *Anatomy. Descriptive and surgical*, 15th edition. USA: Barnes and Noble Books, 1995.

Iurlaro S, Beghi E, Massetto N, et al. Does headache represent a clinical marker in early diagnosis of cerebral venous thrombosis? A prospective multicentric study. *Neurol Sci* 2004;25(Suppl 3):S298–9.

Juhl S, Shorsh K, Videbaek H, Binzer MN. Concomitant arterial and venous thrombosis in a body builder with severe hyperhomocysteinemia and abuse of anabolic steroids. *Ugeskr Laeger* 2004;166(40):3508–9.

Kieslich M, Porto L, Lanfermann H, Jacobi G, Schwabe D, Bohles H. Cerebrovascular complications of L-aspariginase in the therapy of acute lymphoblastic leukemia. *J Pediatr Hematol Oncol* 2003;25(6):484–7.

Krishnan A, Karnad DR, Limaye U, Siddharth W. Cerebral venous and dural sinus thrombosis in severe Falciparum Malaria. *J Infect* 2004;48(1):86–90.

Lalive PH, de Moerloose P, Lovblad K, Sarasin FP, Mermillod B, Sztajzel R. Is measurement of d-dimer useful in the diagnosis of cerebral venous thrombosis? *Neurology* 2003;61(8):1057–60.

Marcucci R, Liotta A, Cellai A, et al. Increased plasma levels of lipoprotein(a) and the risk of idiopathic and recurrent venous thromboembolism. *Am J Med* 2003;115 (8):601–5.

Masjuan J, Pardo J, Callejo JM, Andres MT, Alvarez-Cermeno JC. Tamoxifen: A new high risk factor for cerebral venous thrombosis. *Neurology* 2004;62(2):334–5.

Masuhr F, Mehraein S, Einhaupl K. Cerebral venous and sinus thrombosis. *J Neurol* 2004;251(1):11–23.

Mouraux A, Gille M, Dorban S, Peeters A. Cortical venous thrombosis after lumbar puncture. *J Neurol* 2002;249(9):1313–15.

Oshiro S, Motomura K, Fukushima T. Systemic lupus erythematosus manifesting as subarachnoid hemorrhage induced by cortical venous thrombosis and followed by medial medullary infarction. *No To Shinkei* 2003;55(9):791–5.

Rogers LR. Cerebrovascular complications in cancer patients. *Neurol Clin* 2003;21 (1):167–92.

Rosenstingl S, Ruivard M, Melon E, Schaeffer A, Gouault-Heilmann M. Cerbral-vein thrombosis: Retrospective study of twenty-seven cases. *Rev Med Intern* 2002;23 (12):973–82.

Selim M. *Radiological and laboratory diagnosis of cerebral venous thrombosis. The diagnosis and management of dural sinus and cerebral venous thrombosis.* San Francisco, CA: Education Program Syllabus American Academy of Neurology Meeting, 2004.

Stam J, de Bruijn SF, de Veber G. Anticoagulation for cerebral sinus thrombosis (Cochrane review), issue 2. The Cochrane Library, 2005.

Stolz E, Klotzsch C, Schlachetzki F, Rahimi A. High-dose corticosteroid treatment is associated with an increased risk of developing cerebral venous thrombosis. *Eur Neurol* 2003;49:247–8.

Torbey M. *Cerebral venous thrombosis: A guide to clinical diagnosis. The diagnosis and management of dural sinus and cerebral venous thrombosis.* San Francisco, CA: Education Program Syllabus American Academy of Neurology Meeting, 2004.

Stroke in Consultation

15 Perioperative stroke

Viktor Szeder, Magdy H. Selim, and Michel T. Torbey

With the increase in the number of elderly patients undergoing surgery, neurologists are being consulted more often either to assess stroke risks or to treat patients who develop a stroke in the perioperative period.

Estimated stroke risk – prediction models

Postoperative stroke risk is related to type of surgery performed (Table 15.1). Several groups estimated the risk of stroke during surgical procedure by creating prediction models.

1. Fortescue et al. in a study of 9,498 patients undergoing coronary artery bypass graft (CABG) reported that major adverse outcomes occurred in 7.2 percent, where 2.2 percent were deaths and 2.2 percent were strokes.
   a) Authors created a prediction model based on multiple variables. Each of the 16 identified preoperative risk factors was assigned a score (Table 15.2).
   b) The maximum possible total risk score was 73 points.
   c) The rate of adverse outcome varied from 2.2 for a patient with a low cumulative score, up to 22.3 in patients in the highest risk category.
2. Charlesworth et al. reviewed 33,062 patients undergoing CABG. Strokes occurred at the rate of 1.61 percent.
   a) The authors provided a risk assessment point system that correlated with the risk of stroke (Table 15.3).
   b) Clinical risk score of 5 points had approximate predicted risk of having a stroke about 1 percent, where 8, 9, and 10 points had 2, 3, and 6 percent, respectively.

Prevention of perioperative stroke

Perioperative stroke can be either related to the inherent cerebral and peripheral vascular risks present in the general population or related to the stroke risk associated with a particular procedure.

Table 15.1: Perioperative stroke risk rates for different surgeries

Surgery	Stroke risk (%)
General surgery	0.2
General surgery with or without carotid bruit	0.5
General surgery after prior stroke	2.9
General surgery with carotid stenosis and bruit or prior symptoms	3.6
CABG retrospective studies	1.4
CABG prospective studies	2.0
CABG surgery after prior stroke or TIA	8.5
CABG surgery + valve surgery	4.2–13.0
CABG surgery + unilateral > 50% carotid stenosis	3.0
CABG surgery + bilateral >50% carotid stenosis	5.0
CABG surgery + carotid occlusion	7.0
Surgery with symptomatic vertebrobasilar stenosis	6.0

Note: CABG, coronary artery bypass graft; TIA, transient ischemic attack;
Source: Modified from Blacker et al. (2004).

Table 15.2: Predicting major adverse outcome and stroke post-CABG

Predictor	Points	Predictor	Points
Preoperative creatinine ⩾3.0 mg/dl	12	Age 60–69 years	5
Age ⩾80	11	Preoperative creatinine 1.5–3.0 mg/dl	5
Cardiogenic shock	10	History of stroke or TIA	4
Emergent operation	9	Ejection fraction 30–49%	3
Age 70–79 years	8	History of COPD	3
Prior CABG	7	Female gender	3
Ejection fraction ≤30%	6	History of HTN	2
History of liver disease	6	Urgent operation	2

Score	0–5	6–10	11–15	16–20	21–25	≥26
Risk of major adverse outcome (%)	2.2	4	5.9	10.9	17	22.3
Death (%)	0.4	1	2	3.5	5.5	11.6

Modified from Ref (1)

Table 15.3: Preoperative calculation of risk of stroke in CABG patients

Variable	Stroke risk score
Age 55–59	1.5
Age 60–64	2.5
Age 65–69	3.5
Age 70–74	4
Age 75–79	4.5
Age ≥80	5.5
Female	1
DM	1.5
Vascular disease	2
Renal failure or creatinine ≥2 mg/dl	2
Ejection fraction ≤40%	1.5
Urgent surgery	1.5
Emergent surgery	2.5

Source: Modified from Charlesworth et al. (2003).

Antiplatelets in the perioperative period

The role of antiplatelets in stroke prevention is without doubt very important. Aspirin (ASA) and clopidogrel are the most studied agents in the perioperative period. Risk of increased bleeding associated with ASA remains controversial.

CABG PATIENTS

1. Initiation of ASA 325 mg daily as soon as 1 hr following CABG has been associated with improved early and late saphenous vein bypass graft patency.
2. The American College of Chest Physicians (ACCP) recommends lifelong ASA therapy in patients undergoing CABG. ASA 325 mg daily should be started 6 hr after CABG for 1 year.
3. Patients with high risk of stroke should probably remain on ASA preoperatively or definitely started on it postoperatively.

CAROTID ENDARTERECTOMY (CEA) PATIENTS

The role of ASA in stroke prevention is stronger in perioperative period in the setting of CEA.

1. Low dose ASA 75 mg/day reduced the number of postoperative strokes without complete recovery within 1 week, with no significant increase of intraoperative bleeding.

2. These results were confirmed by another randomized clinical trial, where patients scheduled for CEA were randomly assigned 81, 325, 650, or 1,300 mg ASA daily before surgery and continued for 3 months. The risk of stroke, myocardial infarction (MI), and death within 30 days and 3 months of CEA was lower for patients taking 81 mg or 325 mg ASA daily than for those taking 650 mg or 1,300 mg.

As for clopidogrel, it exerts its effect by selectively inhibiting adenosine diphosphate (ADP)-induced platelet aggregation. It is currently used in combination with ASA to decrease thrombotic events in patients with cerebrovascular and coronary artery disease. Although clopidogrel has clear indications for stroke prevention, it is not clear how to manage this medication at the time of surgery. Normal platelet function is restored in about 7 days after discontinuation of clopidogrel.

1. In patients who received clopidogrel and ASA initially in treatment of an acute coronary syndrome (ACS) and subsequently proceeded on to CABG, no excess of major bleeding after surgery was noted if the drug was discontinued more than 5 days before CABG. When clopidogrel was discontinued less than 5 days, risk of major bleeding was higher in the clopidogrel group compared to the ASA group.
2. In the CURE trial, the primary outcome of cardiovascular death, MI, and stroke occurred in 16.2 percent of ASA-treated patients and 14.5 percent of clopidogrel with ASA-treated patients. But the risk of bleeding was higher in the combined treatment group.
3. Studying the reduction of cerebral emboli in patients undergoing CEA using transcranial Doppler, the magnitude of embolization in the first 3 hr after surgery was significantly reduced in patients on 150 mg ASA and 75 mg clopidogrel (2.2 percent) compared with patients on 150 mg ASA and placebo (18.5 percent), representing a 10-fold reduction in the relative risk. However, in the clopidogrel-treated patients, the time from flow restoration to skin closure was significantly increased, although there was no increase in bleeding complications or blood transfusions.

Table 15.4 summarizes the recommendation for perioperative antiplatelets. There is no definite evidence at this stage that ASA-clopidogrel combined is superior to ASA alone. So both choices are at least equally effective.

Anticoagulation in the perioperative period

Although patients with atrial fibrillation and mechanical valves are dependent on anticoagulation to lower their thromboembolic risk, in the perioperative period, this benefit may be outweighed by risk of bleeding.

Table 15.4: Recommendations for antiplatelet use in perioperative period

	CEA	CABG
ASA		
Preoperatively	81–325 mg daily	75–325 mg daily
during surgery	Continue	discontinue at least 5 days before CABG
post operatively	81–325 mg daily	restart 75–325 mg daily 6 hr post-CABG
	or	
ASA/clopidogrel		
Preoperatively		
ASA	150 mg daily for 4 weeks before	75–325 mg daily
Clopidogrel	75 mg 12 hr before CEA	Load: 300 mg + maintenance: 75 mg daily
During surgery	Continue antiplatelets	Discontinue at least 5 days before CABG
Postoperatively		
ASA	150 mg daily	150 mg daily restart 6 hr post-CABG
Clopidogrel	75 mg daily	75 mg daily restart 6 hr post-CABG

Note: CEA, carotid endarterectomy; CABG, coronary artery bypass graft; ASA, aspirin.

1. There is lack of well-designed studies or reports on large populations for accurate risk quantification for patients temporarily discontinuing anticoagulation for surgery.
2. A systematic review of 31 studies examining the perioperative management and outcomes of patients receiving long-term oral anticoagulation found a stroke risk of 0.4 percent.
3. Warfarin cessation for endoscopy in patients with atrial fibrillation increases the risk of stroke to 1.06 percent within 30 days postprocedure.
4. Some procedures, such as colonoscopy or minor surgeries, may be performed while warfarin is continued, provided that the INR in the perioperative period is between 1.5 and 2.0.
5. Abrupt cessation of warfarin therapy is not without risk. This may result in a hypercoagulable state associated with thromboembolic event. The American College of Cardiology, in association with the

American Heart Association Task Force on Practice Guidelines and the ACCP, recommend this:

a) Bridging anticoagulant therapy with heparin or low molecular weight heparin (LMWH) should be considered for the majority of patients who require temporary interruption of warfarin therapy.

Preoperative anticoagulant management is essential in order to limit postoperative complications.

1. In patients who are receiving warfarin therapy with a target INR of 2.0–3.0, stopping warfarin 5 days before surgery will ensure a normal INR at the time of surgery.
2. Elderly patients may require a longer time for the INR to normalize after warfarin is stopped.
3. If INR target was 2.5–3.5, it is reasonable to stop warfarin 6 days before surgery.
4. INR testing should be performed on the day before surgery to ensure that it is normal.
5. If INR>1.5 on the day before surgery, low dose oral vitamin K (1–2 mg) will ensure a normal INR at the time of surgery.
6. Postoperative resumption of warfarin will depend on the type of surgery performed.

Treatment of stroke in the perioperative period

Thrombolytics

IV rt-PA. Acute ischemic stroke after cardiac and vascular operations is a devastating complication. Although intravenous (IV) recombinant tissue plasminogen activator (rt-PA) has been approved for use in acute ischemic stroke within the first 3 hr, *its use in postoperative patients has been contraindicated*.

IA rt-PA. Intraarterial (IA) thrombolysis is reasonably safe. In acute stroke within 12 days of cardiac operation, IA thrombolysis within 6 hr of stroke symptoms onset was performed. Neurologic improvement occurred in 38 percent of patients.

IA rt-PA appears to be safe in selected patients undergoing CEA. In one study all patients who underwent thrombectomy and urokinase demonstrated significant improvement over their preexploration state.

Although there is scarcity of studies reporting the use of thrombolytics in the perioperative period, IA route appears to be safe in selected patients.

Transarterial embolectomy

This newly developed technique has the potential of playing an important role in a subset of patients in whom emboli do not respond to thrombolysis.

1. In one study, mechanical embolectomy was used as first treatment and emboli were extracted with a vascular retrieval snare in five patients. The procedure was found to be safe and reproducible.
2. In another study, Kerber et al. used a snare in five patients who failed thrombolysis. In all five patients recanalization was achieved with subsequent improvement in neurological status in four or five patients. So this technique appears to be promising and may be a practical choice for patients in the perioperative period.

Prophylactic neuroprotection

Despite advances in perioperative care, postoperative stroke incidence has not changed significantly. Prophylactic neuroprotection appears to be a very attractive choice.

ß–ADRENERGIC RECEPTORS (ßAR) ANTAGONISTS

These agents are known to have benefits during cardiac and noncardiac surgery; they have shown to reduce the incidence of MI and postoperative arrhythmias.

Patients who use βAR antagonists also have a substantial reduction in the incidence of postoperative neurologic complications.

STATINS

Kertai et al. demonstrated that a combination of statin and beta-blocker use in patients with abdominal aneurysm surgery is associated with a reduced incidence of perioperative mortality. Furthermore, short-term treatment with atorvastatin significantly reduces the incidence of major cardiovascular events after vascular surgery.

⟾ Statin (atorvastatin, simvastatin, pravastatin, lovastatin, fluvasatin) for at least 1 week prior to CEA or combined CEA with CABG reduced the odds of perioperative stroke threefold and death fivefold.

These studies demonstrate that the concept of neuroprotection may be more successful in the perioperative setting and should be investigated more.

Carotid stenosis and specific surgeries

It is not uncommon as a stroke consultant to be asked "whether a patient with carotid stenosis undergoing surgery should have his carotid fixed prior to surgery." Certainly the answer will depend on the type of surgery.

Carotid stenosis and general surgery

1. The incidence of perioperative stroke in patients undergoing general surgery performed under general anesthesia is less than 0.5 percent.
2. Carotid stenosis is associated with a 3.6 percent risk of stroke.
3. Greater degree of stenosis is not associated with an increased risk.
4. No evidence to mandate prophylactic CEA for patient undergoing general surgery.
5. Intracranial angioplasty and stenting are associated with stroke and death rate ranging between 4 and 40 percent.
   a) The stroke risk associated with intracranial stenting or angioplasty exceeds the perioperative risk for general surgery in asymptomatic and symptomatic patients.
6. Recommendations are summarized in Table 15.5.

Table 15.5: Recommendations for carotid stenosis management before general surgery

If extracranial or intracranial stenosis asymptomatic no indication for CEA or stenting prior to surgery.
If extracranial stenosis symptomatic CEA or stenting is indicated prior to surgery.
If intracranial stenosis symptomatic surgery should be delayed for about a month and intraoperative hypotension should be avoided.

Source: Modified from Kerber et al. (2002).

Carotid stenosis and CABG

Studies have shown that the risk of stroke during CABG is high in patients with symptomatic carotid stenosis. However, the role of asymptomatic carotid disease as a cause of perioperative stroke remains uncertain Table 15.6.

1. The risk of perioperative stroke in asymptomatic patients increases with severity of carotid stenosis.
2. Risk of stroke in patients undergoing first-time CABG increased with severity of carotid stenosis ranging from zero percent in patients without stenosis to 3.2 percent in those with >70 percent stenosis and 27.3 percent in those with carotid occlusion.

There is no consensus regarding the potential benefit of CEA for asymptomatic disease prior to CABG. Data at best is conflicting.

1. Hines et al. in a retrospective analysis did not find any increased risk of stroke from either prophylactic CEA or combined CEA+CABG. The

Table 15.6: Recommendations for carotid stenosis management before CABG

When both coronary and extracranial carotid stenosis exist symptomatic
  lesions should be treated first in a staged procedure
If both lesions where symptomatic combined approached could be
  used. Consider carotid stenting for carotid disease
Patients with unilateral asymptomatic carotid disease ($\leq$75% stenosis)
  combined procedure should not be done
For patients with unilateral asymptomatic carotid disease ($\leq$80% stenosis)
  it is not clearly established which is the best approach

Source: Modified from Gavaghan et al. (1991) and Kerber et al. (2002).

authors concluded that patients with 80–99 percent carotid stenosis undergoing CEA prior to or in conjunction with CABG have a decreased incidence of postoperative stroke.

2. In a prospective study by Bilfinger et al., the risk of postoperative stroke was higher in patients undergoing combined CABG/CEA compared to CABG alone.

Table 15.6 summarizes our recommendations for management of carotid stenosis in CABG patients.

Bibliography

Barkhoudarian G, Ali MJ, Deveikis J, Thompson BG. Intravenously administered abciximab in the management of early cerebral ischemia after carotid endarterectomy: Case report. *Neurosurgery* 2004;55:709.

Bilfinger TV, Reda H, Giron F, et al. Coronary and carotid operations under prospective standardized conditions: Incidence and outcome. *Ann Thorac Surg* 2000;69:1792–8.

Blacker DJ, Flemming KD, Link MJ, Brown RD, Jr. The preoperative cerebrovascular consultation: Common cerebrovascular questions before general or cardiac surgery. *Mayo Clin Proc* 2004;79:223–9.

Bonow R, Carabello B, De Leon A, et al. ACC/AHA guidelines for the management of patients with valvular heart disease. A report of the American College of Cardiology/American Heart Association Task Force on Practice Guidelines (Committee on Management of Patients with Valvular Heart Disease). *JACC* 1998;32:1558–65.

Cartier R, Hamani I, Leclerc Y, Hebert Y. Influence of carotid atheroma on the neurologic status after myocardial revascularization. *Ann Chir* 1997;51:894–8.

Charlesworth DC, Likosky DS, Marrin CA, et al. Northern New England Cardiovascular Disease Study Group. Development and validation of a prediction model for strokes after coronary artery bypass grafting. *Ann Thorac Surg* 2003;76:436–43.

Chimowitz MI. Angioplasty or stenting is not appropriate as first-line treatment of intracranial stenosis. *Arch Neurol* 2001;58:1690–2.

Douketis J. Perioperative anticoagulation management in patients who are receiving oral anticoagulant therapy: A practical guide to clinicians. *Thromb Res* 2003;108:3–13.

Dunn AS, Turpie AG. Perioperative management of patients receiving oral anticoagulants: A systematic review. *Arch Intern Med* 2003;163:901–8.

Durazzo AE, Machado FS, Ikeoka DT, et al. Reduction in cardiovascular events after vascular surgery with atorvastatin: A randomized trial. *J Vasc Surg* 2004;39:967–75; discussion 975–6.

Evans BA, Wijdicks EF. High-grade carotid stenosis detected before general surgery: Is endarterectomy indicated? *Neurology* 2001;57:1328–30.

Fortescue EB, Kahn K, Bates DW. Development and validation of a clinical prediction rule for major adverse outcomes in coronary bypass grafting. *Am J Cardiol* 2001;88:1251–8.

Gavaghan TP, Gebski V, Baron DW. Immediate postoperative aspirin improves vein graft patency early and late after coronary artery bypass graft surgery. A placebo-controlled, randomized study. *Circulation* 1991;83:1526–33.

Gerraty RP, Gates PC, Doyle JC. Carotid stenosis and perioperative stroke risk in symptomatic and asymptomatic patients undergoing vascular or coronary surgery. *Stroke* 1993;24:1115–18.

Greer DM, Buonanno FS. Perioperative stroke risk assessment and management. In KL Furie, PJ Kelly (eds), *Current clinical neurology: Handbook of stroke prevention in clinical practice*. Totowa, NJ: Humana, 2002:243–53.

Hines GL, Scott WC, Schubach SL, et al. Prophylactic carotid endarterectomy in patients with high-grade carotid stenosis undergoing coronary bypass: Does it decrease the incidence of perioperative stroke? *Ann Vasc Surg* 1998;12:23–7.

Kerber CW, Barr JD, Berger RM, Chopko BW. Snare retrieval of intracranial thrombus in patients with acute stroke. *J Vasc Interv Radiol* 2002;13:1269–74.

Kertai MD, Boersma E, Westerhout CM, et al. A combination of statins and beta-blockers is independently associated with a reduction in the incidence of perioperative mortality and nonfatal myocardial infarction in patients undergoing abdominal aortic aneurysm surgery. *Eur J Vasc Endovasc Surg* 2004;28:343–52.

Lindblad B, Persson NH, Takolander R, Bergqvist D. Does low-dose acetylsalicylic acid prevent stroke after carotid surgery? A double-blind, placebo-controlled randomized trial. *Stroke* 1993;24:1125–8.

Mangano DT, Layug EL, Wallace A, Tateo I. Effect of atenolol on mortality and cardiovascular morbidity after noncardiac surgery. Multicenter Study of Perioperative Ischemia Research Group. *N Engl J Med* 1996;335:1713–20.

McGirt MJ, Perler BA, Brooke BS, et al. 3-hydroxy-3-methylglutaryl coenzyme A reductase inhibitors reduce the risk of perioperative stroke and mortality after carotid endarterectomy. *J Vasc Surg* 2005;42:829–36.

Moazami N, Smedira NG, McCarthy PM, et al. Safety and efficacy of intraarterial thrombolysis for perioperative stroke after cardiac operation. *Ann Thorac Surg* 2001;72:1933–7; discussion 1937–9.

Parikh S, Cohen JR. Perioperative stroke after general surgical procedures. *NY State J Med* 1993;93:162–5.

Payne DA, Jones CI, Hayes PD, et al. Beneficial effects of clopidogrel combined with aspirin in reducing cerebral emboli in patients undergoing carotid endarterectomy. *Circulation* 2004;109:1476–81.

Taylor DW, Barnett HJ, Haynes RB, et al. Low-dose and high-dose acetylsalicylic acid for patients undergoing carotid endarterectomy: A randomised controlled trial. ASA and Carotid Endarterectomy (ACE) Trial Collaborators. *Lancet* 1999;353:2179–84.

Wallace A, Layug B, Tateo I, et al. Prophylactic atenolol reduces postoperative myocardial ischemia. McSPI Research Group. *Anesthesiology* 1998;88:7–17.

Wikholm G. Transarterial embolectomy in acute stroke. *AJNR Am J Neuroradiol* 2003;24:892–4.

Winkelaar GB, Salvian AJ, Fry PD, et al. Intraoperative intraarterial urokinase in early postoperative stroke following carotid endarterectomy: A useful adjunct. *Ann Vasc Surg* 1999;13:566–70.

Yusuf S, Zhao F, Mehta SR, et al. Effects of clopidogrel in addition to aspirin in patients with acute coronary syndromes without ST-segment elevation. *N Engl J Med* 2001;345:494–502.

16 Stroke on OB/Gyn wards

Ann K. Helms

Introduction

Stroke, although rare during pregnancy, is a much-feared complication, not only due to concern for the long-term outcome of the mother, but also for the fetus. Additionally, practitioners often feel especially challenged by questions of safety and efficacy of diagnostic modalities and therapeutic options in a pregnant woman. This chapter attempts to clearly present the types and causes of stroke during pregnancy and the peripartum period, as well as discuss options for diagnosis and treatment in such cases.

Ischemic stroke related to pregnancy

All forms of stroke, including ischemic strokes, intracerebral hemorrhage (ICH), subarachnoid hemorrhage (SAH), and cerebral venous thrombosis are seen during and shortly after pregnancy. Thankfully, stroke during pregnancy and the peurperium is not common. Early epidemiologic studies reported an incidence of 3–5 ischemic strokes per 100,000 births. Interestingly, nearly half were in the postpartum period, and the rest clustered in the latter half of pregnancy. Several more recent studies have shown that, in fact, the incidence of ischemic stroke during pregnancy is not increased over the baseline rate of stroke in young women. The first several weeks postpartum, however, are associated with a higher risk of stroke than is seen in the general population of young women.

Hemorrhagic strokes related to pregnancy

ICH, in contrast, is more frequent during pregnancy, when ICH is as frequent as ischemic stroke, whereas cerebral infarctions make up the bulk of strokes in nonpregnant patients. Postpartum, ICH rates are even higher. SAH is also much more common during the peurperium and postpartum period.

Increased rates of hemorrhagic strokes are seen in the following cases:

1. ICH due to pregnancy-induced hypertension.
2. ICH or SAH due to increased rates of bleeding of vascular malformations such as arteriovenous malformations and aneurysms.
3. Arteriovenous malformation (AVMs) have increased rates of bleeding throughout pregnancy.
4. AVMs tend to bleed from the venous side likely due to increased blood volume.
5. Aneurysms have increased bleed rates during the last half of pregnancy.

Causes of pregnancy related stroke

It is important to state that pregnancy, in and of itself, does not cause strokes. In fact, most strokes occurring during pregnancy and the peurperium are not due to pregnancy-specific causes, but are similar in etiology to strokes seen in nonpregnant young patients (see Table 16.1). Additionally, it is important to emphasize that strokes during and around pregnancy, whether due to pregnancy-specific causes or not, usually present no differently from strokes in the general population.

Hemostatic, hemodynamic, and hormonal changes during pregnancy

The increased rate of certain types of stroke during pregnancy and of all strokes postpartum would suggest that underlying metabolic changes are contributing to the development of strokes. Changes in the levels of numerous hemostatic factors contribute to a mild hypercoagulable state during pregnancy (see Table 16.2).

Additionally, hormonal changes are felt to contribute to the development of acquired activated protein C resistance in some cases. Also, hemodynamic shifts, including increased blood volume, with subsequent increased venous BP and cardiac output may also contribute to certain types of stroke associated with pregnancy. These changes return to normal within several weeks after delivery, correlating with the period of increased stroke risk peripartum. Finally, certain pregnancy-related complications, including hypertension, dehydration, infection, and cesarean delivery have been found to increase the risk of stroke as well.

Unique causes of pregnancy related stroke

There are only a few clinical entities specific to pregnancy and the postpartum state that can cause strokes. There are several others that, while not exclusively seen in pregnancy, are more commonly associated with pregnancy and the puerperium (see Table 16.1). Despite the fact that most are rare, they must be considered in any pregnant or postpartum woman with

Table 16.1: Causes of stroke in young people

	Neurologic Deficits	
	Nonhemorrhagic	
Hemorrhagic	**Ischemic**	**Nonischemic**
Pregnancy unrelated	Pregnancy unrelated	Eclampsia
Hypertension	Traditional risk factors	Postpartum cerebral angiopathy
Bleeding diatheses	Cardioembolism	
Aneurysm	PFO	
AVM/vascular malformation	Hypercoagulable state	
Drug abuse: Amphetamines, cocaine	Genetic	
	Hyperhomocysteinemia	
Pregnancy related	Sickle Cell Disease	
Eclampsia	Acquired	
Choriocarcinoma	Antiphospholipid Antibody Syndrome	
Postpartum cerebral angiopathy	Vasculitis	
Cerebral venous thrombosis	Vascular trauma/ dissection	
Hypertension		
Aneurysm	Pregnancy related	
AVM/vascular malformation	Cardioembolism	
	PFO	
	Peripartum cardiomyopathy	
	Air embolism	
	Amniotic fluid embolism	
	Eclampsia	

stroke symptoms since the presentation of strokes does not differ between pregnancy-specific and pregnancy unrelated causes. The management, however, can be very different.

Preeclampsia and eclampsia

Preeclampsia and eclampsia are cited in many series as the most common cause of strokes associated with pregnancy. Preeclampsia is characterized by the development after 20 weeks gestation of hypertension (>140/90) and

Table 16.2: Changes in hemostatic factors during pregnancy	
Coagulation factors	
Clotting factors I, V, VII, VIII, IX, X	Increased
von Willebrand factor	Increased
Fibrinogen	Increased
Thrombin	Increased
Coagulation inhibitors	
Protein S	Decreased
Fibrinolytic Factors	
Tissue plasminogen activator	Increased
Plasminogen activator inhibitor	Increased
Tissue factor pathway inhibitor	Increased

proteinuria (>300 mg/day). It occurs in 5–8 percent of all pregnancies, but 14–20 percent of primigravidas. Eclampsia is diagnosed when coma or seizures develop. Neurologic abnormalities, including headache, mental status changes, as well as focal deficits, frequently involving visual dysfunction, are seen. Occasionally, strokes, both ischemic and hemorrhagic, do occur causing permanent deficits.

Imaging in preeclampsia and eclampsia

Older studies attributed high rates of ischemic strokes during pregnancy to preeclampsia and eclampsia. Interestingly, the majority of patients only had temporary neurologic symptoms and later studies found such patients to have normal diffusion-weighted magnetic resonance imaging (MRI). Thus, these were felt to represent vasogenic edema and have been categorized as reversible leukoencephalopathy rather than stroke. A minority of patients with permanent deficits did have restricted diffusion on MRI scans, and can be categorized as ischemic stroke.

1. Preeclampsia – Hypertension (HTN) and proteinuria >20 weeks gestation
2. Eclampsia – preeclampsia plus coma or seizure
3. Reversible neurologic findings are common
   a) T2 hyperintensities on MRI, DWI negative
4. Ischemic stroke is rare
   a) T2 hyperintense, DWI positive
5. ICHs are seen
   a) CT or MRI positive for blood.

In contrast, eclampsia is the most common cause of ICH during pregnancy and the peurperium. This appears to be due to the same vascular pathology caused by chronic hypertension in nonpregnant patients.

Treatment of preeclampsia and eclampsia

1. Definitive treatment is by delivery of fetus and placenta.
2. Supportive care includes controlling BP until delivery can be done.
   a) Can help prevent ICH.
   b) American College of Obstetrics and Gynecology (ACOG) recommends keeping DBP <105–110.
   c) Use labetolol or hydralazine IV.
   d) Continue to monitor postpartum as risks persist for several weeks.

There are no recommendations for a maximum systolic BP, although a recent study found that 100 percent of women with prehemorrhage monitoring had a systolic BP of 155 mmHg or greater, leading the authors to suggest treatment be directed for systolic BP less than 155 mmHg.

Cardioembolism is the most common cause of strokes associated with pregnancy

Most cardioembolic strokes during and after pregnancy are due to pre-existing disease such as prosthetic heart valves, cardiac arrhythmia, or rheumatic heart disease, which is still common in many parts of the world. Transthoracic echocardiography should pose no risk during pregnancy, although there has been suggestion that the use of saline contrast to evaluate for right to left shunting may be problematic. Some researchers fear that the introduction of bubbles could result in emboli to the placenta and harm to the fetus. To our knowledge there have been no reports published documenting any harm from saline contrast during pregnancy. Additionally, at our center we have performed a number of transcranial Doppler studies with saline contrast to evaluate for patent foramen ovale in pregnant women with no adverse effects. Transesophageal echocardiography has been performed safely during pregnancy and has been used in place of fluoroscopy to guide cardiac procedures in pregnant women.

Paradoxical embolism

Paradoxical embolism through a patent foramen ovale is also seen in non-pregnant young patients. However, the increased rate of venous thrombosis, combined with the changing intrathoracic pressures during pregnancy and delivery increase the potential for right to left shunting during pregnancy and delivery. The most likely manifestation of this phenomenon is the paradoxical embolization of a deep venous thrombosis through a patent foramen ovale causing ischemic stroke. Additionally, air or amniotic fluid can occasionally embolize as well.

Air or amniotic fluid embolism

Air embolism is a rare but serious complication of obstetrical procedures; it has been reported during cesarean section, hysteroscopy, and pregnancy terminations. There are also isolated reports of fatal air embolism from sexual activity, particularly orogenital sex during pregnancy.

➤ Air enters via venous circulation
➤ Paradoxical embolization to arterial circulation can occur
➤ Hemodynamic collapse is most common
➤ Neurologic deficits develop if cerebral embolism occurs, this is rare in isolation
➤ Stabilize the patient hemodynamically first
➤ Administer hyperbaric oxygen therapy as soon as possible

Embolism of amniotic fluid is more common, but still quite rare. It occurs most frequently during or shortly after labor and has also been reported during cesarean sections and therapeutic abortions, as well as rarely from abdominal trauma or uterine rupture.

1. in 8–80,000 pregnancies.
2. High mortality, 61–86 percent.
3. Usually presents with respiratory distress or cardiovascular collapse.
4. Can also see coagulopathy or seizures.
5. Focal neurologic deficits can be due to hypoperfusion or thrombosis or hemorrhage.
6. Neurologic deficits are not usually seen in isolation.
7. Diagnosis of exclusion.
8. Treatment involves cardiovascular and respiratory support as well as correction of coagulopathy.

PERIPARTUM CARDIOMYOPATHY

Peripartum cardiomyopathy is a syndrome of heart failure specifically associated with pregnancy. It causes decreased ejection fraction that can lead to intracardiac thrombi and embolic strokes in up to 10 percent of patients. The major features are listed below:

➤ Unexplained heart failure
➤ Last month of pregnancy or first 5 months postpartum
➤ Unclear etiology, possibly postviral autoimmune
➤ Develops in 1 out of 3,000–4,000 pregnancies
➤ Much more common in Haiti, 1 in 350
➤ High mortality rate, up to 18 percent in U.S. studies
➤ Around half recover good function (EF>50 percent)
➤ Up to 10 percent require a heart transplant
➤ High recurrence rate in subsequent pregnancies

The management of peripartum cardiomyopathy is primarily supportive.

1. Monitor for arrhythmias
   a) patients may require a pacemaker or defibrillator.
2. Anticoagulate (INR 2–3) to prevent further emboli while the low ejection fraction persists
3. Deliver only for obstetric reasons
   a) delivery does not improve ejection fraction.
4. Discourage subsequent pregnancy
   a) high rate of recurrence.

POSTPARTUM CEREBRAL ANGIOPATHY

Postpartum cerebral angiopathy is a poorly understood rare entity that can cause cerebral infarction and ICH associated with pregnancy. It is felt by some to be a subset of reversible cerebral segmental vasoconstriction syndrome.

1. vasculopathy of large- and medium-sized cerebral blood vessels;
2. etiology is not clear
   a) bromocriptine, ergotamine, and sympathomimetics reported as precipitating factors;
3. intimal hyperplasia without inflammation seen in one autopsy;
4. usually presents within a few weeks postpartum
   a) headaches, often thunderclap;
   b) hypertension;
   c) seizures;
   d) visual field deficits;
   e) focal deficits from infarction or hemorrhage;
5. diagnosis by angiography showing segmental narrowing;
6. MRI can show T2 hyperintensity without restricted diffusion similar to eclampsia;
7. CSF is normal or has moderate pleocytosis;
8. course is benign compared to other forms of cerebral vasculopathy
   a) rarely recurs after discontinuing therapy;
   b) more aggressive cases have been reported;
9. no agreed upon treatment
   a) steroids and magnesium have been used;
   b) patients rarely require more aggressive immunosuppression;
   c) control hypertension to avoid hemorrhage;
10. must rule out other forms of vasculitis
    a) ANA, ESR, HIV, hepatitis panel, complement levels, anticardiolipin antibodies, and lupus anticoagulant.

CHORIOCARCINOMA

Choriocarcinoma is a human chorionic gonadotropin-secreting tumor that develops through malignant transformation of trophoblastic cells usually of fetal origin. It is most frequently seen associated with molar pregnancies, but has been described during normal pregnancies as well. The tumor can arise during pregnancy, or up to years afterward. Metastasis of cancer cells to the brain can lead to subarachnoid or ICHs. Intravascular metastasis may cause aneurysm formation.

⭢ occurs in 1 of 20,000–50,000 pregnancies
⭢ more common in very young or very old mothers
⭢ 2–19 percent of women with molar pregnancy will develop chorio-carcinoma
⭢ brain metastasis occurs in 3–28 percent
⭢ usually presents with vaginal bleeding or symptoms of metastasis
⭢ can present with neurologic deficits due to ischemia or hemorrhage
⭢ treatment is with chemotherapy, and/or surgical resection of tumor

PITUITARY INFARCTION

Ischemic necrosis of the pituitary, or Sheehan's syndrome, can occur in the postpartum period in women who have excessive hemorrhaging and hypotension during or after delivery. The anterior pituitary is enlarged during pregnancy that somehow makes it more prone to infarction in a period of hopovolemic shock. This syndrome is only rarely seen unassociated with pregnancy:

1. occurs in less than 1 percent of women with severe postpartum hemorrhage;
2. often delayed presentation;
3. most frequently presents with inability to lactate and no return of menses;
4. leads to varying degrees of pituitary dysfunction including
   a) hypothyroidism
   b) hypogonadism
   c) hypotension and hyponatremia
   d) weight loss, nausea, abdominal pain, poor appetite
   e) diabetes insipidus
5. can be fatal if not treated;
6. see low pituitary hormone levels with high hypothalamic releasing factors;
7. MRI shows an empty sella;
8. treatment is supportive with pituitary hormone replacement.

Pituitary apoplexy occurs when there is significant hemorrhage into a pre-existing pituitary adenoma. Although the enlargement of the pituitary during pregnancy may make this more likely than in a nonpregnant woman, the requirement for a baseline pituitary adenoma makes it a quite rare occurrence. Presentation is with headache, oculomotor palsies, and hypopituitarism.

DIFFERENTIAL DIAGNOSIS

Stroke mimics should always be considered in patients presenting with stroke symptoms. These include metabolic derangements such as hypo- or hyperglycemia, electrolyte imbalances, migraine, and psychogenic disorders. Seizures can not only cause focal deficits independently, but can also be a secondary effect of a stroke. In patients who have received epidural or spinal anesthesia, spinal cord or peripheral nerve pathology should also be considered.

CEREBRAL IMAGING IN PREGNANCY

For initial imaging of the pregnant woman with suspected stroke, most researchers recommend MRI over CT scanning, although neither should be used unless necessary. CT used to be preferred in cases of suspected hemorrhage, although newer MRI sequences are as sensitive as CT in the detection of intracranial blood. Gadolinium contrast medium should be avoided as it crosses the placenta and has unknown effects on the fetus.

MRI versus CT as initial evaluation of suspected stroke in pregnancy

1. CT
   a) limited but quantifiable risk of ionizing radiation to fetus
      i) <1 mrad to uterus with CT of head;
      ii) concern for teratogenicity and oncogenicity;
   b) inferior to MRI in ability to detect early ischemia;
   c) superior or equivalent to MRI in detection of hemorrhage.
2. MRI
   a) superior in the detection of early ischemia and posterior fossa disease;
   b) can differentiate nonischemic changes (eclampsia) from stroke;
   c) no ionizing radiation;
   d) no clear teratogenicity in second and third trimesters;
   e) theoretical concern (based on animal data) of ocular abnormalities and low birth weight if used in first trimester.

Vascular imaging in pregnancy

Vascular imaging is also a concern. When possible, carotid ultrasound and transcranial Doppler studies should be used to evaluate cerebral and cervical vessels. If this is not sufficient, such as in suspected aneurysm or vasculitis, angiography may be necessary.

1. MR angiography.
2. Does not require contrast administration.
3. Same theoretical risks as with MRI.
4. Resolution is limited to larger vessels in circle of Willis
   a) cannot see vasculitis
   b) may miss small aneurysm or AVM.
5. CT angiography.
6. Ionizing radiation as above, comparable dose to digital subtraction angiography.

7. Small risk of treatable fetal hypothyroidism due to contrast during third trimester.
8. Resolution is limited to larger vessels in circle of Willis
   a) cannot see vasculitis
   b) may miss small aneurysm or AVM.
9. Digital subtraction angiography.
10. If fluoro time is limited, radiation dose to fetus is the same as a brain CT.
11. Small risk of treatable fetal hypothyroidism due to contrast during third trimester.
12. Highest resolution
    a) necessary to diagnose vasculitis, small aneurysms, or distal AVMs.

As with parenchymal imaging, MRA is the study of choice in most cases. If contraindications to MR exist or vasculitis is suspected, digital subtraction angiography should be the initial choice.

Treatment of pregnancy related ischemic stroke

In general, treatment of pregnant patients with ischemic stroke should be similar to nonpregnant patients, but care is necessary regarding choice of thrombolysis and antithrombotic medications. One aspect of treatment, however, that does require extra consideration in pregnancy is the use of thrombolytic therapy. The safety of tPA during pregnancy is not established, although there are several reports of its successful use in pregnant women for several indications including stroke. One might assume that the intraarterial route for thrombolysis might be safer given the lower doses used and the local administration, although this too is not established. Regardless, tPA should not be denied simply due to a pregnant state, although the risks and benefits should be carefully weighed and discussed. Until further research suggests otherwise, the choice for IV versus IA should be as in any patient based on clinical criteria, timing, and availability of resources.

Antithrombotic medication

There is no consensus on which antithrombotic to use for stroke prophylaxis during pregnancy. In cases of heart valve replacement, the high risk of stroke requires the use of prophylactic anticoagulation. Unfortunately, the use of warfarin during pregnancy is associated with a 6.4 percent rate of congenital abnormalities, which can be reduced but not eliminated by substituting subcutaneous heparin for weeks 6–12 of gestation. In the United States, the usual practice is to substitute subcutaneous heparin or low molecular weight heparin either for the whole pregnancy, or during the first trimester with subsequent return to warfarin for the rest of gestation. Recently, the American Stroke Association published recommendations regarding stroke prophylaxis in pregnant women. Their recommendations for women with high-risk thromboembolic conditions, such as heart valve replacement or coagulopathy are for any of the following three options:

1. Adjusted-dose unfractionated heparin (UFH) throughout pregnancy subcutaneously with APTT monitoring.
2. Adjusted-dose low molecular weight heparin (LMWH) with factor Xa monitoring throughout pregnancy, or
3. UFH or LMWH until week 13, followed by warfarin until the middle of the third trimester, when UFH or LMWH is then reinstituted until delivery

For other pregnant patients with history of stroke, a balance needs to be found between the risks and inconvenience of anticoagulation and the risks of aspirin exposure to the fetus. The ASA statement on stroke treatment suggests that for pregnant women with lower risk conditions, UFH or LMWH should be used during the first trimester, followed by low dose aspirin for the remainder of the pregnancy.

1. Aspirin
   a) pregnancy category D;
   b) increased risk of neural tube defects, gastroschisis, cleft palate with first trimester exposure;
   c) doses less than 150 mg/day may be safe in the second and third trimesters;
   d) concern for bleeding in mother and fetus.
2. Clopidogrel
   a) not well studied in pregnancy;
   b) pregnancy category B;
   c) one report of successful pregnancy on clopidogrel;
   d) concern for bleeding in mother and fetus.
3. Aggrenox (aspirin/dypiridamole)
   a) not well studied in pregnancy;
   b) pregnancy category D due to aspirin component;
   c) concern for bleeding in mother and fetus.
4. Warfarin
   a) pregnancy category X;
   b) first trimester use associated with fetal warfarin syndrome: nasal hypoplasia, stippled cartilage on x-ray, optic atrophy, cataracts, growth and mental retardation, and microcephaly;
   c) during the last two trimesters, growth retardation and brain abnormalities have been observed;
   d) risk of embryopathy lower with doses <5 mg/day;
   e) concern for bleeding in mother and fetus.

5. Heparin
   a) pregnancy category C;
   b) no teratogenicity;
   c) concern for bleeding in mother and fetus.
6. Low molecular weight heparin
   a) pregnancy category B;
   b) similar concerns to heparin.

Treatment of pregnancy related hemorrhagic stroke

Management of ICHs should be the same in pregnant as in nonpregnant patients. In cases of AVM, most authors recommend that treatment of the AVM be based solely on neurosurgical concerns. Delivery by cesarean section is probably not necessary unless warranted by obstetric concerns. For treatment of SAH due to aneurysm rupture, clipping can be performed, but endovascular treatment has been advocated more recently. In the case of labor occurring in a patient with an unsecured aneurysm, delivery by cesarean section should be strongly considered with simultaneous or postpartum treatment of the aneurysm.

Outcomes

Outcomes in pregnancy-related stroke are varied for both mother and baby. In one study, half of survivors recovered completely and half had mild to moderate deficits. In the same study, however, there was a 12 percent fetal death rate, and 35 percent of infants were delivered prematurely, with 65 percent of infants requiring delivery by cesarean section.

Conclusion

Stroke can be a complication of pregnancy and the peurperium and its prompt diagnosis and proper treatment can limit morbidity and mortality to both mother and child. Appropriate evaluation and correct diagnosis of the contributing causes are also essential as knowledge of the etiology will affect how a woman should be managed and how she should be counseled about her future stroke risk, in general as well as with subsequent pregnancies.

Bibliography

American College of Obstetricians and Gynecologists. Diagnosis and management of preeclampsia and eclampsia. ACOG practice bulletin no. 33. *Obstet Gynecol* 2002;99:159–67.

Anonymous. Low dose aspirin in pregnancy and early childhood development: Follow up of the Collaborative Low Dose Aspirin Study in Pregnancy. CLASP Collaborative Group. *BJOG* 1995;102:861–8.

Batman PA, Thomlinson J, Moore VC, Sykes R. Death due to air embolism during sexual intercourse in the puerperium. *Postgrad Med J* 1998 Oct;74(876):612–3.

Brenner B. Haemostatic changes in pregnancy. *Thromb Res* 2004;114:409–14.

Brick JF. Vanishing cerebrovascular disease of pregnancy. *Neurology* 1988;38 (5):804–6.

Chan WS, Anand S Ginsberg J. Anticoagulation of pregnant women with mechanical heart valves: A systematic review of the literature. *Arch Intern Med* 2000;160:191–6.

Cross JN, Castro PO Jennett WB. Cerebral strokes associated with pregnancy and the puerperium. *BMJ* 1968;3:214–18.

Davies S. Amniotic fluid embolus: A review of the literature. *Can J Anesth* 2001;48:88–98.

De Wilde JP, Rivers AW, Price DL. A review of the current use of magnetic resonance imaging in pregnancy and safety implication for the fetus. *Prog Biophys Mol Biol* 2005;87:335–53.

Dietrich MF, Miller KL, King SH. Determination of potential uterine (conceptus) doses from axial and helical CT scans. *Health Phys* 2005;88(Suppl 1):S10–13.

Elkayam U, Akhter MW, Singh H Khan, S, Bitar, F, Hameed A., Shotan A. Pregnancy–associated cardiomyopathy. Clinical characteristics and a comparison between early and late presentation. *Circulation* 2005;222:2050–5.

Elkayam U, Tummala PP, Rao K, Akhter MW, Karaalp IS, Wani OR, Hameed A, Gviazda I Shotan A. Maternal and fetal outcomes in women with peripartum cardiomyopathy. *NEJM* 2001;344:1567–71.

Fett JD. Peripartum cardiomyopathy. Insights from Haiti regarding a disease of unknown etiology. *Minn Med* 2002;85:46–8.

Filkins J, Kaleklkar MB, Chambliss MJ. Unexpected death due to gestational choriocarcinoma: A report of two cases. *Am J Forensic Med Pathol* 1998;19:387–90.

Finnerty JJ, Chisholm CS, Chapple H, Login IS, Pinkerton JV. Cerebral arteriovenous malformation in pregnancy: Presentation and neurologic, obstetric, and ethical significance. *Am J Obstet Gynecol* 1999;181:296–303.

Fleyfel M, Bourzoufi K, Huin G, Subtil D Puech F. Recombinant tissue type plasminogen activator treatment of thrombosed mitral valve prosthesis during pregnancy. *Can J Anaesthesia* 1997;44:735–8.

Ford RF, Barton JR O'Brien JM, Hollingsworth PW. Demographics, management, and outcome of peripartum cardiomyopathy in a community hospital. *Am J Obstet Gynec* 2000;182:1036–8.

Fox MW, Harms RW, Davis DH. Selected neurologic complications of pregnancy. *Mayo Clin Proc* 1990;65:1595–618.

Geocadin RG, Razumovsky AY, Wityk RJ, Bhardwaj A Ulatowski JA. Intracerebral hemorrhage and postpartum cerebral vasculopathy. *J Neurol Sci* 2002;205:29–34.

Granier I, Garcia E, Geissler A, Boespflug, Gasselin J. Postpartum cerebral angiopathy associated with administration of sumatriptan and dihydroergotamine – a case report. *Intensive Care Med* 1999;23:532–4.

Heinrichs WL, Fong P, Flannery M. Midgestational exposure of pregnant BALB/c mice to magnetic resonance imaging conditions. *Magn Reson Imaging* 1988;6:305–11.

Hellgren M. Hemostasis during normal pregnancy and peurperium. *Semin Thromb Hemost* 2003;29:125–30.

Hunt H, Shifrin B, Suzuki K. Ruptured berry aneurysms and pregnancy. *Obstet Gynecol* 1974;43:827–36.

Imperiale TF, Stollenwerk–Petrulis A. A meta–analysis of low dose aspirin for the prevention of pregnancy–induced hypertensive disease. *JAMA* 1991;266:260–4.

Jaigobin C Silver FL. Stroke and pregnancy. *Stroke* 2000;31:2948–51.

Janssens E, Hommel M, Monier–Vehier M, Lecterc, Masgent B Leys D. Postpartum cerebral angiopathy possibly due to bromocriptine therapy. *Stroke* 1995;26: 128–30.

Jeng J-S, Tang S-C, Yip P-K. Stroke in women of reproductive age: Comparison between stroke related and unrelated to pregnancy. *J Neurol Sci* 2004;221:25–9.

Kaiser RT. Air embolism death of a pregnant woman secondary to orogenital sex. *Acad Emerg Med* 1994 Nov–Dec;1(6):555–8.

Kittner SJ, Stern BJ, Feeser BR, Hebel JR, Nagey DA, Buchholz DW, Earley CJ, Johnson CJ, Macko RF, Sloan MA, Wityk RJ, Wozniak MA. Pregnancy and the risk of stroke. *N Engl J Med* 1996;335:768–74.

Klinzing P, Markert UR, Liesaus K, Peiker G. Case report: Successful pregnancy and delivery after myocardial infarction and essential thrombocythemia treated with clopidrogel. *Clin Exp Obstet Gynecol* 2001;28(4):215–16.

Konstantinopoulos PS, Mousa S, Khairallah R, Mtanos G. Postpartum cerebral angiopathy: An important diagnostic consideration in the postpartum period. *Am J Obstet Gynecol* 2004:191:375–377.

Kovacs K. Sheehan syndrome. *Lancet* 2003:361(9356):520–2.

Koželj M, Novak–Antolič Z, Grad A Peternel P. Patent foramen ovale as a potential cause of paradoxical embolism in the postpartum period. *Eur J Obstet Gynecol Reprod Biol* 1999;84:55–7.

Kozer E, Nikfar S, Costei A, Boskovic R, Nulman I Koren G. Aspirin consumption during the first trimester of pregnancy and congenital anomalies: A meta–analysis. *Am J Obstet Gynecol* 2002;187:1623–30.

Lanska DJ, Kryscio. Risk factors for peripartum and postpartum stroke and intracranial venous thrombosis. *Stroke* 2000;31:1274–82.

Lidegaard O. Oral contraception and risk of a cerebral thromboembolic attack: Results of a case–control study. *BMJ* 1993;306:956–63.

Martin JN, Thigpen BD, Moore RC, Rose CH, Cushman J May W. Stroke and severe preeclampsia and eclampsia: A paradigm shift focusing on systolic blood pressure. *Obstet Gynecol* 2005;105:246–54.

Momma F, Beck H, Miyamoto T, Nagao S. Intracranial aneurysm due to metastatic choriocarcinoma. *Surg Neurol* 1986;25:74–6.

Mushkat Y, Luxman D, Nachum Z, David MP Melamed Y. Gas embolism complicating obstetric or gynecologic procedures. Case reports and review of the literature. *Eur J Obstet Gynecol Reprod Biol* 1995;63(1):97–103.

Picone O, Castaigne V, Ede C Fernandez H. Cerebral metastatses of a choriocarcinoma during pregnancy. *Obstet Gynecol* 2003;102:1380–3.

Piotin M, de Souza Filho CB, Kothimbakam R, Moret J. Endovascular treatment of acutely ruptured intracranial aneurysms in pregnancy. *Am J Obstet Gynecol* 2001;185:1261–2.

Rankin SC. CT angiography. *Eur Radiol* 1999;9:297–310.

Sacco RL, Adams A, Albers G, Alberts MJ, Benavente O, Furie K, Goldstein LB, Gorelick P, Halperin J, Harbaugh R, Johnston SC Katzan, I, Kelly–Hayes, M, Kenton EJ, Marks M, Schwamm LH Tomsick T. Guidelines for prevention of stroke in patients with ischemic stroke or transient ischemic attack: A statement for healthcare professionals from the American Heart Association/American Stroke Association Council on Stroke. *Stroke* 2006;37;577–617.

Sadasivan B, Malik G, Lee C Ausman J. Vascular malformations and pregnancy. *Surg Neurol* 1990;305–313.

Salonen RH, Lichtenstein P, Bellocco R Petersson, Cnattingius S. Increased risks of circulatory diseases in the late pregnancy and puerperium. *Epidemiology* 2001;12 (4):456–60.

Salvatore De Santo L, Romano G Della Corte A, Tizzano F, Petraio A, Amarelli C, De Feo M, Dialetto G, Scardone M, Cotrufo M. Mitral mechanical replacement in young rheumatic women: Analysis of long–term survival, valve–related complications, and pregnancy outcomes over a 3707–patient–year follow–up. *J Thorac Cardiovasc Surg* 2005;130:13–19.

Sánchez–Luceros A, Meschengieser SS, Marchese C, Votta RC, Casais PD, Woods AI, Nadal MV, Salviu MJ Lazzari MA. Factor VIII and von Willebrand factor changes during normal pregnancy and puerperium. *Blood Coagul Fibrinolysis* 2003;14:647–51.

Schaefer PW. Diffusion–weighted imaging as a problem–solving tool in the evaluation of patients with acute strokelike syndromes. *Top Magn Reson Imaging* 2000;11:300–9.

Schumacher B, Belfort MA, Card RJ. Successful treatment of acute myocardial infarction during pregnancy with tissue plasminogen activator. *Am J Obstet Gynecol* 1997;176:716–19.

Schwartz RB. Neuroradiographic imaging: Techniques and safety considerations. *Adv Neurol* 2002;90:1–8.

Semple PL, Denny L, Coughlan M Soeters R. & Van Wijk L. The role of neurosurgery in the treatment of cerebral metastases from choriocarcinoma: A report of two cases. *Int J Gynecol Cancer* 2004;14:157–61.

Shah AK, Whitty JE. Brain MRI in peripartum seizures: Usefulness of combined T2 and diffusion weighted MR imaging. *J Neurol Sci* 1999;166:122–5.

Sharshar T, Lamy C, Mas JL. Incidence and causes of strokes associated with pregnancy and puerperium. A study of public hospitals of Ile de France. Stroke in Pregnancy Study Group. *Stroke* 1995;26:930–6.

Singhal AB. Postpartum angiopathy with reversible posterior leukoencephalopathy. *Arch Neurol* 2004;61:411–16.

Tyndall DA, Sulik KK. Effects of magnetic resonance imaging on eye development in the C57BL/6J mouse. *Teratology* 1991;43:263–75.

Weatherby SJ, Edwards NC, West R, Heafield MTE, Good outcome in early pregnancy following direct thrombolysis for cerebral venous sinus thrombosis. *J Neurol* 2003;250:1372–3.

Weinmann H, Brasch RL, Press W, Wesbey GE Characteristics of gadolinium–DTPA complex: A potential NMR contrast agent. *AJR* 1984;142:619–624.

Wiebers DO, Whisnant JP. The incidence of stroke among pregnant women in Rochester, Minn, 1955 through 1979. *JAMA* 1985;254:3055–7.

Wilterdink JL, Feldman E. Intracranial hemorrhage. *Adv Neurol* 2002;90:63–74.

Witlin AG, Mattar F, Sibai BM. Cerebrovascular disorders complicating pregnancy – beyond eclampsia. *Am J Obstet Gynecol* 2000;183:83–8.

17 Stroke on pediatric wards

Marta Lopez Vicente, Santiago Ortega-Gutierrez, and Michel T. Torbey

Stroke is an important cause of mortality and chronic morbidity in children ranking among the top 10 causes of death in children. The incidence of pediatric stroke varies from 1.3 to 13 per 100,000 children per year.

1. In children, the rate of stroke is higher in males than in females and in African Americans compared to Caucasians.
2. Most strokes occur in the distribution of the middle cerebral artery.

Etiology

The etiology of pediatric stroke is much more diverse than in adults (Table 17.1). Sickle cell disease (SCD), moyamoya disease, and hyperhomocystenemia are the most frequent.

SCD

This is an autosomal recessive disorder secondary to a mutation in the sixth position of the β-globin chain where valine is substituted for glutamic acid. Clinical presentation is age dependent:

➠ Ischemic stroke is more frequent between 2 and 5 years old.
➠ Hemorrhagic stroke (HS) is more frequent around 20–30 years old.

Moyamoya disease

This is a progressive intracranial vasculopathy leading to stenosis or occlusion in the terminal portions of the internal carotid artery (ICA) and the proximal anterior cerebral artery (ACA), middle cerebral artery (MCA), or both, reducing cerebral perfusion.

1. Etiology is unknown.
2. Ten percent of cases are familiar.
3. Chromosomes 3p, 17q25, and 6 are involved in this disease.

Table 17.1: Etiology of pediatric stroke

Ischemic	Hemorrhagic
Cardiac disease	Genetic vasculopathy
Congenital heart disease	Arteriovascular malformation
Rheumatic heart disease	Intracranial aneurysm
Cardiomyopathy	Angiomas
Endocarditis/myocarditis	Ehler-Darlos syndrome
Dysrythmias	Neurocutaneous disorders
Hematological disorders	Moyamoya syndrome
Hemoglobinopathy (SCD)	Fibromuscular dysplasia
Polycytemia	Fabry's disease
Thrombocytosis	Hematological disorders
Leukemia/lymphoma	Hemoglobinopathy
Coagulopathies	Platelet disorders
Protein C/S deficiency	Coagulopathy
Antithrombin III deficiency	Hypofibrinogenemia
Anticardiolipin antibodies	Trauma
Lupus anticoagulant	Hypertension
Factor V Leiden mutation	Congenital adrenal
Disseminated intravascular	hyperplasia
coagulation	Stimulant drug use
Oral contraceptive pills	Coartation of the aorta
Metabolic	
Mitochondrial disorders	
Homocystinuria/hyperhomo-	
cysteinemia	
Fabry's disease	
Dyslipidemias	
Vasculopathy	
Moyamoya syndrome	
Fibromuscular dysplasia	
Neurocutaneous disorders	
Vasculitis	
Connective tissue diseases	
Henoch-Schonlein purpura	
Polyarteritis nodosa	
Kawasaki's disease	
Hypertension	
Infection	
Meningitis, Varicella	
Idiopathic	

Table 17.2: Disorders associated with moyamoya disease

Chromosomal disorders
  Down syndrome
  Noonan syndrome
  William syndrome
  Alagille syndrome
  Oteogenesis imperfecta

Hematologic disorders
  Sickle cell disease
  Fanconi anemia
  Paroxismal nocturnal
    hemoglobinuria
  Hereditary spherocytosis
  β-Thalassemia

Hypercoagulable states
  Protein C/S deficiency
  Lupus anticoagulant
  Factor V Leiden mutation
  Antiphospholipid antibodies
  Hemophilia A
  Plasminogen deficiency

Autoimmune disorders
  Systemic lupus erythematosus
  Graves' thyrotoxicosis
  Ulcerative colitis

Cardiac abnormalities
  Bicuspid aortic valve
  Coartation of aorta

Metabolic disease
  Diabetes
  Hyperphosphatasia
  Homocystinuria
  Glycogen storage disease type Ia
  Primary oxalosis

Neurocutaneous disorders
  Neurofibromatosis
  Tuberous sclerosis
  Facial angioma
  Microcephalic osteodysplasia
  Primordial short stature
    type 2 with café-au-lait spots
  Livedo reticularis

4. Associated with specific ethnic group such as Japanese.
5. Coexists with other genetic diseases such as trisomy 21 or SCD.
6. Different geographic disease pattern:
   a) In Asia, moyamoya disease is most commonly a primary disorder.
   b) In the United States and Europe, it is more often associated with other conditions (Table 17.2).

Hyperhomocysteinemia

Classic homacysteinemia is an autosomal recessive disorder of methionine metabolism. Cystathionine synthetase deficiency is the most common enzyme defect. Reduction in the activity of the 5,10-methylene tetra-hydrofolate reductase gene results in reduction of 5-methyl tetrahydrofolate needed for the conversion of homocysteine to methionine resulting in hyperhomocysteinemia.

⇒ Elevated homocysteine levels appears to be a risk factor for stroke
⇒ Vitamin supplements appear to reduce homocysteine levels

Pathophysiology

Pediatric stroke can be either ischemic or hemorrhagic. Although 44–61 percent of strokes are ischemic, HS occurs much more frequently in children than in adults.

1. The mechanisms by which acute ischemic stroke (AIS) occurs in children include
   a) thromboembolism from intracranial or extracranial vessels or from the heart (more frequent);
   b) acute, transient, or progressive arteriopathy;
   c) other rare causes.
2. HS is associated with vascular malformation, coagulopathy, malignancy, and trauma.

Clinical presentation

The clinical presentation of stroke in children varies according to age, underlying cause, and stroke location.

1. Focal neurological deficits are the most common presentation of AIS in older children. Hemiparesis can be seen in 45–100 percent of patients.
2. In the first year of life, typical presentation is seizure (20–30 percent), lethargy, and/or apnea, often without focal neurological deficits.
3. In HS, the most common presentation is headache, vomiting, and altered level of consciousness.

Diagnosis

Establishing a stroke diagnosis in children can be quite challenging due to the vague clinical presentation. In most situations a careful family and birth history should be obtained to assess risk factors such congenital heart disease, thrombophilic states, sickle cell anemia, or a previously diagnosed arteriovenous malformations (AVM) The evaluation should include questions about any history of head or neck trauma, unexplained fever or recent infection (varicella in the last 12 months), vasculitis, drug ingestion, blood disorder, and associated headache. Table 17.3 reviews the differential diagnosis of stroke in children.

Laboratory screening

1. It should include complete blood count with iron, folate, CBC, folate, serum electrolytes and urine drug screen, ESR and ANA.

> **Table 17.3:** Differential diagnosis
>
> Hemiplegic migraine
> Cerebral abscess
> Encephalitis
> Traumatic extradural or intradural hematoma
> Cerebral tumor
> Epilepsy
> Malingering/conversion disorder
> Multiple sclerosis
> Acute disseminated encephalomyelitis

2. Children suspected to have a *hypercoagulable disorder* should be screened for prothrombotic abnormalities:
   a) PT, PTT, INR, protein C and protein S, antithrombin III, heparin cofactor II
   b) plasminogen, von Willebrand antigen, Factor VIII, Factor XII, Factor V Leiden
   c) activated protein C resistance, prothrombin 20210 gene, total homocysteine
   d) Lp (a) lipoprotein and antiphospholipid antibodies such as lupus coagulant and cardiolipin antibodies.
3. Children suspected to have a *metabolic disorder* should have serum and cerebrospinal fluid (CSF) lactate and pyruvate, organic acid in urine, and serum amino acids and ammonia levels measured.
4. More extensive diagnostic testing such as lipid profile, HIV testing, and hemoglobin electrophoresis are indicated in children with no identifiable cause of stroke (Table 17.4).

Neuroimaging

COMPUTED TOMOGRAPHY (CT)/MAGNETIC RESONANCE IMAGING (MRI)

1. Although CT should be initially obtained as a quick screening study, the best first imaging method to determine stroke is MRI.
2. The gold standard for the definite assessment of cerebral vasculature is cerebral angiography.
   a) It is recommended in any child with an unexplained infarct or hemorrhage not elucidated by MRI or MR angiography (MRA) to R/O vasculitis or vascular abnormalities.
   b) In moyamoya disease, angiography provides the definitive diagnosis. Typical finding consist of bilateral stenosis of the ICA and the

Table 17.4: Diagnostic evaluation of pediatric stroke

First line: 24–48 hr of admission

⮞ CT/MRI of brain	⮞ Liver function test
⮞ Complete blood count	⮞ Chest x-ray
⮞ PT/PTT	⮞ ESR, ANA
⮞ Electrolytes, Ca, Mg, Phos, glucose, renal function studies (BUN, creatinine)	⮞ Urinalysis, urine drug screen
	⮞ EKG

Second line: after 48hr as indicated

	Screening metabolic disorders
Echocardiogram	Serum amino acids, urine for organic acids
Holter monitoring	Serum lactate/pyruvate
TCD and/or carotid Doppler	Plasma ammonia levels
MRA	Lipid profile
EEG	Urine and serum homocysteine
Hypercoagulable evaluation	Blood culture
Antithrombin III activity assay	Hemoglobin electrophoresis
Protein C and S activity assay	Complement profile
Factor V mutation	VDRL
Antiphospholipid antibodies	HIV testing
Anticardiolipin lupus coagulant	Rheumatoid factor
	Lumbar puncture

development of collateral network with the appearance of the typical pattern known as "puff of smoke."

TRANSCRANIAL DOPPLER (TCD)

1. Established as a level I test for patient with sickle cell.
2. In normal children, the velocity in the MCA is on average close to 90 cm/s. In SCD children, the velocity is in a range of 130–140 cm/s.
   a) Velocities >170 cm/s are associated with increased risk of stroke. Children with velocities >200 cm/s have a stroke risk of >10 percent per year.
   b) The current recommendation is to periodically evaluate SCD children between 2 and 16 years using TCD and initiate chronic transfusion therapy in patient with high TCD velocity (Figure 17.1).

Treatment

The goal of stroke treatment is to limit infarct size, improve outcome, and prevent recurrence. The acute management of children with stroke includes

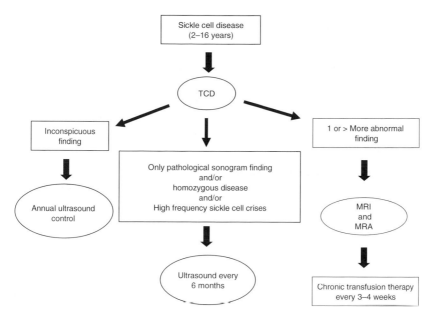

Figure 17.1 Algorithm of primary prevention of sickle cell disease.

evaluation of airway and cardiovascular status, aggressive treatment of infection, fever, hypo-hypertension, hypovolemia, and hypo-hyperglycemia (Figure 17.2).

1. Seizure activity should be controlled with appropriate agents, such as benzodiazepines, Phenobarbital, or phenytoin.
2. In case of intracranial hypertension, mannitol in bolus doses of 0.25–0.5 g/kg is indicated. Mild hyperventilation (pCO_2 of 30–35 mmHg) can be employed in acute herniation syndromes.

Antithrombotic and anticoagulants

Accumulating experience with antithrombotic and anticoagulant treatment in children suggests that these agents can be used safely, although more studies are necessary to provide more information about their indication, efficacy, and adequate dosage (Table 17.5).

1. Anticoagulation with low molecular weight heparin (LMWH) is increasingly used as the first choice for acute treatment in children with AIS.
   a) Its indications are arterial dissection, coagulations disorders, cardioembolic origin, and children with progressive or additional neurology deficit not caused by cerebral hemorrhage.

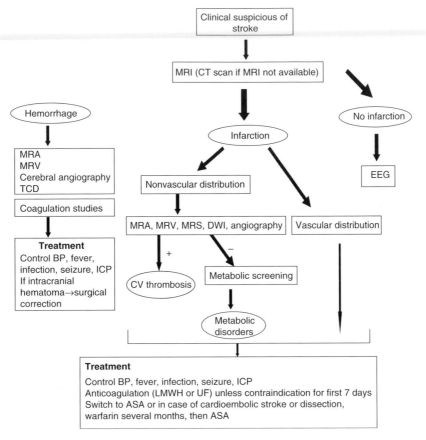

Figure 17.2 Algorithm of diagnosis and treatment of pediatric stroke. MRI, magnetic resonance imaging; CT scan, computed tomography; MRA, magnetic resonance angiography; TCD, transcranial Doppler; MRS, magnetic resonance spectroscopy; DWI, diffusion-weight imaging; BP, blood pressure; ICP, intracranial hypertension; CV thrombosis, cerebral venous thrombosis; EEG, electroencephalogram; ECG, electrocardiogram.

  b) Hemorrhage is a potential side effect of LMWH but to date there are no reported cases in children.
  c) Loading dose of heparin is 75 U/kg intravenously followed by 20 U/kg/hr for children over 1 year of age (or 28 U/kg/hr below 1 year of age). Target PTT 60–85.
  d) LMWH can be given to children subcutaneously in two divided doses of 1 mg/kg/dose (or 1.5 mg/kg every 12 hr in neonates).
2. Long-term anticoagulation with warfarin is indicated in congenital or acquired heart disease, severe hypercoagulable states, arterial dissection and recurrence of AIS, or transient ischemic attacks while on aspirin treatment. INR should be 2–3.

Table 17.5: Drugs used in pediatric stroke

Drug	Dosage	Monitoring
Antiplatelet		
Aspirin (ASA)	Acute 3–5 mg/kg/day Prophylaxis: 1–3 mg/kg/day	Optional. PFA-100
Anticoagulants		aPTT, platelet count,
Heparin unfractionated	20 U/kg/hr (>1 year)	antifactor Xa assay
LMWH	28 U/kg/hr (<1 year)	INR: 2–3
Warfarin	1.0 mg/kg/hr (>1 year) 1.5 mg/kg/hr (<1 year) Individual dosage	If mechanical heart valves INR: 2.5–3.5
Thrombolysis		
r-tPA	0.11 – 0.5 mg/kg (IV)	

3. Although Aspirin (ASA) and dipirydamole are the most common antiplatelets used in children, there are no controlled trials on the use of ASA or other antiplatelets agents.
   a) Children taking ASA could have an increased risk of developing Reye's syndrome. No reported cases in the literature.
   b) Daily ASA dose of 2–3 mg/kg/day can cause an antiplatelet effect. It is not clear whether this dose is clinically effective.

Thrombolytics

The use of thrombolytic therapy is controversial in pediatric stroke. Most of the children are diagnosed outside the 3-hr window established for adult stroke, making them poor candidates to this therapy. Some studies have demonstrated that therapy with r-tPA could be effective in children even with lower doses than in adults. It is necessary more studies about the efficacy of thrombolysis in pediatric stroke but it may be safely administered in select pediatric patients.

Specific SCD treatment options

1. Acute exchange transfusion remains the main therapy for acute stroke in SCD. This therapy improves tissue perfusion and oxygenation. Furthermore, it reduces the percentage of HbS.
2. Rate of stroke recurrence in SCD is 47–93 percent. The most effective way to prevent secondary stroke in SCD is through chronic transfusion

therapy every 3–4 weeks. This chronic treatment reduces the relapse rate to 13 percent.

3. The standard recommendation is to maintain HbS percentage less than 30 percent for the initial 3 years of an acute event.

4. A potential complication associated with chronic transfusion is iron overload. Chelation with deferoxamine is usually recommended when serum ferritin levels are more than 5,618 pmol/l.

   a) The initial dose is 50 mg/kg daily for several days to weeks.

5. Hydroxyurea (HU) has been studied as an alternative therapy in patients for whom chronic transfusion therapy is not a possible choice.

   a) HU leads to HbF induction, improves the red blood cell deformability, reduces the irreversibly sickled cell fraction, and is associated with improvements in erythrocyte survival.

   b) The dosage starts at 15–20 mg/kg/day and escalates by 5 mg/kg/day every 8 weeks as tolerated, up to a maximum of 30 mg/kg/day.

   c) Maximal benefits of HU are not achieved until after at least 6 months of treatment.

   d) Although HU therapy is escalated to maximum tolerated dosage, monthly transfusions are continued, and the transfused volume is slightly reduced.

6. In case of iron overload, phlebotomy is very well tolerated, with blood removal of 10 ml/kg every 2–4 weeks while maintaining a hemoglobin concentration above 8 g/dl.

7. Bone marrow transplantation may be curative for SCD patients and is potentially an option for stroke prevention.

   a) Survival has been in the 90 percent range and event-free survival about 85 percent, although posttransplant hemorrhage and/or seizure have been reported in a few cases.

   b) There is no clear consensus on the indications for its use in SCD, but it could be an option for some patients, especially for those who are at a higher significant adverse effect, including stroke.

Moyamoya disease treatment

Surgery is also the best treatment for moyamoya disease because of its progression despite medical treatment. Revascularization surgery provides more blood flow reducing ischemic symptoms and improving neurological outcome. Different surgical procedures have been used as follows:

1. *Direct revascularization* such as superficial temporal-middle cerebral artery bypass.

2. *Indirect revascularization* such as encephaloduroarteriosynangiosis (EDAS), pial synangiosis, and indirect revascularization using omental flaps. These indirect methods are preferred in children.

Stroke among children is a rare disease; however, it has been associated with high mortality and morbidity rate. It is very important to keep a high index of suspicion in a child who arrives at the emergency department with unexplained neurological symptoms. Improvement in imaging techniques have allowed physicians to quickly diagnose and understand the mechanisms of stroke in children. However, more studies are necessary to determine the different options of treatment and the possible prevention of these episodes.

Bibliography

Adams RJ, Ohene-Frempong K, Wang W. Sickle cell and the brain. *Hematology* 2001;31–46.

Adams RJ. Stroke prevention and treatment in sickle cell disease. *Arch Neurol* 2001;58:565–8.

Calder K, Kokorowski P, Tran T, Henderson S. Emergency department presentation of pediatric stroke. *Pediatr Emerg Care* 2003;19:320–8.

Carlin TM, Chanmugan A. Stroke in children. *Emerg Med Clin N Am* 2002;20:671–85.

Carlson MD, Leber S, Deveikis J, Silverstein FS. Successful use of rt-PA in pediatric stroke. *Neurology* 2001;57:157–8.

Gebreyohanns M, Adams RJ. Sickle cell disease: Primary stroke prevention. *CNS Spectrums* 2004;9:445–9.

Gosalakkal JA. Moyamoya disease: A review. *Neurol India* 2002;50:6–10.

Gruber A, Nasel C, Lang W, Kitzmuller E, Bavinzski G, Czech T. Intra-arterial thrombolysis for the treatment of perioperative childhood cardioembolic stroke. *Neurology* 2000;54:1684–6.

Hartfield DS, Lowry NJ, Keene DL, Yager JY. Iron deficiency: A cause of stroke in infants and children. *Pediatr Neurol* 1997;16:50–3.

Husson B, Rodesch G, Lasjaunias P, Tardieu M, Sébire G. Magnetic resonance angiography in childhood arterial brain infarcts. A comparative study with contrast angiography. *Stroke* 2002;33:1280–5.

Kirkham FJ. Is there a genetic basis for pediatric stroke? *Curr Opin Pediatr* 2003;15:547–58.

Kirkham FJ. Stroke in childhood. *Arch Dis Child* 1999;81:85–9.

Kirton A, Wong JH, Mah J, Ross BC, Kennedy J, Bell K, Hill MD. Successful endovascular therapy for acute basilar thrombosis in an adolescent. *Pediatrics* 2003;112(3 Pt 1):248–51.

Lanthier S, Carmant L, David M, Larbrisseau A, de Veber G. Stroke in children: The coexistence of multiple risk factors predicts poor outcome. *Neurology* 2000;54:371–8.

Lynch JK, Hirtz DG, DeVeber G, Nelson KB. Report of the National Institute of Neurological Disorders and Stroke workshop on perinatal and childhood stroke. *Pediatrics* 2002;109:116–23.

Lynch JK. Cerebrovascular disorders in children. *Curr Neurol Neurosci Rep* 2004;4:129–38.

Miller ST, Marcklin EA, Pegelow CH, et al. Silent infarction as a risk factor for overt stroke in children with sickle cell anemia: A report from the cooperative study of sickle cell disease. *J Pediatr* 2001;139:385–90.

Nestoridi E, Buonanno FS, Jones RM, et al. Arterial ischemic stroke in childhood: The role of plasma-phase risk factors. *Curr Opin Neurol* 2002;15:139–44.

Nowak-Gottl U, Gunther G, Kurnik K, Strater R, Kirkham F. Arterial ischemic stroke in neonates, infants, and children: An overview of underlying conditions, imaging methods, and treatment modalities. *Semin Thromb Hemost* 2003;29:405–14.

Pegelow CH, Wang W, Granger S, et al. Silent infarcts in children with sickle cell anemia and abnormal cerebral artery velocity. *Arch Neurol* 2001;58:2017–21.

Prengler M, Pavlakis SG, Prohovnik I, Adams RJ. Sickle cell disease: The neurological complications. *Ann Neurol* 2002;51:543–52.

Riebel TKebelmann-Betzing C, Gotze R Overberg US. Transcranial Doppler ultrasound in neurologically asymptomatic children and young adults with sickle cell disease. *Eur Radiol* 2003;13:563–70.

Scothorn DJ, Price C, Schwartz D, et al. Risk of recurrent stroke in children with sickle cell disease receiving blood transfusion therapy for at least five years after initial stroke. *J Pediatr* 2002;140:348–54.

Seibert JJ, Glasier CM, Kirby RS, et al. Transcranial Doppler, MRA, and MRI as a screening examination for cerebrovascular disease in patients with sickle cell anemia: An 8-year study. *Pediatr Radiol* 1998;28:138–42.

Strater R, Kurnik K, Heller C, Schobess R, Luigs P, Nowak-Gottl U. Aspirin versus low-dose low-molecular-weight heparin: Antithrombotic therapy in pediatric ischemic stroke patients: A prospective follow-up study. *Stroke* 2002;33:1947–8.

Venkataraman A, Kingsley PB, Kalina P, et al. Newborn brain infarction: Clinical aspects and magnetic resonance imaging. *CNS Spectr* 2004;9:436–44.

Ware RE, Zimmerman SA, Schultz WH. Hydroxyurea as an alternative to blood transfusions for the prevention of recurrent stroke in children with sickle cell disease. *Blood* 1999;94:3022–6.

Ware RE, Zimmerman SA, Sylvestre PB, et al. Prevention of secondary stroke and resolution of transfusional iron overload in children with sickle cell anemia using hydroxyurea and phlebotomy. *J Pediatr* 2004;145:346–52.

Yoshida Y, Yoshimoto T, Shirane R, Sakurai Y. Clinical course, surgical management, and long-term outcome of moyamoya patients with rebleeding after an episode of intracerebral hemorrhage. An extensive follow-up study. *Stroke* 1999;30:2272–6.

Prevention of First and Recurrent Stroke

18 Antithrombotic therapies

Mark Alberts

Introduction

Antiplatelet therapy has been a medical mainstay for the prevention of ischemic stroke since the 1970s when a Canadian study first reported that high-dose aspirin (ASA) was safe and effective for the prevention of strokes after patients had a transient ischemic attack (TIA). Since then considerable new knowledge has emerged about the efficacy of various doses of ASA and new agents have been developed that inhibit or affect various processes in the platelet aggregation pathway.

This chapter reviews several topics, including (1) platelet physiology as it relates to clotting, (2) the pharmacology of commonly used antiplatelet agents, (3) clinical efficacy studies of antiplatelets (AP) agents as they relate to cerebrovascular disease, (4) the merging concept of ASA resistance, and (5) recent and ongoing clinical studies that may affect the use of AP agents.

Platelet physiology

Platelets are derived from the cytoplasm of megakaryocytes in the bone marrow. They circulate in search of areas of damaged endothelium, whereupon their normal function is to form a barrier to bleeding by binding fibrinogen, which is converted to fibrin, thereby forming a hemostatic plug. This occurs in several steps (Figure 18.1):

- Adhesion
- Activation
- Secretion
- Aggregation (clot formation)

A host of receptors and proteins are involved in these processes, including von Willebrand's factor (which if deficient can lead to a bleeding diathesis). Each represents a potential candidate for inhibition by an antiplatelet agent.

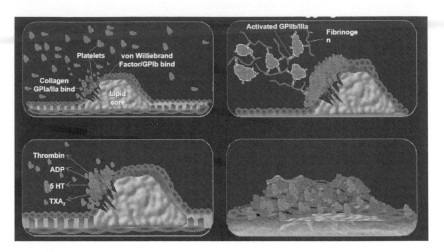

Figure 18.1 Pictorial depiction of four main steps in platelet-mediated clot formation: (a) platelet adhesion, (b) activation, (c) aggregation, and finally (d) platelet plug (clot) formation (Schafer, 1996).

Of particular importance are thromboxane A2 (TBXA2), ADP, and the glycoprotein IIb/IIIa receptor.

1. Thromboxane A2 is produced as the final product in the metabolism of arachidonic acid via cyclooxygenase. It is a powerful stimulus that further amplifies the platelet binding to a local stimulus.
2. There are two cyclooxygenase systems involved in clotting:
   a) Cyclooxygenase 1 (COX-1) resides in the platelets and is involved in the clotting processes outlined above. COX-1 can be inhibited by low-dose aspirin as well as high-dose aspirin.
   b) Cyclooxygenase 2 is synthesized in platelets and has natural anti-platelet properties, as well as being a vasodilator. COX-2 can be inhibited by high-dose aspirin. The COX system is discussed in more detail below.
3. ADP is a powerful agonist of platelet activation, and its release and binding to ADP receptors stimulates a secondary wave of platelet activation.
4. The glycoprotein IIb/IIIa receptor is the final common pathway in the formation of a platelet clot. Once it is stimulated, it undergoes a conformational change and binds fibrinogen, which is then converted to insoluble fibrin, thereby forming a definitive platelet plug (clot), which prevents further local bleeding in most cases.

The normal process of clot formation becomes pathogenic when it occurs due to stimulation by an atherosclerotic plaque or a foreign body such as an endovascular device (catheter, stent).

1. In the case of atherosclerosis, the irregular surface of the plaque serves as a stimulus to precipitate platelet adhesion, activation, and subsequent thrombus formation.
2. The subsequent atherothrombotic lesion can cause an ischemic stroke or TIA by occluding a blood vessel or by acting as a source of an artery-to-artery embolism that then occludes a downstream vessel.

Certain aspects of the atherosclerotic plaque may play important roles in causing platelet adhesion. Two processes of particular importance are shear stress and inflammation:

1. Normal vessels have shear stress rates that range from 470 to 4,700. However, vessels with severe degrees of narrowing have shear rates of 50,000 or more. Such high shear rates can lead to platelet adhesion by stimulating the von Willebrand's factor/glycoprotein Ib pathways.
2. Inflammatory ligands such as CD40 in some atherosclerotic lesions may also serve as powerful stimulators for platelet attraction and activation.

Mechanisms of action for antiplatelet agents

As discussed above, there are several important processes in the platelet activation cascade that have been targeted for inhibition as a means to achieve an antiplatelet effect. These include cyclooxygenase, the ADP receptor, the glycoprotein IIb/IIIa receptor, and several others.

Aspirin is the most commonly used antiplatelet agent, due mostly to its long history of efficacy and safety, its availability over the counter, and its low cost.

1. ASA works by irreversibly binding to a serine residue of the cyclooxygenase-1 enzyme in the platelet, thereby rendering it inactive.
2. By reducing the formation of TBXA2, ASA prevents platelet activation to some degree as well as blocking vasoconstriction (which is also partially mediated by TBXA2).
3. The antiplatelet effects of ASA usually begin within a few minutes of ingestion and become maximal within a few hours.
4. Enteric coated preparations of ASA may have a lag in achieving peak antiplatelet effects in some people, due to delayed absorption.
5. Low doses of ASA inhibit COX-1 in most people.
6. Higher doses of ASA inhibit COX-2, which is located in the vascular endothelium. COX-2 metabolizes the formation of prostacyclin that tends to inhibit platelet aggregation and cause vasodilatation.
7. Thus, higher doses of ASA may not achieve an enhanced antiplatelet effect due to the inhibition of prostacyclin formation.

8. COX-2 can be made constantly by the vascular endothelium, so its inhibition is not permanent as is the case for COX-1 (which is made in platelets).
   a) By inhibiting COX-2, high-dose ASA can also inhibit or reduce inflammation, which is likely important in some cases of unstable atherosclerotic plaques.
9. To what extent different doses of ASA achieve (or fails to achieve) inhibition of COX-1 and/or COX-2 in different people may form one basis for ASA resistance (discusses later).

Blockade of the ADP receptor is achieved by using thienopyridines such as clopidogrel (and ticlopidine, which is rarely used now).

1. These agents work by irreversibly blocking the P2Y12 ADP receptor on the platelet's surface.
2. Clopidogrel is rapidly transformed via the liver to an active metabolite, although the exact nature of this metabolite remains unclear.
3. Clopidogrel also inhibits other platelet constituents such as platelet ligand PD40, and it may also have an anti-inflammatory effect on some atherosclerotic plaques.
4. Platelet inhibition takes longer with clopidogrel than with ASA; maximal inhibition typically takes 5–7 days unless a loading dose is used (loading doses of clopidogrel for cerebrovascular disease is not currently FDA approved).

Dipyridamole is a unique antiplatelet agent that is now used as an extended-release formulation combined with low-dose (25mg) ASA (Aggrenox).

1. The mechanisms of action of dypyridamole in terms of its antiplatelet effect remain uncertain.
2. Possible factors that may lead to its antiplatelet effects include increasing intracellular cyclic-AMP, increasing prostacyclin levels, and enhancing the effects of nitric oxide perhaps by affecting NO-synthetase.
3. It may also improve the rheology of platelets by reducing blood viscosity.
4. It also has some vasodilatory effects and can lower blood pressure by a small amount.

Clinical efficacy studies

Aspirin

There have been dozens of clinical studies of ASA as an antiplatelet agent for the prevention of ischemic atherothrombotic vascular events. We review

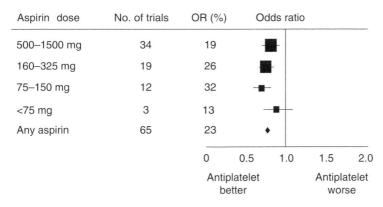

Aspirin dose	No. of trials	OR (%)	Odds ratio
500–1500 mg	34	19	
160–325 mg	19	26	
75–150 mg	12	32	
<75 mg	3	13	
Any aspirin	65	23	

0   0.5   1.0   1.5   2.0

Antiplatelet   Antiplatelet
better   worse

Figure 18.2 Meta-analysis results showing the efficacy of different aspirin doses and dose ranges for the prevention of vascular events. The vast majority of these studies compared a dose of aspirin to placebo, not to other aspirin doses.

some of the key studies to provide some context and a frame of reference for comparing ASA to other agents for mostly secondary stroke prevention:

1. The Canadian study is a seminal one for the use of ASA in cerebrovascular disease. This study showed that high-dose ASA (1,300 mg/day) was effective in preventing strokes in patients with a recent TIA. The efficacy appeared to be greater in men than in women, but this was likely an artifact explained by the small number of women in the study.
2. Following the Canadian study, there were a series of additional studies that tested lower doses of ASA, mostly for secondary prevention of vascular events after a stroke or TIA. Many were done in Europe such as the Dutch TIA study and the Swedish Aspirin Low Dose Trial (SALT).
   a) All showed efficacy for low-dose ASA, even down to 30 mg/day.
   b) In general, these studies found relative risk reductions in the range of 15–20 percent for secondary prevention of ischemic stroke.
3. Two large international studies, the Chinese Aspirin Stroke Trial (CAST) and the International Stroke Trial (IST) studied low-dose ASA as an acute stroke therapy.
   a) These studies found that ASA in doses of 81–325 mg/day started within 48 hr of an ischemic stroke and continued for at least 2 weeks reduced the risk of recurrent stroke or vascular death by 9–10 patients per every 1,000 treated.
4. Further studies and large meta-analyses all showed consistent benefit for various doses of ASA in preventing vascular events (typically stroke, MI, or vascular death) in a variety of high-risk populations (see Figure 18.2). These included patients with acute coronary syndromes, history of myocardial infarction (MI), stroke, TIA, and other high-risk groups.
5. As a group, antiplatelet agents reduced the risk of recurrent stroke in patients with prior stroke or TIA, with a relative risk reduction of 15–20

Table 18.1: Aspirin for primary prevention of stroke and vascular events

Study	Stroke endpoint	MI endpoint	All CV events
WHS	0.84 (0.70–1.01)	1.03 (0.84–1.25)	0.91 (0.80–1.03)
Total women	0.83 (0.70–0.97)	1.01 (0.84–1.21)	0.88 (0.79–0.99)
PHS	1.22 (0.93–1.59)	0.58 (0.47–0.71)	0.86 (0.71–0.96)
Total men	1.13 (0.96–1.59)	0.68 (0.54–0.86)	0.86 (0.78–0.94)

Notes: Results are listed as odds ratios with 95% confidence intervals in parentheses. WHS, Women's Health Study; PHS, Physicians Health Study. Stroke endpoint includes all strokes.
Source: Results adapted from Berger et al. (2006).

percent, and odds ratio reduction of 23–25 percent, and an absolute risk reduction of 24–27 fewer events per 1,000 treated patients.

6. Aspirin alone showed a more modest benefit in stroke patients, with risk reductions in the range of 15–20 percent when used for secondary prevention.

Interest in primary prevention of ischemic stroke led to two large studies: the Physicians Health Study (PHS) and the Women's Health Study (WHS). Both examined low-dose ASA (75–100 mg) given every other day to healthy men (for the PHS) and healthy women (WHS). The results were clear, yet somewhat perplexing.

1. In the PHS, ASA was effective in preventing MIs, but did not show efficacy for the prevention of strokes; in fact, it increased the risk of a hemorrhagic stroke by a small amount.
2. The WHS found just the opposite; namely ASA prevented ischemic strokes in women, but did not prevent MIs (see Table 18.1).

Clopidogrel

Clopidogrel has been studied in a number of trials for stroke prevention. The seminal trial CAPRIE examined a mixed population of about 19,000 patients with symptomatic ischemic vascular disease and compared clopidogrel 75 mg/day to aspirin 325 mg/day.

1. Overall it found a relative risk reduction (RRR) of 8.7 percent (absolute benefit of 0.5 percent) for the prevention of stroke, MI, and vascular death for clopidogrel versus aspirin. This benefit was enhanced in patients with diabetes and a prior history of stroke or MI (absolute risk reduction of 3 percent, RRR 14 percent).
2. Clopidogrel was extremely well tolerated, with fewer major bleeds and GI complications when compared to ASA.

In an effort to further enhance the efficacy of clopidogrel over ASA, a number of studies using combination therapy (clopidogrel + ASA) have been conducted and completed in stroke patients.

1. The first large trial, MATCH, enrolled patients with recent stroke or TIA who also had other vascular risk factors (diabetes, prior events, etc.).
   a) Patients in MATCH got randomized to clopidogrel 75 mg/day monotherapy versus clopidogrel + ASA 75 mg/day.
   b) Overall there was a nonsignificant RRR of 6.4 percent in favor of combination therapy vs clopidogrel monotherapy for the endpoint of stroke, MI, VD, or rehospitalization for a vascular cause.
   c) The combination group had higher rates of life-threatening hemorrhages and moderate hemorrhages compared to clopidogrel monotherapy.
2. The most recent study of combination therapy with clopidogrel was CHARISMA, which compared ASA + clopidogrel versus ASA alone in patients with either symptomatic atherothrombotic vascular disease (about 12,000 patients) and those with just a number of vascular risk factors (about 3,000 patients).
   a) As designed, CHARISMA was really a mixed study, with most patients being symptomatic (prior stroke, coronary syndrome, limb ischemia, etc.), and a minority being asymptomatic but with some combination of vascular risk factors. Therefore, it was really a study of secondary prevention combined with some primary prevention.
   b) The dose of aspirin could vary between 75 and 325 mg/day in CHARISMA.
   c) For the primary end point of stroke, MI, and vascular death, there was a nonsignificant RRR of 7.1 percent ($p = 0.22$) that favored combination therapy.
   d) The major benefit was seen in the secondary prevention group, where the RRR was a significant 12 percent ($p = 0.046$).
   e) The primary prevention group appeared to have worse outcomes on combination therapy. This was largely due to significant differences in the event rates for the symptomatic and asymptomatic groups, as well as different treatment effects in these two patient groups.
   f) There was more severe and moderate bleeding (as defined by the GUSTO criteria) in the combination group versus ASA monotherapy.

At this time, based on all of the available data, the combination of ASA + clopidogrel cannot be recommended as first-line therapy for patients with ischemic stroke. There are a number of ongoing studies that are investigating this combination in various groups of patients with ischemic stroke; results should be available in the next 2–4 years.

Loading doses of clopidogrel are widely used in patients with ACS and those undergoing coronary stenting as well as carotid stenting.

⬛➡ The safety and efficacy of clopidogrel loading doses for acute ischemic
stroke is currently unproven.

Aspirin and extended-release dipyridamole

The combination of low-dose ASA (25 mg) combined with a slow-release
formulation of dipyridamole (200 mg) is marketed as Aggrenox, a capsule
dosed bid. It is FDA approved for the secondary prevention of stroke in
patients with stroke or TIA. It has been studies in two large trials: ESPS-2
and ESPIRIT.

1. In ESPS-2, the combination reduced the risk of stroke by 37 percent
   versus placebo and 23 percent versus low-dose ASA. Of note was a
   discontinuation rate of 25 percent in patients taking combination
   therapy, due largely to headaches and GI upset.
2. The other large trial was ESPIRIT, which enrolled patients with recent
   ischemic strokes.
   a) Patients were randomized to low-dose ASA, warfarin, or ASA
      combined with dipyridamole.
   b) Interestingly, clinician could decide the dose of ASA and the dose
      and formulation of dipyridamole in the ESPIRIT trial.
   c) Overall, about 83 percent of patients took medications that were
      similar to or identical to Aggrenox.
   d) ESPIRIT showed a benefit for combination therapy versus low-dose
      ASA for the end point of stroke, MI, and vascular death, with an
      RRR of 12 percent, which was just significant.
   e) Interestingly, the on-treatment analysis of ESPIRIT showed less
      efficacy than the intention-to-treat analysis. This is potentially
      important, since about 20 percent of patients discontinued com-
      bination therapy, although no information was provided about
      which medication they changed to.
   f) Major bleeding was not a problem with combination therapy. The
      results of the warfarin group of ESPRIT has not been reported at
      this time.

Uncertainty remains about whether clopidogrel or ASA + ER-DP is more
efficacious for the secondary prevention of stroke. Hopefully this question will
be answered by the PRoFESS trial, which randomized stroke patients to
clopidogrel 75 mg/day versus ASA + ER-DP (Aggrenox). This is an event-
driving trial, and the results may be known soon after this book is published.

Aspirin resistance

The clinical issue of aspirin resistance is one of the more controversial
entities in vascular medicine. Numerous studies have shown fairly clearly
that a significant minority of patients who are taking aspirin will not exhibit

the expected antiplatelet effects. I term this "aspirin resistance," while aspirin failure defines a patient who has an ischemic vascular event while taking aspirin.

1. Thus, not all patients who are aspirin resistant will be aspirin failures, and only some of the patients who are aspirin failures will be found to have aspirin resistance.
2. Various studies have reported rates of aspirin resistance ranging from 5 percent up to almost 50 percent. These rates vary depending upon the population under study, the dose of aspirin, and how aspirin resistance is defined.

Over the past 5 years a number of point-of-care testing devices and paradigms have been developed and approved by the FDA for detecting the antiplatelet effects of aspirin. Serum and urinary thromboxane B2 have also been used as surrogate markers for aspirin resistance. Although there is no well-defined "gold standard" for aspirin resistance in terms of either testing method or results, it is nonetheless encouraging that most large series have reported rates of aspirin resistance in the range of 15–25 percent.

Does aspirin resistance predict an increased risk of ischemic vascular events such as stroke, MI, or vascular death? Here the data is also fairly consistent.

1. Several studies have shown that patients who are aspirin resistant do have higher rates of vascular events.
2. A subset of patients from the HOPE study found a clear relationship between urinary TBXB2 and the risk of a vascular event.
3. A study of cardiovascular patients found that the risk of a vascular event was 24 percent in aspirin-resistant patients versus 10 percent in aspirin-responsive patients.
4. Our own study of patients with an acute ischemic stroke or TIA found that 47 percent of such patients were aspirin resistant.

What causes aspirin resistance? Numerous explanations have been put forth, and I suspect that there are different reasons in different patients.

1. In some cases, the dose of aspirin may simply be inadequate to effectively block the patients. This is supported in an analysis done by the ATC, which found that there was a dose-effect relationship between aspirin dose and clinical efficacy, with higher doses of aspirin associated with improved efficacy.
2. In other cases, formulation of aspirin may be important. Some studies have shown that enteric coated aspirin may not be absorbed as well as uncoated aspirin, leading to a suboptimal antiplatelet effect.
3. Other factors such as altered metabolism, genetics, and diet may also be important (see Table 18.2).
   a) Several studies, including our own, have shown that older women are more likely to have aspirin resistance.

Table 18.2: Potential causes of aspirin resistance

Poor bioavailability
    Inadequate absorption
    Underdosing
Altered metabolism of aspirin
    Different sites of action
Alternative pathways for platelet activation
    ADP receptor, fibrinogen receptor
Increased platelet production/turnover
    Seen in various disease states
Tachphylaxis to effects of aspirin
    May develop after 6–12 months
Genetic factors
    Various polymorphisms in receptors

Table 18.3: One approach to deciding which antiplatelet agents to use for different circumstances. Other approaches are also valid, and this will certainly vary depending upon the clinical scenario, individual patient factors, and physician preferences

Antiplatelet theraphy
    ASA, or Clopidogrel, or Aggrenox all acceptable
    See current guidelines
When to use Clopidigrel?
    ASA failures, ASA allergy, headaches, PAD
    High-risk: DM, old CAD, recent stent (carotoid, coronary)
When to use Aggrenox?
    No HA, No CAD, Young, sturdy stomaches
    When to use ASA + Clopidogrel?
    Recent CAD, ACS, poststent (carotid or coronary)
    Failed all monotherapies??
    ?Mirror CHARISMA population??

To date no study has shown that altering aspirin dose or formulation to maintain an effective antiplatelet response results in reduced rates of ischemic events. Such studies will be needed before we can say that aspirin should be administered as a dose-adjusted medication, with the dose being altered to maintain a specific level of antiplatelet effect.

Conclusions

Antiplatelet therapy is a mainstay for stroke prevention, particularly secondary prevention. Different antiplatelet agents have various mechanisms of action that may enhance their efficacy in some cases. Numerous studies have proven the efficacy of these agents, yet their benefit is often quite modest. Combination therapy also holds promise, although this may depend on the combinations used in different patient populations. In some cases combination therapy has an increased risk of bleeding. The issue of aspirin resistance is receiving increased attention. Whether dose-adjusted aspirin therapy will be an effective approach for alleviating aspirin resistance remains to be proven.

My general approach to the use of antiplatelet agents in patients with stroke/TIA for secondary prevention is shown in Table 18.3. Obviously this is a broad perspective, and I always individualize treatment based on specific patient characteristics, medical issues, socioeconomic factors, and the overall clinical scenario.

Bibliography

Berger JS, Roncaglioni MC, Avanzini F, et al. Aspirin for the primary prevention of cardiovascular, events in women and men: a six-specific metaanalysis of randomized controlled trials. JAMA 2006; 295(3):306–13. Diener HC, Ringleb P. Antithrombotic secondary prevention after stroke. *Curr Treat Options Neurol* 2001;3:451–62.

Diener HC. Antiplatelet drugs in secondary prevention of stroke: Lessons from recent trials. *Neurology* 1997;49:S75–81.

Halkes PH, van Gijn J, Kappelle LJ, Koudstaal PJ, Algra A. Aspirin plus dipyridamole versus aspirin alone after cerebral ischaemia of arterial origin (ESPRIT): Randomised controlled trial. *Lancet* 2006;367:1665–73.

Helgason CM, Bolin KM, Hoff JA, et al. Development of aspirin resistance in persons with previous ischemic stroke. *Stroke* 1994;25:2331–6.

Sacco RL, Adams R, Albers G, et al. Guidelines for prevention of stroke in patients with ischemic stroke or transient ischemic attack: A statement for healthcare professionals from the American Heart Association/American Stroke Association Council on Stroke: Co-sponsored by the Council on Cardiovascular Radiology and Intervention: The American Academy of Neurology affirms the value of this guideline. *Stroke* 2006;37:577–617.

Sandercock P. Antiplatelet therapy with aspirin in acute ischaemic stroke. *Thromb Haemost* 1997;78:180–2.

Sandercock PA, van den Belt AG, Lindley RI, Slattery J. Antithrombotic therapy in acute ischaemic stroke: An overview of the completed randomised trials. *J Neurol Neurosurg Psychiatry* 1993;56:17–25.

Schafer AI, Antiplatelets therapy. *Am J Med.* 1996; 101(2): 199–209.

Teal PA. Recent clinical trial results with antiplatelet therapy: Implications in stroke prevention. *Cerebrovasc Dis* 2004;17(Suppl 3):6–10.

van Gijn J, Algra A. Aspirin and stroke prevention. *Thromb Res* 2003;110:349–53.

19 Surgical and endovascular therapies

Nazli Janjua, Ammar Alkawi, Jawad F. Kirmani, and Adnan Qureshi

Introduction

Surgical and endovascular treatment of stroke can be classified in many ways: primary versus secondary stroke prevention and treatment of acute stroke, extracranial versus intracranial treatment, and standard of care versus experimental treatment lacking support level I evidence. We consider the combined approach to stroke patients according to extracranial versus intracranial disease, special instances of acute treatment, and prevention of cardioemboli where surgical intervention may be performed.

Extracranial carotid disease

Cervical internal carotid artery (ICA) stenosis

Surgical treatment of severe symptomatic cervical ICA stenosis is supported by level I evidence. Excellent surgical expertise is essential as well as adequate patient selection. These are identified by the criteria as follows:

1. Noninvasive imaging (MRA, CTA, carotid Duplex, or ultrasound) reveals moderate-severe stenosis of the carotid artery that is clinically symptomatic.
2. Obtain other sources of noninvasive imaging and verify the initial findings. Do both studies corroborate each other? If yes, consider conventional angiography and proceed with neurosurgical or vascular surgical consultation for possible CEA.

Many surgeons are comfortable operating on the basis of noninvasive imaging, though the degree of carotid stenoses in the North American Symptomatic Carotid Endarterectomy Trial (NASCET) and European Carotid Surgery Trial (ECST) was based on selective angiography.

1. The stenosis is symptomatic and is
   a) moderate (50–69 percent). Surgical therapy offers a 5-year absolute risk (AR) reduction of 6.5 percent over medical therapy and can be advised if exceptional surgical experience is available.

  b) severe (70–99 percent): these patients derive the most benefit from CEA; AR reduction of 11–17 percent after or at 2–3 years.
2. The stenosis is asymptomatic and is over 59 percent as measured by arteriography; CEA may be considered, particularly among men.
3. If the patient has significant medical comorbidity (e.g., age over 80 years, severe cardiac or pulmonary disease, contralateral carotid occlusion, contralateral laryngeal nerve palsy, prior radiation therapy or surgery to the neck, recurrent stenosis after prior CEA), consider carotid stent supported angioplasty (CAS). The risk of perioperative myocardial infarction (MI), stroke, and death among patients treated with CAS versus CEA is 12.2 versus 20 percent.
4. Ongoing analyses are underway comparing the efficacy of CAS versus CEA, and a number of registries are actively enrolling patients to evaluate the efficacy of various stent devices (Table 19.1).

Carotid occlusion

External carotid artery (ECA)-ICA bypass was performed for symptomatic carotid occlusion in the past, but poor results from the Cooperative Study on External-Internal Carotid (EC-IC) Bypass led to discontinuation of this procedure. However, it is thought that patient selection for EC-IC bypass in the cooperative study was suboptimal for identifying candidates most likely to benefit from surgery, and interest in this procedure has again been raised under the auspices of the Carotid Occlusion Surgery Study (COSS), which randomizes patients to medical treatment versus superficial temporal artery (STA)-middle cerebral artery (MCA) bypass.

1. Patients may be considered for the COSS study if they are found to have ICA occlusion and have had an ipsilateral stroke or TIA within the past 120 days *and*
   a) if the patient has positron emission tomography (PET) evidence of elevated oxygen extraction fraction (OEF) uptake in the ipsilateral hemisphere *and*
   b) the patient is able to consent. (Complete inclusion and exclusion criteria are summarized in Table 19.2)

Pre- and postoperative management

Most surgical preoperative management maintains patients on an anti-platelet regimen such as aspirin prior to CEA.

Postoperative complications of CEA include reperfusion hemorrhage, wound dissection and hemorrhage, other surgical/anesthetic-related complications, and restenosis or occlusion of the treated ICA. CAS may also be complicated by reperfusion hemorrhage.

Table 19.1: Carotid stent registries

Registry	Device/sponsor	Comments/enrolment
ARCHeR	AccuLink stent with and without distal protection device (DPD), AccuNet/Guidant	3 trials: (1) w/o DPD, (2) with DPD, (3) equivalency study for second generation device 581 patients in 3 trials
BEACH	Wallstent, with FilterWire EX DPD/Boston Scientific	Symptomatic ICA stenoses >50% or asymptomatic >80% 747 patients
CABERNET	NexStent, EPI Filter DPD/Boston Scientific/EndoTex	Symptomatic stenoses >/= 50%; asymptomatic >/= 80% by ultrasound or 60% by angiogram 454 patients
CARESS[a]	Device unspecified/ISIS	Symptomatic stenoses >/=50%, asymptomatic >/= 75%, showed equivalency in 30 day stroke/ death rates between CEA vs CAS. 439 patients.
CREATE[b]	Protégé, with Spider DPD/ev3	symptomatic stenosis >/= 50%, asymptomatic >/=70%, among high risk patients (age>75 years, LVEF<35%, or prior CEA). Feasibility of device trial. 30 patients
GCASR[c]	Any device	Voluntary international registry 12,392 procedures involving 11,243 patients
MAVErIC	Exponent/Medtronic	Efficacy of device trial Planned enrollment 350 patients

PASCAL	Exponent, any device/Medtronic	Safety and efficacy of device
		Planned enrollment of 100 patients
SECuRITY	Xact stent/Abbot	Safety and efficacy of device
SHELTER	Wallstent/Boston Scientific	Safety and efficacy of device
		Planned enrollment of 400 patients

Notes: ARCHeR, ACCULINK for Revascularization of Carotids in High-Risk Patients; BEACH, Boston Scientific EPI-A Carotid Stenting Trial for High Risk Surgical Patients; CABERNET, Carotid Artery Revascularization Using the Boston Scientific FilterWire and the EndoTex NexStent; CARESS, Carotid Revascularization with Endarterectomy or Stenting Systems; CREATE, Carotid Revascularization With ev3 Arterial Technology Evolution; LVEF, left ventricular ejection fraction; GCASR, Global Carotid Artery Stent Registry; MAVErIC, Medtronic AVE Self-Expanding Carotid Stent System with Distal Protection in the Treatment of Carotid Stenosis; PASCAL, Performance and Safety of the Medtronic AVE Self-Expandable Stent in Treatment of Carotid Artery Lesions; SECuRITY, Registry Study to evaluate the Neuroshield Bare-Wire Cerebral Protection System and X-Act Stent in patients at high risk for Carotid Endarterectomy; SHELTER, Stenting of High Risk Patients Extracranial Lesions Trial with Emboli Removal.

[a] Results published in *J Endovasc Ther* 2003;10:1021–30.
[b] *Catheter Cardiovasc Interv* 2004;63:1–6.
[c] *Catheter Cardiovasc Interv* 2003;60:259–266.

Table 19.2: Carotid occlusion surgery Study inclusion/exclusion criteria

Inclusion	Exclusion
Age 18–85 years and legally an adult	Nonatherosclerotic carotid vascular disease
Angiographically demonstrated ICA occlusion	Blood dyscrasias (polycythemia vera, essential thrombocytosis, sickle cell SS or SC disease)[5]a
Contralateral ICA stenosis $\leq$ 50%	Known cardiac disease likely to cause cerebral ischemia (infective endocarditis, left atrial or ventricular thrombus, sick sinus syndrome, myxoma, cardiomyopathy with ejection fraction < 25%)[6]b
TIA or other stroke with a Barthel Index score of 12–20 within the past 120 days	Other nonatherosclerotic condition likely to cause focal cerebral ischemia
PET-measured elevated oxygen extraction fraction (OEF) in the hemisphere distal to the occluded ICA Ipsilateral:contralateral OEF ratio in the middle cerebral artery territory >1.130 determined from the ratio image of $O^{15}O$ / $H_2{}^{15}O$ counts.	Subsequent cerebrovascular surgery planned that might alter cerebral hemodynamics or stroke risk (contralateral ICA or CCA CEA or CAS, ipsilateral ECA CEA or CAS, carotid stump closure, VA or basilar artery angioplasty, any arterial grafting procedures to the carotid or vertebral arteries)
Competent to give informed consent	Other neurological disease that would confound follow-up assessment
	Pregnancy
Geographically accessible and reliable for followup	Any condition likely to lead to death within 2 years
	Any condition that in the participating surgeon's judgment makes the participant an unsuitable surgical candidate
	Concurrent participation in any other experimental treatment trial

Participation within the previous 12 months in any experimental study that included exposure to ionizing radiation

Acute, progressing or unstable neurological deficit (neurological deficit must be stable for 72 hr prior to the performance of PET)

If supplemental arteriography is required, allergy to iodine or x-ray contrast media serum creatinine >3.0 mg/dl or other contraindication to arteriography

Allergy or contraindication to aspirin

Medical indication for treatment with anticoagulant drugs, ticlopidine, clopidogrel or other antithrombotic medications such that these medications cannot be replaced with aspirin in the perioperative period as deemed necessary by the COSS neurosurgeon if the participant is randomized to surgical treatment

Uncontrolled diabetes mellitus (FBS > 300 mg%/16.7 mmol/l) unless controlled within the 120-day period of stroke/TIA

Uncontrolled hypertension (systolic BP>180, diastolic BP >110 mmHg) unless controlled within the 120 day period of stroke/TIA

Uncontrolled hypotension (diastolic < 65 mmHg) unless controlled within the 120-day period of stroke/TIA

Notes: [a] The following conditions are *not exclusions*: anticardiolipin antibodies, lupus anticoagulant, protein S, C, or antithrombin III deficiency, Factor V Leiden, or other causes of activated protein C resistance, prothrombin gene mutations.
[b] The following conditions are *not exclusions*: atrial fibrillation, patent foramen ovale, atrial septal aneurysm.
Source: http://www.cosstrial.org/coss/inEx.asp, accessed September 6, 2005.

1. Reperfusion hemorrhage occurs with reestablishment of normal blood flow through a chronically ischemic hemisphere. This may result in intracerebral hemorrhage (ICH). This may be best avoided by
   a) intensive care monitoring with frequent neurological checks to assess for change in clinical status that may indicate developing ICH or restenosis. Patients may present with focal deficits or seizures (with reperfusion injury/ICH);
   b) blood pressure monitoring postoperatively to avoid extreme hypertension.
2. Patients s/p CAS often require dual antiplatelet therapy for a minimum of 3–6 weeks after which time they should be maintained on at least one antiplatelet agent, for example, aspirin.
3. Wound hemorrhage may lead to tracheal obstruction, and if this occurs, the following steps should be undertaken:
   a) urgent stabilization of the airway by means of an endotracheal tube;
   b) urgent surgical reexploration to identify and stabilize any source of arterial hemorrhage.
4. Anesthetic complications not particular to neurological issues are beyond the scope of this text but may include neuromuscular and allergic reactions to anesthetics and adverse cardiopulmonary events.

Intracranial atherosclerosis

Intracranial carotid occlusion

Progressive vasculopathies leading to occlusion of the intracranial ICA and MCA, such as Moya-moya disease, have also been successfully treated with bypass procedures including

1. STA-MCA bypass (see above under heading "Carotid occlusion")
2. *Encephaloduroarteriosynangiosis (EDAS)* involves dissecting a scalp artery over a course of several inches and then making a small temporary opening in the skull directly beneath the artery. The artery is then sutured to the surface of the brain and the bone replaced.
3. Galeoduroencephalosynangiosis is a procedure in which multiple small holes (burr holes) are placed in the skull to allow for growth of new vessels into the brain from the scalp.
4. Encephalomyosynangiosis is a procedure in which the temporalis muscle is dissected and through an opening in the skull placed onto the surface of the brain.

Intracranial atherosclerosis

Studies to evaluate the natural history of intracranial atherosclerosis are underway. At this time, endovascular (or surgical) therapy is not known to be more efficacious than medical therapy. However, it may be considered in unusual circumstances of extreme symptomatic atherosclerosis, recurrent stroke despite maximal medical therapy, and in the setting of acute stroke, which will be considered separately. PTA is considered a mainstay of treatment for severe, refractory cerebral vasospasm following aneurysmal subarachnoid hemorrhage, thus a wealth of feasibility data for this treatment modality already exists, though efficacy data in the form of randomized clinical trials is lacking.

Deployment of small-sized balloon expandable coronary stents has been performed safely in the intracranial vasculature and with technical success. Stent deployment has thus far been best described in proximal circle of Willis vessels (e.g., carotid terminus, M1 stem), though primary angioplasty has been reported and has been found successful in more distal vessels such as divisional branches of the MCA and the A2 segment. As with other treatments of the extracranial carotid (ECA) and vertebral arteries (VA), adequate patient selection and excellent technical capabilities are essential.

Patient selection should identify those with the following criteria:

1. a high-grade proximal intracranial vessel (e.g., ICA terminus, M1 stem) exists *and*
2. there is evidence of decreased cerebral perfusion by CT, MRI, or SPECT *and/or*
3. there is no cerebrovascular reserve as demonstrated by CO_2 or acetazolamide transcranial Doppler (TCD) study, *and/or*
4. recurrent strokes in relation to the diseased vessel have occurred, despite maximal medical therapy.

Intraprocedural management

Intraprocedural complications may involve thromboembolic events. Immediate treatment with intravenous (IV) glycoprotein (GP) IIb/IIIa inhibitors or fibrinolytics is usually employed to treat in situ or in stent restenosis or occlusion. Mechanical thrombectomy with snare devices has been reported in distal MCA vessels.

Postprocedure management

1. Reperfusion hemorrhage is a potential complication following EC-IC bypass procedures or other arteriosynangiotic procedures. Monitoring for these events and management of complications is as for postoperative management of extracranial carotid revascularization procedures.
2. Postprocedure management should include diligent ICU observation with frequent neurologic checks to assess for any change in neurological status that may indicate restenosis or occlusive events.
3. Early imaging with CT should be undertaken or patients experiencing a change in their neurologic status to assess for hemorrhage that may occur in patients receiving antiplatelets, anticoagulants, or fibrinolytics, or acute and evolving stroke.

4. Immediate angiography may be needed in patients with symptoms of acute stroke after PTA/stent placement who suffer a neurological deterioration, and endovascular treatments of acute stroke (see below) may be considered.

Extracranial VA origin disease

VA stent supported angioplasty

Though there is no standardized evidence mandating revascularization for symptomatically stenosed extracranial VA, the wealth of evidence supporting treatment of carotid origin disease has raised interest in treatment of atherosclerotic vertebral ostia. Surgical treatment of VA origin disease is technically challenging and rarely if ever performed; however, endovascular access to the VA origin is less problematic and is a lower risk procedure compared to surgery as well as to other intracranial neuroendovascular procedures, and individual series reporting excellent technical success of these procedures have been published. A review of the Cochrane database for primary percutaneous transluminal angioplasty (PTA) and stenting found evidence for feasibility of angioplasty of the VA, though efficacy could not be well established. Treatment of symptomatic VA origin disease, recurrent despite maximal medical therapy, can therefore be considered if

1. the stenotic VA is the dominant VA *or*
2. a posterior inferior cerebellar artery (PICA) stroke has occurred ipsilateral to the stenotic VA origin in question.

Postoperative management

As with CAS, patients should be maintained on double antiplatelet therapy. Reperfusion injury is less well described, and likely less common, in the posterior circulation territory compared with the anterior circulation territory.

An algorithm of management for patients presenting with subacute strokes and TIAs referable is shown in Figure 19.1.

Endovascular treatments of acute stroke

Though there is no approved treatment for patients arriving beyond 3 hr after the onset of an acute ischemic stroke, intraarterial (IA) thrombolysis or mechanical thrombectomy may be performed in centers where neurointerventional capabilities exist.

Intraarterial thrombolysis

Patients may be considered for IA thrombolysis using prourokinase (proUK), recombinant alteplase (rt-PA), or reteplase if:

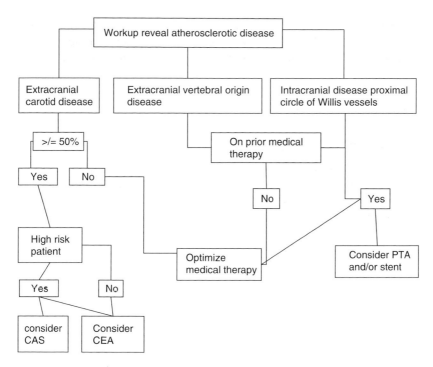

Figure 19.1 Algorithm of management for subacute stroke/TIA.

1. They are within 6 hr of an acute ischemic stroke and brain imaging (e.g., CT) is negative for ICH.
2. Other relative contraindications, which should be weighed on an individual basis, include renal insufficiency, contrast allergy, other severe medical comorbidity, including malignant hypertension, which may increase the risk of ICH with selective thrombolytic therapy.
3. Selected patients may be considered for "bridging" therapy with a lower dose IV rt-PA and additional IA thrombolysis if they have National Institutes of Health Stroke scale scores ≥10.

Mechanical thrombectomy

Patients arriving within 8 hr may also be considered for mechanical thrombectomy using the Food and Drug Administration (FDA)-approved Merci ™ Concentric Retrieval Device (Concentric Medical, Mountainview, CA, Figure 19.2) if:

1. They are within 8 hr of an acute ischemic stroke and are not candidates for intravenous (IV) rt-PA *or*
2. They fail to improve after IV rt-PA and are still within 8 hr of acute ischemic stroke. (Multi-Merci trial)

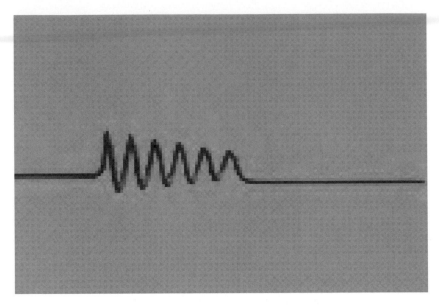

Figure 19.2 Merci ™ Concentric Retrieval Device for mechanical thrombectomy in acute stroke.

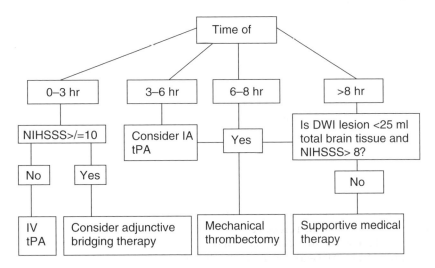

Figure 19.3 Algorithm of management for acute stroke patients.

3. As with IA thrombolysis, other relative contraindications, which should be weighed on an individual basis, include renal insufficiency, contrast allergy, other severe medical comorbidity, including malignant hypertension, which may increase the risk of ICH with selective thrombolytic therapy.

4. For patients arriving outside of 8 hr, therapy must be individualized according to the presence or absence of ischemic changes seen on cerebral imaging, degree of territory involved (e.g., posterior circulation), and degree of neurological deficit. Patients with a National Institutes of Health stroke scale score ≥ 8 and a diffusion weighted magnetic resonance image volume of injury ≤ 25 ml may represent a group of patients at high risk for neurological worsening and may represent a subgroup worthy of revascularization therapies.

An algorithm of management for patients presenting with acute stroke is shown in Figure 19.3.

Secondary prevention of cardioembolic sources of stroke

A significant association between the presence of patent foramen ovale (PFO) and right-to-left intracardiac shunts and cryptogenic strokes among young patients (generally under 40 years) has been demonstrated. There is currently no evidence to suggest that these patients would benefit from anticoagulation therapy or surgical closure of their PFOs.

Bibliography

Adams H P Jr, Brott T G, Furlan A J, et al. Guidelines for thrombolytic therapy for acute stroke: A supplement to the guidelines for the management of patients with acute ischemic stroke. A statement for healthcare professionals from a special writing group of the stroke council, American Heart Association. *Circulation* 1996;94:1167–74.

American Society of Interventional and Therapeutic Neuroradiology. Mechanical and pharmacologic treatment of vasospasm. *AJNR Am J Neuroradiol* 2001;22(8 Suppl):S26–7.

Barnett H J, Taylor D W, Eliasziw M, et al. Benefit of carotid endarterectomy in patients with symptomatic moderate or severe stenosis. North American Symptomatic Carotid Endarterectomy Trial Collaborators. *N Engl J Med* 1998;339:1415–25.

Carotid Occlusion Surgery Study. *Proceedings of the 28th International Stroke Conference*. Phoenix, AZ, February 2003.

Crawley F, Brown M M. Percutaneous transluminal angioplasty and stenting for vertebral artery stenosis. *Cochrane Database Syst Rev* 2000;(2):CD000516.

Davalos A, Blanco M, Pedraza S, et al. The clinical-DWI mismatch: A new diagnostic approach to the brain tissue at risk of infarction. *Neurology* 2004;62:2187–92.

del Zoppo G J, Higashida R T, Furlan A J, Pessin M S, Rowley H A, Gent M. PROACT: A phase II randomized trial of recombinant pro-urokinase by direct arterial delivery in acute middle cerebral artery stroke. PROACT investigators. Prolyse in acute cerebral thromboembolism. *Stroke* 1998;29:4–11.

Di Tullio M, Sacco R L, Gopal A, Mohr J P, Homma S. Patent foramen ovale as a risk factor for cryptogenic stroke. *Ann Intern Med* 1992;117:461–5.

Emergency interventional stroke therapy: A statement from the American Society of Interventional and Therapeutic Neuroradiology and Society of Cardiovascular and Interventional Radiology. *J Vasc Intervent Radiol* 2001;12:143.

Endarterectomy for asymptomatic carotid artery stenosis. Executive Committee for the Asymptomatic Carotid Atherosclerosis Study. *JAMA* 1995;273:1421–8.

European Carotid Surgery Trialists' Collaborative Group. Randomised trial of carotid endarterectomy for recently symptomatic carotid stenosis: Final results of the MRC European carotid surgery trial (ECST). *Lancet* 1998;351:1379–87.

Failure of extracranial-intracranial arterial bypass to reduce the risk of ischemic stroke. Results of an international randomized trial. The EC/IC Bypass Study Group. *N Engl J Med* 1985;313:1191–200.

Feldmann E, Wilterdink J, Kosinski A, Sarafin J, Thovmasian N. Stroke Outcomes and Neuroimaging of Intracranial Atherosclerosis (SONIA). *Proceedings of the 28th International Stroke Conference*. American Stroke Association, Phoenix, AZ, February, 2003.

Furlan A, Higashida R, Wechsler L, et al. Intra-arterial prourokinase for acute ischemic stroke. The PROACT II study: A randomized controlled trial. Prolyse in acute cerebral thromboembolism. *JAMA* 1999;282:2003–11.

Gobin Y P, Starkman S, Duckwiler G R, et al. MERCI 1: A phase 1 study of mechanical embolus removal in cerebral ischemia. *Stroke* 2004;35:2848–54.

Hobson R W. CREST (Carotid Revascularization Endarterectomy versus Stent Trial): Background, design, and current status. *Semin Vasc Surg* 2000;13:139–43.

http://cpmcnet.columbia.edu/dept/nsg/PNS/moyamoya.html, accessed September 2, 2005.

IMS study investigators. Combined intravenous and intra-arterial recanalization for acute ischemic stroke: The Interventional Management of Stroke Study. *Stroke* 2004;35:904–11.

Karapanayiotides T, Meuli R, Devuyst G, et al. Postcarotid endarterectomy hyperperfusion or reperfusion syndrome. *Stroke* 2005;36:21–6.

Kawaguchi T, Fujita S, Hosoda K, et al. Multiple burr-hole operation for adult moyamoya disease. *J Neurosurg* 1996;84:468–76.

Lechat P, Mas J L, Lascault G, et al. Prevalence of patent foramen ovale in patients with stroke. *N Engl J Med* 1988;318:1148–52.

Lin Y H, Juang J M, Jeng J S, Yip P K, Kao H L. Symptomatic ostial vertebral artery stenosis treated with tubular coronary stents: Clinical results and restenosis analysis. *J Endovasc Ther* 2004;11:719–26.

Polin R S, Coenen V A, Hansen C A, et al. Efficacy of transluminal angioplasty for the management of symptomatic cerebral vasospasm following aneurysmal subarachnoid hemorrhage. *J Neurosurg* 2000;92:284–90.

Qureshi A I, Suri M F, Siddiqui A M, et al. Clinical and angiographic results of dilatation procedures for symptomatic intracranial atherosclerotic disease. *J Neuroimaging* 2005;15:240–9.

Ross I B, Shevell M I, Montes J L, et al. Encephaloduroarteriosynangiosis (EDAS) for the treatment of childhood moyamoya disease. *Pediatr Neurol* 1994;10:199–204.

Smith W S, Sung G, Starkman S, et al., MERCI trial investigators. Safety and efficacy of mechanical embolectomy in acute ischemic stroke: Results of the MERCI trial. *Stroke* 2005;36:1432–8.

SSYLVIA study investigators. Stenting of Symptomatic Atherosclerotic Lesions in the Vertebral or Intracranial Arteries (SSYLVIA): Study results. *Stroke* 2004;35:1388–92.

Straube T, Stingele R, Jansen O. Primary stenting of intracranial atherosclerotic stenoses. *Cardiovasc Intervent Radiol* 2005;28:289–95.

Webster M W, Chancellor A M, Smith H J, et al. Patent foramen ovale in young stroke patients. *Lancet* 1988;2:11–12.

Yadav J S, Wholey M H, Kuntz R E, et al., Stenting and angioplasty with protection in patients at high risk for endarterectomy investigators. Protected carotid-artery stenting versus endarterectomy in high-risk patients. *N Engl J Med* 2004;351: 1493–501.

20 Stroke risk factors: Impact and management

Laura Pedelty and Philip B. Gorelick

Introduction

Stroke is a major cause of death and disability worldwide. An estimated 700,000 new or recurrent strokes and 275,000 stroke deaths occur annually in the United States (American Heart Association, 2005). Despite the common nomenclature "cerebrovascular accident" or CVA, stroke is not an "accident": there are well-documented modifiable and nonmodifiable risk factors that lead to this disease. With its high prevalence and associated social and economic burden, and its association with well-documented and modifiable risk factors, stroke is especially well suited to preventive strategies. Improved control of modifiable risk factors could potentially decrease the burden of cardiovascular disease and stroke in the United States by over $13 billion Table 20.1 lists important known risk factors for stroke. Nonmodifiable risk factors for stroke include age, race/ethnicity (blacks and Hispanics), sex (male), and family history. Although these factors are not amenable to intervention or modification, their recognition is important so that individuals at higher risk can be identified for vigilant monitoring and management of other, potentially modifiable risk factors. This chapter focuses on key modifiable antecedent factors that predispose to stroke, and outlines preventive treatment options. Seven modifiable risk factors are considered here: hypertension, hyperlipidemia, atrial fibrillation, diabetes mellitus, smoking, hyperhomocysteinemia, and alcohol. Carotid stenosis and cardiac disease are treated in other chapters.

Hypertension

Hypertension is the most important modifiable risk factor for stroke. Because hypertension has a high relative risk and high prevalence in the population, its population attributable risk (PAR, a measure that explains the estimated proportion of disease attributable to a specific risk factor) is high: for hypertension, the PAR for stroke is about 25 percent and may be as

---

Table 20.1: Nonmodifiable and well-documented modifiable risk factors for stroke (Goldstein et al., 2001)

Nonmodifiable risk factors
Age
Race (blacks and Hispanics)
Sex (men)
Family history of stroke/TIA

Well-documented modifiable risk factors
Hypertension
Smoking
Diabetes mellitus
Asymptomatic carotid stenosis
Sickle cell disease
Hyperlipidemia
Atrial fibrillation

Less well-documented or potentially modifiable risk factors
Obesity
Physical inactivity
Alcohol use ≥5 drinks/day
Hyperhomocysteinemia
Drug abuse
Hypercoagulable
Oral contraceptive use
Inflammatory processes

---

high as 50 percent. Other key aspects of the epidemiological relationship between hypertension and stroke are listed below:

1. All forms of hypertension (systolic, diastolic, or combined systolic and diastolic) increase stroke risk.
2. Hypertensive individuals are about 3–4 times more likely to experience stroke than nonhypertensive individuals.
3. Borderline hypertensive individuals are about 1.5 times more likely to experience stroke than nonhypertensive individuals.
4. Hypertension is a risk factor for stroke in all geographic regions and among all ethnic groups studied.
5. Elevated systolic blood pressure may be a better predictor of stroke risk than elevated diastolic blood pressure.
6. Most strokes occur among those with only mild hypertension, pre-hypertension, or even normal blood pressure.
7. A continuous relationship between the risk of stroke and blood pressure exists, which can be demonstrated as low as 115/75 mmHg.
8. Because of this continuum of risk between blood pressure and stroke, we are now shifting our emphasis to absolute blood pressure level

rather than a threshold of risk associated with a specific blood pressure level (e.g., ≥140/90 mmHg).

9. Clinical trials have shown that blood pressure lowering results in
substantial reduction of stroke risk. Some blood pressure lowering
agents (e.g., angiotensin-converting enzyme inhibitors, ACE-Is,
angiotensin receptor blockers, ARBs) may have beneficial effects
independent of blood pressure lowering.

10. For stroke prevention, getting blood pressure to goal is important. For
those at highest risk of stroke, lifestyle and pharmacological management are recommended and for those at lowest risk, lifestyle
management is recommended as the first treatment of choice. Nonhypertensive individuals may benefit from blood pressure lowering to
reduce stroke risk.

11. More epidemiological study is needed to clarify the relationships.

Prevention of stroke by treatment of blood pressure

We recommend following the JNC 7 guidelines for blood pressure management to reduce stroke risk. The goal is to reach a blood pressure of less
than 140/90 mmHg for most individuals and a goal of less than 130/80
mmHg in those individuals who have diabetes mellitus or chronic kidney
disease, with even lower blood pressure targets in some individuals with
heart failure or other conditions that require more extreme blood pressure
lowering. Figure 20.1 is a simple algorithm for blood pressure management
utilizing lifestyle and pharmacological interventions and is consistent with
JNC 7 recommendations. Table 20.2 summarizes five key points regarding
the chronic management of blood pressure following stroke.

Table 20.2: Answers to five key questions about chronic management
of blood pressure after stroke (Pedelty and Gorelick, 2004)

1. *When is it safe to lower blood pressure after an acute ischemic stroke?*
There are not yet definitive data to guide this decision. Informal discussion
with experts suggests that blood pressure lowering may begin from 7 days
to up to a month's time after acute ischemic stroke. Instituting therapy
earlier within this window may be beneficial in maximizing compliance:
patients counseled and treated closer to the time of the event may be
more likely to receive and be compliant with treatment, while delayed
institution of therapy may risk losing the patient to timely followup, with
a consequent increased risk of recurrent stroke. While documenting stable
collateral blood flow before beginning to lower the blood pressure has
clear theoretical benefits, in most clinical settings, stability of collateral
flow is difficult to determine, and we continue to be guided by clinical
experience and expert opinion.

Studies are ongoing to determine if blood pressure lowering or elevation
is beneficial in the acute phase immediately after ischemic stroke.

2. *What is the target blood pressure goal and how soon should it be reached?* Definitive evidence to guide precise blood pressure targets for chronic management after ischemic stroke has not been established, nor has the time at which the target blood pressure goal should be reached. We recommend following the JNC 7 guidelines (blood pressure target <140/90 mmHg for most patients and <130/80 mmHg for patients with diabetes mellitus or chronic kidney disease). JNC 7 guidelines recommend follow-up of blood pressure control at approximately monthly intervals in uncomplicated patients until blood pressure reaches the target value, and at 3–6 month intervals thereafter.

3. *Which agent or agents is most effective?* Overview analyses suggest that all major classes of blood pressure lowering medication decrease the risk of a first stroke. Therefore, the choice of agent may be irrelevant unless there is a compelling indication for a specific agent or class of agents. The JNC 7 guidelines review compelling indications according to drug class or specific medication. At present, an ACE-I (perindopril) in combination with a diuretic (indapamide) has been shown to reduce the risk of recurrent stroke. ARBs may also reduce the risk of recurrent stroke.

4. *Will blood pressure lowering precipitate stroke?* In most patients, lowering blood pressure will result in fewer first or recurrent strokes. The concern that blood pressure lowering might lead to cerebral hypoperfusion and stroke, especially in the elderly, generally has not proven to be true. Several studies have now shown that high risk individuals without hypertension may benefit from blood pressure lowering to reduce first or recurrent stroke risk.

5. *Should blood pressure be lowered once there is cognitive impairment or dementia?* This question has not been fully resolved. Some epidemiological data suggest that once there is cognitive impairment, it may be better to gently elevate blood pressure. The issue needs to be studied in a large-scale clinical trial setting. However, if there is no cognitive impairment, blood pressure lowering is protective, resulting in fewer cases of Alzheimer's disease and fewer cases of vascular dementia.

Hyperlipidemia

Disorders of lipids and lipoproteins relatively well studied in stroke include abnormalities of total cholesterol, low density lipoproteins (LDLs), high density lipoproteins (HDLs), lipoprotein (a) (Lp[a]), and triglycerides. Epidemiological studies are not fully consistent with regard to the relationship between lipids and lipoproteins and stroke risk. Key epidemiological relationships between the various lipid and lipoprotein disorders in stroke are summarized below:

1. Increasing total cholesterol level seems to be associated with increased risk of ischemic stroke.
2. Low HDL-cholesterol may be a risk factor for ischemic stroke but the relationship of elevated LDL-cholesterol to stroke remains uncertain.
3. Lp(a) may be a risk factor for ischemic stroke.
4. Elevated levels of triglycerides may be a risk factor for ischemic stroke; however, the relationship may be confounded by its link to the metabolic syndrome (obesity, hyperglycemia, and dyslipidemia).
5. Statins lower the risk of stroke especially in individuals with coronary heart disease (CHD).
6. There may be a continuum of risk in the relationship of total cholesterol to stroke in individuals with CHD, with a reduction of stroke risk irrespective of cholesterol level.
7. Statins lower the systemic inflammatory marker high-sensitivity C-reactive protein (hs-CRP) and the vascular inflammatory marker lipoprotein-associated phospholipase A2 (Lp-PLA2). Whether lowering of these inflammatory markers is in fact protective against cardiovascular events remains to be determined.
8. More epidemiological study is needed to clarify the relationships.

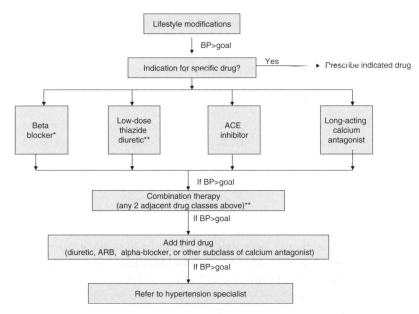

Figure 20.1 A simple algorithm for choosing antihypertensive drug therapy to prevent a first stroke (Elliot WJ et al. 2002) (*) An initial beta-blocker is not recommended for hypertensive patients over age 60. An ARB may be considered as initial therapy. (**) JNC 7 guidelines recommend a thiazide-type diuretic for most patients (Chobanian et al., 2003). [After Elliot et al. (2002). Reproduced with permission].

Treatment recommendations

The guidelines of the Expert Panel on Detection, Evaluation, and Treatment of High Blood Cholesterol in Adults and its subsequent update provide specific recommendations for stroke risk reduction. With regard to cerebrovascular disease and stroke, specific treatment recommendations are made for CHD risk equivalents, which include symptomatic carotid artery disease.

For patients with baseline LDL-cholesterol ≥130 mg/dl, intensive lifestyle therapy is recommended, including (1) reduced intake of saturated fats (less than 7 percent of total calories) and cholesterol (<200 mg/day), (2) consideration of plant stanols/sterols and increased viscous fiber (10–25 g/day) to enhance LDL lowering, and (3) consideration of weight reduction and increased physical exercise, along with maximum control of other risk factors (e.g., hypertension). Most patients with CHD risk equivalents such as symptomatic carotid artery disease, for example, will require an LDL-lowering drug to achieve the target LDL-cholesterol goal (<100 mg/dl).

For patients with LDL-cholesterol levels of 100–129 mg/dl, recommendations are to (1) initiate or intensify lifestyle and/or drug therapies to lower LDL-cholesterol; (2) focus on weight reduction and increased physical activity in individuals with metabolic syndrome; (3) intensify LDL-lowering treatment as well as treatment for other lipid and nonlipid risk factors; and (4) treat elevated triglyceride or low HDL-cholesterol (e.g., nicotinic acid or fibrates).

The update to the NCEP 2001 statement includes lower LDL-cholesterol targets based on risk assessment (e.g., a target of <70 mg/dl instead of <100 mg/dl for those at very high risk as a reasonable option). Such intensive lipid lowering therapy with statin agents has become a new trend in cardiovascular disease prevention.

The Heart Protection Study demonstrated reductions in coronary events as well as revascularization in patients with preexisting cerebrovascular disease, irrespective of baseline cholesterol level, with institution of statin therapy. However, among these same patients with preexisting cerebrovascular disease, there was no evident reduction in stroke incidence. The question, therefore, remains whether we should initiate statin therapy in all patients with stroke, but no history of CHD or other major indication for statins (e.g., diabetes mellitus). The Stroke Prevention by Aggressive Reduction in Cholesterol Levels (SPARCL) trial is testing this important question in a randomized clinical trial designed to prevent recurrent stroke. Results presented at the European Stroke Congress in May 2006 showed a reduced risk of stroke, major coronary events, CHD, and revascularization events in the atorvastatin (80 mg/day) treatment group compared to controls.

Atrial fibrillation

Atrial fibrillation is an important risk factor for stroke, especially among the elderly . Key epidemiological relationships between atrial fibrillation and stroke are reviewed below:

1. Nonvalvular atrial fibrillation (NVAF) increases the risk of stroke by about six times.
2. NVAF is the most common cause of cardioembolic stroke.
3. Valvular atrial fibrillation increases the risk of stroke by about 17 times.
4. It is estimated that over 2 million Americans have atrial fibrillation, about 60,000 strokes are attributable to this arrhythmia, and in individuals ≥80 years of age, about 25 percent of strokes is caused by atrial fibrillation.
5. Strokes associated with atrial fibrillation may be associated with higher mortality, larger size, and more disability.
6. Antithrombotics remain the key method for stroke reduction as rhythm control may not reduce stroke risk.
7. The administration of warfarin is associated with an estimated 60–70 percent reduction of stroke, whereas aspirin is associated with an estimated 20 percent reduction of stroke.
8. In clinical trials, the risk of major hemorrhage for individuals treated with warfarin is generally low (about 1.0–1.5 percent/year).

Treatment recommendations

The decision about which patient to treat and which antithrombotic agent to use to treat the patient with atrial fibrillation is based on risk stratification schemes. The SPAF III group has identified individuals with NVAF at low risk for stroke (about 1 percent/year), who may be candidates for aspirin therapy, in distinction to a population at much higher risk (8 percent/year) in whom warfarin therapy should be considered. According to this scheme, low risk NVAF patients include those under age 75 with no history of any of the following: (1) hypertension, (2) recent congestive heart failure, (3) left ventricular fractional shortening of ≤25 percent, (4) previous thromboembolism, or (5) systolic blood pressure >160 mmHg. Table 20.3 illustrates two commonly employed risk stratification schemes and recommendations; recently, the CHADS2 scheme has become popular.

Based on individual risk assessment (see Table 20.3), warfarin remains the treatment of choice for most patients with atrial fibrillation for stroke prevention. Rate control in conjunction with anticoagulant therapy is not inferior to rhythm control in preventing stroke and other cardiovascular complications of NVAF. Still, only about one-half of eligible individuals with

Table 20.3: Risk stratification schemes for treatment of atrial fibrillation in stroke prevention

CHADS$_2$ scheme

Point assignment according to condition
Congestive heart failure, Hypertension, Age >75 years, Diabetes
   mellitus: 1 point each Stroke or TIA: 2 points for either type of event

CHADS2 score	Treatment recommendation
0 (low risk or stroke rate about 1%/year)	Aspirin 75–325 mg/day
1 (low risk or stroke rate about 1.5%/year)	Aspirin 75–325 mg/day
2 (moderate risk or stroke rate about 2.5%/year)	Warfarin or aspirin
3 (high risk or stroke rate about 5%/year)	Warfarin
>/=4 (very high risk or stroke rate about >7%/year)	Warfarin

For warfarin use, the INR target is 2.0–3.0; some recommend an INR target of 1.6–2.5 for those >75 years of age. Any individual with atrial fibrillation and prior stroke or TIA should be considered high risk and treated with warfarin.

ACCP 2004 recommendations (56)

Risk level	
High: age >75 or any history of	Warfarin, INR 2.5 (range 2–3)
prior ischemic stroke	
TIA	
systemic embolism	
moderate-severe impairment of LV function and/or CHF	
history of HTN	
DM	
Intermediate: age 65–75, no other	Warfarin, INR 2.5 (range 2–3)
risk factors	or aspirin 325 mg/day
Low: age <65, no other risk factors	Aspirin 325 mg/day

atrial fibrillation receive anticoagulation therapy, and of these, only about one-half have INR values maintained in the optimal therapeutic range. Better education of physicians and patients about the benefits and risks of warfarin therapy in atrial fibrillation, along with support systems such as anticoagulation clinics, could optimize the use of warfarin.

Diabetes mellitus

An estimated 13.9 million Americans carry a diagnosis of diabetes mellitus, and an additional 5.9 million may be undiagnosed. Patients with diabetes are more likely to have other risk factors such as hypertension and dyslipidemia; however, diabetes carries an increased risk of stroke even after adjustment for these and other factors. In addition:

1. Both Type I and Type II diabetes are associated with increased risk of stroke.
2. Atherothrombotic infarcts are more common and more severe in patients with diabetes, and hyperglycemia and diabetes are associated with increased mortality and morbidity after stroke.
3. The impact is especially large for young patients with diabetes: 76 percent of stroke patients in the age group 35–44 have diabetes.
4. The prevalence of diabetes is higher (22 percent or five times that of the population at large) among ethnic minorities including African Americans and Hispanic Americans, and stroke risk is especially high for these populations.
5. Diabetics with hypertension are at particularly high risk for stroke, and aggressive management of blood pressure reduces risk in diabetics even more markedly than in nondiabetics.
6. Hyperglycemia in the absence of diabetes is associated with a prothrombotic state and an adverse lipid profile (the metabolic syndrome).
7. Intensive treatment of diabetes results in a decrease in microvascular complications (retinopathy, peripheral neuropathy, nephropathy), but a decrease in macrovascular complications such as stroke has not been demonstrated definitively.

Treatment recommendations

Because of the high risk of stroke in this population, and because of demonstrated efficacy of aggressive management of comorbid risk factors, the American Diabetes Association recommends stringent control of glucose, blood pressure, and cholesterol, with a target Hgb A1C <7.0 percent, SPB <130, DPB <80, LDL-cholesterol <100, triglycerides <150, and HDL >40. Use of an ACE inhibitor may be associated with decreased carotid IMT. The 2006 American Heart Association/American Stroke Association guidelines for the prevention of ischemic stroke recommend, in addition to a blood pressure target of <130/80 mmHg, that adults with diabetes, especially those with other risk factors, should receive a statin agent for prevention of a first stroke and consideration of an ACE inhibitor or ARB.

Smoking

Despite a widespread public health campaign, a substantial proportion of the population continues to smoke cigarettes. Cigarette smoking may increase the risk of stroke and other vascular disease through several mechanisms, including increased viscosity and fibrinogen levels, vascular endothelial damage, increased platelet aggregation, and vasoconstriction. Current epidemiological studies suggest that

1. cigarette smokers comprise 25 percent of the population in the United States. The proportion is higher in minority populations, including African Americans.
2. Cigarette smoking is associated with a 1.5–2-fold increase in the risk of stroke, including subarachnoid hemorrhage, ischemic stroke, and, in some but not all studies, intracerebral hemorrhage.
3. Cigarette smoking increases stroke risk in a dose-dependent fashion: the risk of stroke rises with the number of cigarettes smoked, and heavy smokers are at about twice the risk of stroke as light smokers.
4. Even passive smoking, that is, environmental exposure to cigarette smoke in nonsmokers, may increase the risk of progression of atherosclerosis and stroke.
5. Women who smoke are at higher risk than men who smoke.
6. Smoking cessation is effective in stroke prevention: the risk of stroke declines to that of nonsmokers within 5 years of cessation, though heavy smokers may never return fully to baseline risk.

Treatment recommendations

All patients who smoke should be counseled about the risks and urged, along with their family members, to stop. Patients should not be encouraged to take up other forms of tobacco (pipes, cigars, snuff, chewing tobacco), as these carry health risks as well. Replacement nicotine – in the form of gum, transdermal patch, inhaler, or nasal spray – is effective in aiding smoking cessation, as is bupropion. Other adjuvant therapies, including acupuncture and hypnotism, have less well-demonstrated efficacy.

Hyperhomocysteinemia

Homocysteine is a sulfur-containing amino acid formed in the metabolism of methionine from dietary protein. It is metabolized through pathways dependent on folate, vitamin B6 (pyridoxine), vitamin B12 (cobalamine), and betaine. Markedly elevated levels of homocysteine (>100 uM/l) are seen in homocystinuria, an autosomal recessive syndrome of abnormalities in the enzyme cystathionine beta-synthase that is characterized by early and severe central and peripheral arterial and venous thrombosis. Milder elevations (>13 uM/l) are also associated with increased risk of vascular events including stroke; the mechanism is unclear, but may depend on promotion of atherosclerosis through oxidative stress, platelet and coagulation factor activation, and endothelial dysfunction and vascular smooth muscle proliferation. Other epidemiological aspects of homocysteine in stroke include the following:

1. Mild hyperhomocysteinemia is seen in 5–10 percent of the general population in the United States. Homocysteine levels increase with age, and 30–40 percent of the elderly population have mildly to moderately increased homocysteine levels (15–100 uM/l).
2. Methylenetetrahydrofolate reductase (MTHFR 677 C→T) polymorphism, present in ~15 percent of the population, is associated with elevated homocysteine levels and increased risk of stroke.
3. Elevated homocysteine is associated with cerebral venous occlusive events and small-vessel disease and microangiopathic stroke as well as large-artery atherosclerotic stroke.
4. Elevated homocysteine levels are associated with carotid atherosclerosis and intimomedial thickness in a dose-dependent fashion.
5. Lower homocysteine levels are associated with lower risk of stroke (odds ratio 0.81).
6. Up to two-thirds of patients with hyperhomocysteinemia have low B12, B6, and/or folate levels.
7. Vitamin supplementation with B-complex vitamins (B6, B12, folate) is associated with reduction in serum homocysteine levels and, in one study, decreased progression of atherosclerotic plaque.
8. A large randomized controlled trial demonstrated effective lowering of plasma homocysteine with B-complex vitamin supplementation, but no reduction in recurrent stroke other studies are underway.

Treatment recommendations

Homocysteine is emerging as a risk marker for cerebrovascular disease, including stroke; its relationship to progression of atherosclerosis and stroke, however, may be complex. Treatment with B-complex vitamins is effective in lowering plasma homocysteine, and carries low risk. Thus, a reasonable approach to elevated homocysteine is as follows.

Patients at high risk for hyperhomocysteinemia, including the elderly, those taking medications that interfere with folate metabolism (methotrexate, carbamazepine, phenytoin), and those with inadequate diets, should be considered for screening, as should patients with personal or family histories of cardiovascular or cerebrovascular disease in the young. Two methods for assaying homocysteine exist: total fasting homocysteine and a 4–8 hr postmethionine load assay. Both are associated with increased risk of stroke; the latter method may be more sensitive in detecting patients with mild to moderate impairment of methionine metabolism.

Patients with elevated homocysteine levels should be further screened for B12, B6, and folate deficiency, and low B12 levels should be appropriately investigated and treated.

Primary stroke prevention should stress diet, including consumption of fortified cereals, grains and wheat germ, green leafy vegetables, legumes, fruits, dairy products, meat, poultry, and fish (aiming for the adult RDAs of folate=200 µg men, 180 µg women; B12=2.4 µg, B6= 1.6 mg). The AHA Nutrition Committee recommends a goal homocysteine <10 µM/l . Mild to moderate elevations may be treated with B-complex containing multivitamins (400 mg to 1 g folate, 2–25 mg B6, 6 µg – 0.5 mg B12). Marked elevations (>100 µM/l) should prompt genetic evaluation for homocystinuria.

Alcohol

Although alcohol consumption is associated with stroke risk, its effect is not linear. For ischemic stroke, there is J-shaped risk curve, with low to moderate consumption apparently conferring protection, but with increasing stroke risk at higher consumption levels. Moderate alcohol intake may decrease ischemic stroke risk through modification of the lipid profile (increased HDL fractions) as well as antithrombotic effects. High consumption is associated with hypertension, liver disease, cardiac arrhythmias, coagulopathy, and epilepsy. Other key points regarding the relationship of alcohol to stroke include the following:

1. Moderate consumption of alcohol (1–2 drinks per day) may be associated with a lower risk of ischemic stroke than complete abstinence.
2. The effect of type of alcohol is not clear, though some studies suggest that red wine confers a greater benefit than beer or hard liquor.
3. Higher consumption (e.g., ≥5 drinks/day) is associated with increased risk of stroke.
4. The risk is higher for hemorrhagic than for ischemic stroke.
5. For hemorrhagic stroke, there may be a linear relation to alcohol consumption.

Treatment recommendations

Individuals who drink in moderation (1 drink/day for nonpregnant women; 2 drinks/day for men) need not be counseled to quit, if they continue to drink in moderation. Those who drink more heavily should be counseled to cut back or cease. Because of the high potential for abuse and associated potential morbidities, those who do not drink should not be counseled to adopt a pattern of alcohol consumption.

Conclusion

Stroke is a devastating disease. Identification and management of modifiable risk factors including hypertension, atrial fibrillation, dyslipidemia, diabetes, and lifestyle factors can substantially reduce the burden of stroke at the individual as well as societal level. The practitioner should routinely screen for nonmodifiable as well as modifiable stroke risk factors in order to identify patients at high risk for first or recurrent stroke, and institute a program of education in conjunction with lifestyle changes, and, where indicated, pharmacotherapy. National guidelines for identification and management of major risk factors exist and continue to be informed by ongoing clinical studies.

Bibliography

American Diabetes Association. Standards of Medical Care in Diabetes. *Diabetes Care* 2005;28(s1):s4–36.

American Heart Association. Heart disease and stroke statistics – 2005 update. Dallas, TX: American Heart Association, 2005.

Chobanian A, Bakris G, Black H, et al. The Seventh Report of the Joint National Committee on Prevention, Detection, Evaluation, and Treatment of High Blood Pressure. *Hypertension* 2003;42(6):1206–52.

Elliot WJ, Garg J, Izahar M. Hypertension treatment. In P Gorelick, M Alter (eds), *The prevention of stroke*. New York: Parthenon,2002:163–8.

The Expert Committee on Diabetes. Report of the Expert Committee on Diabetes. *Diabetes Care* 1997;20:1183–97.

Expert Panel on Detection Evaluation and Treatment of High Blood Cholesterol in Adults. Executive Summary of the Third Report of the National Cholesterol Education Program (NCEP) Expert Panel on Detection, Evaluation, and Treatment of High Blood Cholesterol in Adults (Adult Treatment Panel III). *JAMA* 2001;285:2486–497.

Ezekowitz MD, Falk RH. The increasing need for anticoagulation therapy to prevent stroke in patients with atrial fibrillation. *Mayo Clinic Proc* 2004;79:903–4.

Gage BF, van Walraven C, Pearce L, et al. Selecting patients with atrial fibrillation for anticoagulation: Stroke risk stratification in patients taking aspirin. *Circulation* 2004;110(16):2287–92.

Gage BF, Waterman AD, Shannon W, Boechler M, Rich MW, Radford MJ. Validation of clinical classification schemes for predicting stroke: Results from the National Registry of Atrial Fibrillation. *JAMA* 2001;285(22):2864–70.

Goldstein LB, Adams R, Laberts MJ, et al. Primary prevention of ischemic stroke: A guideline from the American Heart Association/American Stroke Association Stroke Council: Cosponsored by the Atherosclerotic Peripheral Vascular Disease Interdisciplinary Working Group; Cardiovascular Nursing Council; Clinical Cardiology Council; Nutrition, Physical Activity, and Metabolism Council; and the Quality of Care and Outcomes Research Interdisciplinary Working Group: The American Academy of Neurology affirms the value of this guideline. *Stroke* 2006 37:1583–633.

Gorelick PB. New horizons for stroke prevention: PROGRESS and HOPE. *Lancet Neurol* 2002a;1:149–56.

Gorelick PB. Stroke prevention therapy beyond antithrombotics: Unifying mechanisms in ischemic stroke pathogenesis and implications for therapy. An invited review. *Stroke* 2002b;33:862–75. A review of new mechanisms of stroke and the role of newer therapeutic agents and their mechanism of action in stroke prevention.

Gorelick PB, Sacco RL, Smith DB, et al. Prevention of a first stroke. A review of guidelines and a multidisciplinary consensus statement from the National Stroke Association. *JAMA* 1999;281(12):1112–20.

Graham IM, Daly LE, Refsum HM, et al. Plasma homocysteine as a risk factor for vascular disease: The European concerted action project. *JAMA* 1997;277 (22):1775–81.

Grundy S, Cleeman J, Merz C, et al. Implications of recent clinical trials for the National Cholesterol Education Program Adult Treatment Panel III guidelines. An update statement to the 2001 NCEP guideline based on new clinical trial information since the publication of the 2001 NCEP guideline.

Heart Protection Study Collaborative Group. Effects of cholesterol–lowering with simvastatin on stroke and other major vascular events in 20,356 people with cerebrovascular disease or other high risk conditions. *Lancet* 2004;363:757–67.

Homocysteine Lowering Trialists' Collaboration. Lowering blood homocysteine with folic acid based supplements: Meta–analysis of randomised trials. *BMJ* 1998;316 (7135):894–8.

The Homocysteine Studies Collaborators. Homocysteine and the risk of ischemic heart disease and stroke: A meta–analysis. *JAMA* 2002;288:2015–22.

Lancaster T, Stead L, Silagy C, Sowden A. Effectiveness of interventions to help people stop smoking: Findings from the Cochrane Library. *BMJ* 2000;321:355–8.

Malinow MR, Bostom AG, Krayss RM. Homocyst(e)ine, diet, and cardiovascular disease. A statement for healthcare professionals from the Nutrition Committee, American Heart Association. *Circulation* 1999;99:178–82.

Pandey D, Gorelick PB. Should statin agents be administered to all patients with ischemic stroke? *Arch Neurol* 2005;62:23–4.

Pedelty LL, Gorelick PB. Chronic management of blood pressure after stroke. *Hypertension* 2004;44:1–5.

Qureshi AI, Suri MF, Kirmani JF, Divani AA. The relative impact of inadequate primary and secondary prevention on cardiovascular mortality in the United States. *Stroke* 2004;35:2346–50.

Reynolds K, Lewis BL, Nolen JD, Kinney GL, Sathya B, He J. Alcohol consumption and the risk of stroke: A meta–analysis. *JAMA* 2003;289:579–88.

Sacco RL, Adams R, Albers G, et al. Guidelines for prevention of stroke in patients with ischemic stroke or transient ischemic attack: A statement for health care professionals from the American Heart Association/American Stroke Association Council on Stroke. *Stroke* 2006;37(2):577–616.

Singer DE, Albers GW, Dalen JE, Go AS, Halperin JL, Manning WJ. Antithrombotic therapy in atrial fibrillation: The seventh AACCP conference on antithrombotic and thrombolytic therapy. *Chest* 2004;126:429–56.

Sloan MA. Primary prevention of stroke by modification of selected risk factors. In S Kasner, P Gorelick (eds), *Prevention and Treatment of ischemic stroke*. Philadelphia: Butterworth Heinemann, 2004: 5–54.

The SPAF III Writing Committee for the Stroke Prevention in Atrial Fibrillation Investigators. Patients with nonvalvular atrial fibrillation at low risk of stroke during treatment with aspirin. Stroke Prevention in Atrial Fibrillation III Study. *JAMA* 1998;279:1273–7.

The Tobacco Use and Dependence Clinical Practice Guideline Panel Staff and Consortium Representatives. A clinical practice guideline for treating tobacco use and dependence: A US Public Health Service Report. *JAMA* 2000;283: 3244–54.

Toole J, Malinow M, Chambless L, et al. Lowering homocysteine in patients with ischemic stroke to prevent recurrent stroke, myocardial infarction, and death: The Vitamin Intervention for Stroke Prevention (VISP) randomized controlled trial. *JAMA* 2004;291(5):565–75.

UK Prospective Diabetes Study Group. Tight blood pressure control and risk of macrovascular and microvascular complications in type 2 diabetes: UKPDS 38. *BMJ* 1998;317:703–13.

Index